IMMUNOLOGY OF DIABETES IV
Progress in Our Understanding

ANNALS OF THE NEW YORK ACADEMY OF SCIENCES
Volume 1079

IMMUNOLOGY OF DIABETES IV

Progress in Our Understanding

Edited by Carani B. Sanjeevi and Toshiaki Hanafusa

Published by Blackwell Publishing on behalf of the New York Academy of Sciences
Boston, Massachusetts
2006

Library of Congress Cataloging-in-Publication Data

Immunology of diabetes IV : progress in our understanding / edited by Carani B. Sanjeevi and Toshiaki Hanafusa.
p. ; cm. – (Annals of the New York Academy of Sciences, ISSN 0077-8923 ; v. 1375)
Includes bibliographical references and index.
ISBN-13: 978-1-57331-641-5 (alk. paper)
ISBN-10: 1-57331-641-5 (alk. paper)
1. Diabetes–Immunological aspects–Congresses. 2. Immunogenetics–Congresses. I. Sanjeevi, C. B. II. Hanafusa, Toshiaki. III. New York Academy of Sciences. IV. Title: Immunology of diabetes 4. V. Title: Immunology of diabetes four. VI. Series.
[DNLM: 1. Diabetes Mellitus, Type 1–genetics–Congresses. 2. Dia- betes Mellitus, Type 1–immunology–Congresses. 3. Diabetes Mellitus, Type 1–prevention & control–Congresses. W1 AN626YL v.1375 2006 / WK 810 I3384i 2006]

RC660.A15I46 2006
616.4'62079–dc22

2006019883

The *Annals of the New York Academy of Sciences* (ISSN: 0077-8923 [print]; ISSN: 1749-6632 [online]) is published 28 times a year on behalf of the New York Academy of Sciences by Blackwell Publishing, with offices located at 350 Main Street, Malden, Massachusetts 02148 USA, PO Box 1354, Garsington Road, Oxford OX4 2DQ UK, and PO Box 378 Carlton South, 3053 Victoria Australia.

Information for subscribers: Subscription prices for 2006 are: Premium Institutional: $3850.00 (US) and £2139.00 (Europe and Rest of World).
Customers in the UK should add VAT at 5%. Customers in the EU should also add VAT at 5% or provide a VAT registration number or evidence of entitlement to exemption. Customers in Canada should add 7% GST or provide evidence of entitlement to exemption. The Premium Institutional price also includes online access to full-text articles from 1997 to present, where available. For other pricing options or more information about online access to Blackwell Publishing journals, including access information and terms and conditions, please visit www.blackwellpublishing.com/nyas.

Membership information: Members may order copies of the *Annals* volumes directly from the Academy by visiting www.nyas.org/annals, emailing membership@nyas.org, faxing 212-888-2894, or calling 800-843-6927 (US only), or +1 212 838 0230, ext. 345 (International). For more information on becoming a member of the New York Academy of Sciences, please visit www.nyas.org/membership.

Journal Customer Services: For ordering information, claims, and any inquiry concerning your institutional subscription, please contact your nearest office:
UK: Email: customerservices@blackwellpublishing.com; Tel: +44 (0) 1865 778315; Fax +44 (0) 1865 471775
US: Email: customerservices@blackwellpublishing.com; Tel: +1 781 388 8599 or 1 800 835 6770 (Toll free in the USA); Fax: +1 781 388 8232
Asia: Email: customerservices@blackwellpublishing.com; Tel: +65 6511 8000; Fax: +61 3 8359 1120
Members: Claims and inquiries on member orders should be directed to the Academy at email: membership@nyas.org or Tel: +1 212 838 0230 (International) or 800-843-6927 (US only).

Printed in the USA.
Printed on acid-free paper.

Mailing: The *Annals of the New York Academy of Sciences* are mailed Standard Rate. **Postmaster:** Send all address changes to *Annals of the New York Academy of Sciences*, Blackwell Publishing, Inc., Journals Subscription Department, 350 Main Street, Malden, MA 01248-5020. Mailing to rest of world by DHL Smart and Global Mail.

Annals are available to subscribers online at the New York Academy of Sciences and also at Blackwell Synergy. Visit www.annalsnyas.org or www.blackwell-synergy.com to search the articles and register for table of contents e-mail alerts. Access to full text and PDF downloads of *Annals* articles are available to nonmembers and subscribers on a pay-per-view basis at www.annalsnyas.org.

The paper used in this publication meets the minimum requirements of the National Standard for Information Sciences Permanence of Paper for Printed Library Materials, ANSI Z39.48_1984.

ISSN: 0077-8923 (print); 1749-6632 (online)
ISBN-10: 1-57331-641-5 (paper); ISBN-13: 978-1-57331-641-5 (paper)

A catalogue record for this title is available from the British Library.

Digitization of the *Annals of the New York Academy of Sciences*

An agreement has recently been reached between Blackwell Publishing and the New York Academy of Sciences to digitize the entire run of the *Annals of the New York Academy of Sciences* back to volume one.

The back files, which have been defined as all of those issues published before 1997, will be sold to libraries as part of Blackwell Publishing's Legacy Sales Program and hosted on the Blackwell Synergy website.

Copyright of all material will remain with the rights holder. Contributors: Please contact Blackwell Publishing if you do not wish an article or picture from the *Annals of the New York Academy of Sciences* to be included in this digitization project.

ANNALS OF THE NEW YORK ACADEMY OF SCIENCES

Volume 1079
October 2006

IMMUNOLOGY OF DIABETES IV

Progress in Our Understanding

Editors
CARANI B. SANJEEVI AND TOSHIAKI HANAFUSA

This volume is the result of a meeting entitled **The 8th Meeting of the Immunology of Diabetes Society,** held on October 6–9, 2005 on Awaji Island, Japan.

CONTENTS

Part III. Latent Autoimmune Diabetes in Adults

Part IV. Animal Models

Part V. T Cells

Part VI. Autoantibodies

Part VII. Genetics

Part VIII. Prediction and Prevention

Financial assistance was received from:

- Japanese Society of the Promotion of Science
- Juvenile Diabetes Research Foundation
- The Federation of Pharmaceutical Manufacturers Association of Japan
- Hyogo International Association
- Japan Diabetes Foundation
- Tsutomu Nakauchi Foundation

Overview

A major focus of the 8th Immunology of Diabetes Society (IDS) meeting was diabetes in Asia, which is believed to be etiologically different from type 1 diabetes in the West. The IDS meets every 18 months, rotating the venue of its meeting among America, Europe, and Asia/Oceania, and the 8th IDS meeting was held in Japan in October 2005.

The first article of this volume establishes the principal theme of the meeting through its description of the formation of the Type 1 Diabetes Genetics Consortium, a worldwide effort to understand the genetic mechanisms underlying the etiopathogenesis of type 1 diabetes. As has always been the case at its meetings, the IDS highlights the standardization workshops it conducts in both antibody and T cell components of the immunology of diabetes. These workshops set the standards for the assays that are used in the world of type 1 diabetes. The second and third chapters contain reports on these workshops.

The second part of the volume contains reports on the genetics and epidemiology of type 1 diabetes in Asia. The contribution of the genetic differences between the Asian and the Caucasian populations in the relatively low incidence of type 1 diabetes in Asia is discussed.

In the third part of this volume, studies are presented on slowly progressive type 1 diabetes (SPIDDM), also called latent autoimmune diabetes in adults (LADA). New diagnostic criteria have been set, and the differences between the Asian and the Caucasian etiologic pathways are addressed.

The rest of the volume is devoted to reviewing the advances in the roles of T cells, antibodies, genetics, animal models, environmental factors, and in the strategies for prediction and prevention. Progress in the vaccine approach is addressed in presentations of the two vaccine candidates, Diamyd and DiaPep 277, currently in Phase III trials. It is hoped that the results from these trials will offer help for some of the problems facing children with newly diagnosed type 1 diabetes. The 9th meeting of the IDS is planned for the fall of 2007 and is tentatively planned to be held in Florida. We hope to see more progress in this rapidly advancing field reported on at that meeting.

—C.B. SANJEEVI
Karolinska Institute, Center for Molecular Medicine, Karolinska Hospital, Stockholm, Sweden

— T. HANAFUSA
Osaka Medical College Osaka, Japan

Ann. N.Y. Acad. Sci. 1079: xv (2006). © 2006 New York Academy of Sciences.
doi: 10.1196/annals.1375.060

The Type 1 Diabetes Genetics Consortium

STEPHEN S. RICH,[a] PATRICK CONCANNON,[b] HENRY ERLICH,[c] CECILE JULIER,[d] GRANT MORAHAN,[e] JORN NERUP,[f] FLEMMING POCIOT,[f] AND JOHN A. TODD[g]

[a]*Wake Forest University School of Medicine, Winston-Salem, North Carolina 27157, USA*

[b]*Benaroya Research Institute, Seattle, Washington 98101, USA*

[c]*Roche Molecular Systems, Alameda, California 94501, USA*

[d]*Pasteur Institute, 75724 Paris Cedex 15, France*

[e]*The Western Australian Institute of Medical Research, Perth WA 6000, Australia*

[f]*Steno Diabetes Center, DK-2820 Gentofte, Denmark*

[g]*JDRF/Wellcome Trust Diabetes Inflammation Laboratory, Cambridge University, Cambridge CB2 2XY, UK*

ABSTRACT: The Type 1 Diabetes Genetics Consortium (T1DGC) is an international, multicenter program organized to promote research to identify genes and their alleles that determine an individual's risk for type 1 diabetes (T1D). The primary goal of the T1DGC is to establish resources and data that can be used by, and that is fully accessible to, the research community in the study of T1D. All the information on T1DGC can be accessed at the following web address: www.t1dgc.org. A resource base of well-characterized families is being assembled that will facilitate the localization and characterization of T1D susceptibility genes. From these families, the T1DGC is establishing banks of DNA, serum, plasma, and cell lines, as well as useful databases. The T1DGC also sponsors training opportunities (bioinformatics) and technology transfer (HLA genotyping).

KEYWORDS: type 1 diabetes; autoantibodies; HLA; families; linkage; genetics

INTRODUCTION

Type 1 diabetes (T1D) is characterized by autoimmune destruction of the pancreatic β cells. It has long been known that the likelihood of a person

Address for correspondence: Stephen S. Rich, Ph.D., Department of Public Health Sciences, Wake Forest University School of Medicine, Winston-Salem, NC 27157. Voice: 336-716-5778; fax: 336-716-5425.

e-mail: srich@wfubmc.edu

Ann. N.Y. Acad. Sci. 1079: 1–8 (2006). © 2006 New York Academy of Sciences.

doi: 10.1196/annals.1375.001

developing T1D is higher the more closely related he or she is to a person with the disease, such that first-degree relatives of cases are at 15 times greater risk of T1D than a randomly selected member of the general population.[1,2] However, monozygotic twins are concordant for T1D at a frequency of approximately 50% and the incidence of T1D has been increasing in Western countries, with a doubling of incidence in the United States over the past 30 years.[3,4] These data suggest that, in addition to a strong genetic component, environmental factors play a key role in influencing the penetrance of the genetically determined events that lead to HLA/autoantibody-associated T1D.

The familial clustering of T1D is influenced by multiple genes, of which at least four together account for about half of the familial aggregation. These four established regions of the genome, for which there is both statistical and replication support, are: the HLA region on 6p21 (including the *HLA-DRB1*, *-DQA1* and *-DRQ1* genes,[5–7] a region 5′ to the insulin gene (*INS*) on chromosome 11p15,[8,9] the CTLA-4 gene (*CTLA4*) region on chromosome 2q31,[10,11] and the protein tyrosine phosphatase-22 (*PTPN22*) gene on chromosome 1p13.[12,13] A fifth region has been implicated, the interleukin-2 receptor alpha (*CD25*) gene on chromosome 10p15,[14] but remains to be replicated by independent studies. Many other genes have been claimed to be associated with T1D (e.g., Refs.15–28); however, with a high false-positive rate in genetics studies of common disease, many of these might not be true effects. Resolution of these potential candidate gene associations will require assembly of large sample sizes to confirm (or refute) their effects. The numerous confirmed regions in the spontaneous mouse model of T1D, the partial explanation of familial clustering, and the small fraction of the human genome investigated using sample sizes appropriate for the risk estimates of the non-HLA genes already discovered, all suggests that many more T1D susceptibility genes remain to be discovered.

The Type 1 Diabetes Genetics Consortium (T1DGC)

The T1DGC is an international effort to identify genes that determine an individual's risk of T1D. Progress toward the goal of gene discovery has been limited by a lack of sufficient clinical and genetic resources. A major effort of the T1DGC is the creation of a resource base of well-characterized families from multiple ethnic groups that will facilitate the localization and characterization of T1D susceptibility genes. Building upon these T1DGC resources, members and collaborators of the T1DGC can undertake positional cloning to identify individual genes that determine susceptibility or protection to T1D.

The T1DGC (http://www.t1dgc.org) was established through the efforts of the National Institute of Diabetes and Digestive and Kidney Diseases (NIDDK) and the Juvenile Diabetes Research Foundation (JDRF). Participation in Consortium activities is available to all investigators who sign a Consortium

Agreement. The Agreement explains the rights and responsibilities of T1DGC members.

The governance of the T1DGC, including scientific agenda, assessment of recruitment, quality control of assays, dissemination of study results, and provision of training and technology transfer, is advised upon by the T1DGC steering committee (see the author list), with from the programmatic advisors (NIDDK, JDRF) and observers (NIAID, NHGRI, Diabetes UK).

A consideration of previous genome scan results for T1D, the contributions of known T1D risk loci to familial clustering of T1D, and the power of affected sib-pair linkage studies, suggested that 4000 affected sib-pair (ASP) families will provide sufficient statistical power to identify chromosome regions with locus-specific genetic risks of $\lambda_s > 1.3$ (where λ_s = expected zero sharing of alleles identical-by-descent of a marker locus/observed; an λ_s value of 1.3 for a causal allele frequency of 0.3 under a multiplicative model would correspond to a relative risk > 2.3, exceeding *PTPN22* and *INS*). This would provide support to begin fine mapping to identify the responsible variants for T1D risk. To reach this goal, the T1DGC initially identified existing resources of ASP families (~1400) with appropriate consents. Efforts are now under way to recruit an additional 2500 ASP families throughout the world.

In order to identify, recruit, and collect the samples and data on 2500 new ASP families, the T1DGC developed four regional networks: North America (NA), Europe (EU), United Kingdom (UK), and Asia Pacific (AP). Recruitment targets vary by network: AP and UK networks are each collecting ~200 ASP families, while EU and NA networks are each collecting 1200 ASP families. Each network has established a recruitment center and staff, and each uses multiple approaches to recruit volunteers. Within each network, field centers identify, ascertain, and collect samples and data from participating families.

The large number of samples and the international locations of the networks have required that the T1DGC establish laboratories in multiple sites. Each network has established a DNA repository (to process samples for DNA, and to provide cell immortalization), an HLA laboratory (to determine classical HLA typing), and an autoantibody laboratory (to characterize plasma from cases). The T1DGC Coordinating Center (at Wake Forest University) has established the system of sample transfer and tracking to the T1DGC laboratories and is the central repository of clinical information and genetic data. The current collection of the T1DGC is shown in TABLE 1. Ultimately, samples and data from the T1DGC network laboratories will be transferred to central NIDDK repositories (data, plasma and serum, and cell lines) from which investigators can make requests.

There have been many challenges to establishing an international consortium. In order to address these, the T1DGC established a committee structure that has developed guidelines for recruitment. The phenotyping committee has developed recommendations for data and specimens to be collected from

TABLE 1. Current sample collection (September, 2005) of the T1DGC

Network	ASP families (participants)	ASP cell line samples	ASP serum samples	ASP plasma samples
Asia Pacific	196 (786)	1,413	3,329	2,654
Europe	496 (2,038)	3,785	9,180	7,407
North America	393 (1,541)	2,570	7,067	5,768
United Kingdom	139 (553)	847	2,652	2,119
Total	1,224 (4,918)	8,615	22,228	17,948

participants, including the definition of T1D as well as the laboratory, physical, and demographic measures. Its members monitor study recruitment and provide guidance to the regional networks in the recruitment of families and also serve as an *ad hoc* eligibility committee when questions of eligibility arise. The ELSI committee drafted a model informed consent template for use by all investigators. Other committees focus on sample collection and analysis (Laboratory, Quality Control), data analysis, and distribution (Bioinformatics, Access) and dissemination of study results (Publications and Presentations).

All samples and data assembled by the Consortium are available to participating Consortium investigators, according to the policies in the T1DGC access policy (found on the T1DGC web site, http://www.t1dgc.org). Samples and data become available to the general research community 1 year after they are available to T1DGC members.

As part of its service and research functions, T1DGC conducts an annual bioinformatics workshop, to provide training in the use of publicly available tools for organization and analyses of genetic data. Consortium members from each network are eligible to participate in these workshops. T1DGC has also sponsored and organized HLA "wet workshops" to disseminate HLA typing methods. Finally, T1DGC laboratories participate in assay standardization efforts. A summary of Consortium activities is provided in TABLE 2.

T1DGC Research Activities

While candidate genes for T1D are the subject of ongoing investigations by many groups, there has previously been little coordinated effort to confirm the validity of a published gene association study, not fully explore the surrounding regions of DNA. The T1DGC has completed an initial genomewide linkage scan with power to detect susceptibility loci with locus-specific genetic risk ratios of $\lambda_S > 1.3$. A combined linkage analysis of four data sets—three previously published collections and one new collection of 254 families—provided a total sample of 1435 families with 1636 affected sib-pairs.[29] In addition to the HLA ($P = 2.0 \times 10^{-52}$), nine non-HLA-linked regions exhibited some evidence of linkage to T1D, including three at (or near) genomewide significance:

TABLE 2. Activities of the T1DGC

Collections
Affected sib-pair families
HLA-A, -B, -C, -DR, -DQ, -DP genotyping
IA-2 and GAD65 autoantibodies
Trio (parents affected child) families of from low prevalence populations
Repositories (Network and NIDDK)
Data
Phenotypic
Genotypic (genomewide linkage scan, candidate gene)
DNA (genomic/whole genome amplified) and cell lines
Serum and plasma samples
Scientific advances
Genomewide linkage scans
MHC fine mapping initiative
Rapid response laboratory for assessment of candidate genes
Technology transfer
HLA genotyping workshops
Bioinformatics workshops
Outreach
Network member meetings
Symposia and scientific sessions

2q31-q33 (*IDDM7*), 10p14-q11 (*IDDM10*), and 16q22-q24. In addition, after taking into account the linkage at the 6p21 (HLA) region, there was evidence supporting linkage for the 6q21 region (*IDDM15*, 19).

Genes in the HLA region (MHC) are recognized to be the major genetic risk factors for T1D susceptibility, as they account for nearly 50% of the genetic risk. However, not all of the T1D susceptibility loci contained in the MHC have been identified or characterized. Mapping and identification of other loci within the HLA region in Caucasian populations has been limited by the extensive linkage disequilibrium in the region and the consequently limited haplotype diversity. In order to address this scientific need, the T1DGC will use its DNA resources to perform high-density genotyping (microsatellite markers and SNPs) in the 4 Mb-interval corresponding to the “classical” HLA region. In combination with the classical HLA typing being done on the same samples, the final data set should provide the opportunity to test hypotheses regarding T1D susceptibility.

Genes other than those in the MHC account for ~50% of the genetic risk for development of T1D; however, these genes are likely to have smaller individual effects. Many genes have been proposed as candidates for contributing to genetic susceptibility of T1D. There is a need to validate these genes and their impact on T1D risk. In order to facilitate evaluation of these candidate genes with larger sample sizes, the T1DGC has established a “rapid response laboratory” and a “molecular technology committee.” The T1DGC rapid response laboratory will provide a mechanism that can facilitate the confirmation of previously published associations, or of associations prior to publication. The T1DGC rapid response laboratory will evaluate candidate genes nominated to the molecular technology committee by Consortium members. The molecular technology committee works with the Consortium members and the rapid response laboratory for SNP selection and characterization of candidate genes using Consortium DNA resources.

SUMMARY

The major goals for the T1DGC are to identify the genes that contribute to the clustering of T1D in families. Previous constraints to understanding the genetic basis of T1D have been the limited number of samples available for analysis, the lack of molecular genetic reagents available to pinpoint susceptibility loci within the human genome, and the limitations of analytic and informatics infrastructure available to understand the genetic data. At present, progress in several of these areas provides new opportunities. The T1DGC has initiated collection of renewable genetic materials for use in family-based linkage and association studies. Despite its high prevalence in Western populations, the T1DGC is planning to collect samples from families of ethnic groups with lower susceptibility to T1D, in order to understand the occurrence of T1D in these populations and help in the identification of the causal variants.

ACKNOWLEDGMENTS

This work was supported by grants to SSR (NIDDK, JDRF), PC (NIDDK, JDRF), and JAT (JDRF, Wellcome Trust.

REFERENCES

1. RICH, S.S. 1990. Mapping genes in diabetes: a genetic epidemiological perspective. Diabetes **39:** 1315–1319.
2. POCIOT, F. & M.F. MCDERMOTT. 2002. Genetics of type 1 diabetes mellitus [Review]. Genes Immun. **3:** 235–249.
3. GREEN, A. & C.C. PATTERSON. 2001. Trends in the incidence of childhood-onset diabetes in Europe 1989–1998. Diabetologia **44**(Suppl 3): B3–B8.
4. FELTBOWER, R.G., P.A. MCKINNEY, R.C. PARSLOW, *et al.* 2003. Type 1 diabetes in Yorkshire, UK: time trends in 0–14 and 15-29-year-olds, age at onset and age-period-cohort modeling. Diabet. Med. **20:** 437–441.
5. NERUP, J., P. PLATZ, O.O. ANDERSEN, *et al.* 1974. HL-A antigens and diabetes mellitus. Lancet **2:** 864–866.

6. Noble, J.A., A.M. Valdes, M. Cook, *et al.* 1996. The role of HLA class II genes in insulin-dependent diabetes mellitus: molecular analysis of 180 Caucasian, multiplex families. Am. J. Hum. Genet. **59:** 1134–1148.
7. Cucca, F., R. Lampis, M. Congia, *et al.* 2001. A correlation between the relative predisposition of MHC class II alleles to type 1 diabetes and the structure of their proteins. Hum. Mol. Genet. **10:** 2025–2037.
8. Bell, G.I., S. Horita, S.J.H. Karam, *et al.* 1984. A polymorphic locus near the human insulin gene is associated with insulin-dependent diabetes mellitus. Diabetes **33:** 176–183.
9. Bennett, S.T., A.M. Lucassen, S.C.L. Gough, *et al.* 1995. Susceptibility to human type 1 diabetes at IDDM2 is determined by tandem repeat variation at the insulin gene minisatellite locus. Nat. Genet. **9:** 284–292.
10. Kristiansen, O.P., Z.M. Larsen & F. Pociot. 2000. CTLA-4 in autoimmune diseases—a general susceptibility gene to autoimmunity? Genes Immun. **1:** 170–184.
11. Ueda, H., J.M.M. Howson, L. Esposito, *et al.* 2003. Association of the T-cell regulatory gene CTLA4 with susceptibility to autoimmune disease. Nature **423:** 506–511.
12. Bottini, N., L. Musumeci, A. Alonso, *et al.* 2004. A functional variant of lymphoid tyrosine phosphatase is associated with type 1 diabetes. Nat. Genet. **36:** 337–338.
13. Smyth, D., J.D. Cooper, J.E. Collins, *et al.* 2004. Replication of an association between the lymphoid tyrosine phosphatase locus (LYP/PTPN22) with type 1 diabetes, and evidence for its role as a general autoimmunity locus. Diabetes **53:** 3020–3023.
14. Vella, A., J.D. Cooper, C.E. Lowe, *et al.* 2005. Localization of a type 1 diabetes locus in the IL2RA/CD25 region by use of tag single-nucleotide polymorphisms. Am. J. Hum. Genet. **76:** 773–779.
15. Davies, J.L., Y. Kawaguchi, S.T. Bennett, *et al.* 1994. A genome-wide search for human type 1 diabetes susceptibility genes. Nature **371:** 130–136.
16. Concannon, P., K.J. Gogolin-Ewens, D.A. Hinds, *et al.* 1998. A second-generation screen of the human genome for susceptibility to insulin-dependent diabetes mellitus. Nat. Genet. **19:** 292–296.
17. Mein, C.A., L. Esposito, M.G. Dunn, *et al.* 1998. A search for type 1 diabetes susceptibility genes in families from the United Kingdom. Nat. Genet. **19:** 297–300.
18. European Consortium for IDDM Genome Studies. 2001. A genomewide scan for type 1 diabetes susceptibility in Scandinavian families: identification of new loci with evidence of interactions. Am. J. Hum. Genet. **69:** 1301–1313.
19. Delepine, M., F. Pociot, C. Habita, *et al.* 1997. Evidence of a non-MHC susceptibility locus in type 1 diabetes linked to HLA on chromosome 6. Am. J. Hum. Genet. **60:** 174–187.
20. Cucca, F., J.V. Goy, Y. Kawaguchi, *et al.* 1998. A male:female bias in type 1 diabetes and linkage to chromosome Xp in MHC HLA-DR3-positive patients. Nat. Genet. **3:** 301–302.
21. Sale, M.M., L.M. Fitzgerald, J.C. Charlesworth, *et al.* 2002. Evidence for a novel type 1 diabetes susceptibility locus on chromosome 8. Diabetes **51**(Suppl 3): S316–S319.

22. LUO, D.F., R. BUZZETTI, J.I. ROTTER, *et al.* 1996. Confirmation of three susceptibility genes to insulin-dependent diabetes mellitus: IDDM4, IDDM5 and IDDM8. Hum. Mol. Genet. **5:** 693–698.
23. MERRIMAN, T., R. TWELLS, M. MERRIMAN, *et al.* 1997. Evidence by allelic association-dependent methods for a type 1 diabetes polygene (IDDM6) on chromosome 18q21. Hum. Mol. Genet. **6:** 1003–1010.
24. MORAHAN, G., D. HUANG, S.I YMER, *et al.* 2001. Linkage disequilibrium of a type 1 diabetes susceptibility locus with a regulatory IL12B allele. Nat. Genet. **27:** 218–221.
25. BOHREN, K.M., V. NADKARNI, J.H. SONG, *et al.* 2004. A M55V polymorphism in a novel SUMO gene (SUMO-4) differentially activates heat shock transcription factors and is associated with susceptibility to type 1 diabetes mellitus. J. Biol. Chem. **279:** 27233–27238.
26. VERGE, C.F., P. VARDI, S. BABU, *et al.* 1998. Evidence for oligogenic inheritance of type 1 diabetes in a large Bedouin Arab family. J. Clin. Invest. **102:** 1569–1575.
25. FIELD, L.L., R. TOBIAS, G. THOMSON, *et al.* 1996. Susceptibility to insulin-dependent diabetes mellitus maps to a locus (IDDM11) on human chromosome 14q24.3-q31. Genomics **33:** 1–8.
28. BUGAWAN, T.L., D.B. MIREL, A.M. VALDES, *et al.* 2003. Association and interaction of the IL4R, IL4, and IL13 loci with type 1 diabetes among Filipinos. Am. J. Hum. Genet. **72:** 1505–1514.
29. CONCANNON, P., H.A. ERLICH, C. JULIER, *et al.* 2005. Type 1 diabetes. Evidence for susceptibility loci from four genome-wide linkage scans in 1,435 multiplex families. Diabetes **54:** 2995–3001.

A Mini Meta-Analysis of Studies on $CD4^+CD25^+$ T cells in Human Type 1 Diabetes

Report of the Immunology of Diabetes Society T Cell Workshop

TIMOTHY I.M. TREE,[a] BART O. ROEP,[b] AND MARK PEAKMAN[a]

[a]*Department of Immunobiology, King's College London, School of Medicine, London SEI 9RT, United Kingdom*

[b]*Department of Immunohaematology and Blood Transfusion, Leiden University Medical Center, 2300 RC Leiden, The Netherlands*

ABSTRACT: Type 1 diabetes mellitus (T1DM) is characterized by a loss of self-tolerance to islet antigens. In health, immunological tolerance is maintained by multiple central and peripheral mechanisms including the action of a specialized set of regulatory T cells characterized by expression of CD4 and CD25 ($CD4^+CD25^+$ Treg). It has been suggested that a defect in this cell population, either numerically or functionally, could contribute to the development of autoimmune diseases, such as T1DM. To investigate this possibility, several research groups have studied the frequency and suppressive capacity of this cell population in individuals with T1DM and, to date, there are four such studies published. We therefore performed a mini meta-analysis to compare the results in the four published studies, account for differences in their findings, and draw a consensus view on the role of this important cell subset in human T1DM.

KEYWORDS: T cell; diabetes; workshop; regulation

INTRODUCTION

Type 1 diabetes mellitus (T1DM) is a chronic, T cell-mediated autoimmune disease that results in the destruction of the insulin-secreting β cells. The pathological mechanisms that lead to disease development are not known with certainty, but there is compelling evidence that the disease is associated with loss of immunological tolerance to self. For example, pancreatic β cell

Address for correspondence: Timothy Tree, Department of Immunobiology, King's College London, 2nd Floor, New Guy's House, Guy's Hospital, London SE1 9RT, UK. Voice: +442071881182; fax: +441883385.
e-mail: timothy.tree@kcl.ac.uk

Ann. N.Y. Acad. Sci. 1079: 9–18 (2006). © 2006 New York Academy of Sciences.
doi: 10.1196/annals.1375.002

destruction is associated temporally with the presence of islet cell autoantibodies directed against the autoantigens insulin, glutamic acid decarboxylase (GAD65), and the islet tyrosine phosphatase, IA-2. Autoreactive T cells recognizing these and other islet autoantigens have been identified and are thought to play a direct role in T1DM immunopathogenesis.[1–3]

T cell tolerance is established centrally in the thymus and further strengthened and maintained through multiple mechanisms of peripheral tolerance.[4] The manifest lack of self-tolerance to β cell autoantigens in patients with T1DM compared with their nondiabetic counterparts could therefore be due, at least in part, to a failure in one or more of these mechanisms. Recent interest has focused on a group of cells residing within the $CD4^+$ T cell population, which may be involved in maintaining peripheral tolerance and preventing organ-specific autoimmune disease, namely the $CD4^+CD25^+$ regulatory T cell (Treg).[5–7] These represent a naturally occurring CD4 T cell population expressing CD25 that arises from the thymus and seeds into the periphery, creating a cohort of cells with profound T cell immunosuppressive qualities. $CD4^+CD25^+$ cells can be detected in peripheral blood in humans, and are able to suppress proliferation and cytokine production from both $CD4^+$ and $CD8^+$ T cells *in vitro* in a cell contact-dependent manner. It is therefore possible that the lack of self-tolerance to islet autoantigens in T1DM may be in part due to a failure of $CD4^+CD25^+$ Treg.

To investigate this possibility, several research groups have studied the frequency and suppressive capacity of this cell population in individuals with T1DM and, to date, there are four such studies published.[8–11] We set out to examine the concordance between these studies and, where differences were identified, to provide possible explanations. The aim of our article was, therefore, to arrive at a consensus view of the role of this important cell subset in human T1DM.

ANALYSIS AND DISCUSSION

Studies Investigating the Role of $CD4^+CD25^+$ Treg in Human T1DM

To date there are four published studies investigating the role of $CD4^+CD25^+$ Treg in human T1DM. In this analysis these papers will be referred to as the New York,[11] Denver,[9] London,[8] and Gainsville[10] studies. We addressed three main areas investigated by these papers, namely the frequency of $CD4^+CD25^+$ T cells in peripheral blood, the phenotype of these cells as defined by the expression of other cellular markers and the suppressive capacity of these cells.

Frequency of $CD4^+CD25^+$ T Cells in Peripheral Blood

All four of the studies addressed the question of whether individuals with T1DM had an altered frequency of circulating T cells expressing CD4 and

CD25 using direct immunofluoresence with specific monoclonal antibodies and flow cytometry. The New York study reported that there were a significantly reduced number of these cells in both new onset (mean 2.6% $\pm$ 0.23, $P < 0.001$) and long-standing T1DM patients (mean 3.7% $\pm$ 0.69, $P < 0.002$) compared to control subjects (mean 6.9% $\pm$ 0.4). In contrast, the three subsequent studies did not observe any significant differences in the frequency of these cells between T1DM patients and control subjects: Denver study T1DM mean 7.4% $\pm$ 1.4, controls mean 7.1% $\pm$ 1.2; London study T1DM mean 18.7% $\pm$ 6.7, controls 16.9% $\pm$ 5.6%; and Gainesville study T1DM mean 13.5% $\pm$ 4.3, controls 14.89% $\pm$ 2.3 (all values are expressed as the percentage of CD4$^+$ lymphocytes coexpressing CD25).

To address this apparent lack of concordance between studies we must consider several potential influencing factors:

Definition of CD4$^+$CD25$^+$/Hi/Bright Populations

It is noteworthy that there is a wide variation in the reported percentage of CD4$^+$ T cells coexpressing CD25. This is largely due to differences in the definition of positivity for CD25 expression. Expression of CD25 does not define a distinct population of CD4$^+$ T cells, but rather it is present as a continuum of expression levels between negative and high expression (FIG. 1). It is believed that regulatory cells express high levels of CD25 and that the CD25 "intermediate" cells may represent recently activated effector T cells. Therefore, a number of criteria have been used to define CD4$^+$CD25$^+$ T cells with regulatory potential including: the use of isotype control antibodies to define a CD4$^+$CD25$^+$ population; the definition of a CD25^{hi} population based on absolute staining intensity; cells expressing a level of CD25 greater than that observed on CD3+CD4– lymphocytes or cells expressing a slightly lower level of CD4. An additional method employed to examine differences is based on assessing the amount of CD25 expressed (measured as the median fluorescence intensity) of the top 5%, 2%, 1%, and 0.5% of CD4$^+$CD25$^+$ T cells. Examples of the gating methods used to define CD25$^+$/hi population are shown in FIGURE 1.

The materials and methods in the New York study do not clarify what definition of positivity was used, making direct comparisons between the studies difficult. However, the Denver, London, and Gainesville studies used all of the above gating definitions and none of these revealed a significant difference between the frequency of CD4$^+$CD25$^+$ cells between T1DM patients and controls. It therefore appears unlikely that a difference in the criteria used to define the cell population can explain the discordance between these studies.

Patient Group Selected

Since CD25 is also expressed upon activated T cells, it is possible that an alteration in the activation state of lymphocytes as part of an ongoing

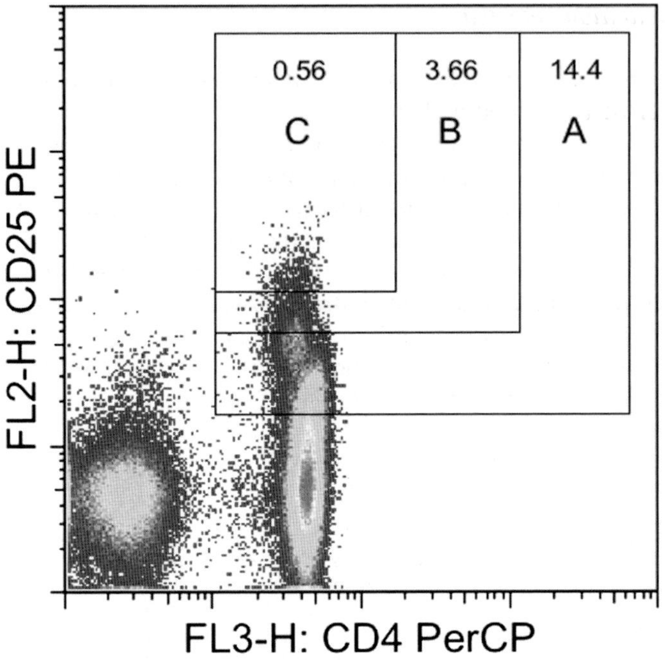

FIGURE 1. Example of the gating methods used to define $CD4^+CD25^+$/hi populations. Lymphocytes identified by their forward and side scatter properties were gated for CD3 expression and then examined for coexpression of CD4 and CD25. Gated regions represent (**A**) $CD4^+CD25^+$ population defined based on 99.5th percentile staining by relevant isotype control antibody, $CD4^+CD25$*hi* populations based upon (**B**) an expression level greater than that observed on CD3+$CD4^-$ lymphocytes and (**C**) expression above a fluorescence intensity of 100. Percentages within the gates represent the percentage of CD3+ $CD4^+$ lymphocytes coexpressing CD25.

autoimmune process may be present at diagnosis and may therefore affect the frequency of cells coexpressing CD4 and CD25. Differences between the New York and other three studies could, therefore, be due to differences in the patient populations studied. The New York study contained both newly diagnosed ($n = 21$) and long-standing ($n = 9$) T1DM patients. In contrast, the Denver study examined only long-standing patients ($n = 17$) and the London study only newly diagnosed patients ($n = 21$). The Gainesville study contained the largest number of T1DM patients ($n = 70$) and examined both long standing and newly diagnosed patients and found no difference in either group. It therefore appears unlikely that the discordance between the New York and other studies lies in the choice of patients.

Control Population Selected

Of particular importance when attempting to identify factors that may contribute to, or be associated with the development of a disease, is the choice of control population with which to compare the patient group. Of particular note in these studies was the age of the populations studied.

The Gainesville study identified a highly significant positive correlation between the frequency of $CD4^+CD25^+$ T cells and age in both the control and T1DM populations ($r = 0.64$, $P < 0.0001$; $r = 0.51$, $P < 0.0001$, respectively). Therefore, in this study, the control populations were selected to be of a similar age to the T1DM populations. Similarly, in the London and Denver study there was no significant difference between the ages of the T1DM and control populations. However, in the New York study there was a significant difference between the age of new onset T1DM patients (mean age 9.4 years $\pm$ 2.2) and the controls (mean age 37 years $\pm$ 5.7). Interestingly, if the data from the Gainesville study were not selected to provide suitable age-matched control populations for the newly diagnosed and long-standing T1DM groups, then T1DM patients appeared to have a reduced frequency of $CD4^+CD25^+$ T cells compared to controls ($P = 0.0006$). This demonstrates the importance of selecting appropriately matched controls for each patient group and may explain the apparent discordance between the studies in terms of the frequency of $CD4^+CD25^+$ T cells detected in newly diagnosed T1DM patients (i.e., the significantly lower level in patients observed in the New York study could be due to comparison with an older control group in which levels are higher by reason of age). Thus the consensus appears to be that there is no significant alteration in the frequency of $CD4^+CD25^+$ T cells in T1DM patients.

Phenotype of $CD4^+CD25^+$ T Cells

In addition to measuring the frequency, the Gainesville and London studies also investigated other phenotypic markers expressed on this population by flow cytometry. The Gainesville study found no significant difference in the percentage of $CD4^+CD25^+$ T cells coexpressing CD62L or the naïve and memory markers CD45RA and CD45R0, respectively. Similarly the London study found no significant difference in the expression of the memory marker CD45R0 or the chronic activation marker HLA-DR. However, in the London study patients with new onset T1DM had a greater percentage of $CD4^+CD25^+$ and $CD4^+CD25^{hi}$ cells coexpressing both the early marker of activation CD69 and the negative costimulatory molecule CTLA-4 (intracellular expression), which is also upregulated upon cellular activation. This suggests that whereas expression of long-term markers of cellular differentiation and activation are not altered within this population, newly diagnosed T1DM patients harbor a higher percentage of very recently activated T cells in the $CD4^+CD25^+$ population. However, it is not possible to determine whether the increase in CD69 and CTLA-4 represents an increase in the number of activated effector or activated regulatory cells.

Suppressive Capacity of $CD4^+CD25^+$ T Cells

The Denver, London, and Gainesville studies all measured the suppressive capacity of the $CD4^+CD25^+$ population using an *in vitro* suppression assay. This assay involves isolation of regulatory ($CD4^+CD25^+$) and responder ($CD4^+CD25–$) cell populations and measurement of the ability of the $CD4^+CD25^+$ cell population to inhibit the activation (measured as proliferation and/or cytokine production) of the responder T cell population. To simplify comparisons between data from the different studies all results are expressed as % suppression defined as the % reduction in the proliferation of the $CD4^+CD25–$ cells when co-cultured with a 1:1 ratio of $CD4^+CD25^+$ T cells (i.e., % suppression = 100—[(cpm in co-cultures/cpm in $CD4^+CD25–$ cultures) × 100]). In the London and Gainesville studies there is a marked difference between T1DM patients and controls with patients having significantly reduced suppressive capacity (London study, mean suppression ± SD: T1DM 25.9% ± 17.9, control 57.3% ± 23.5; $P = 0.007$, Gainesville study median suppression, interquartile range: T1DM 14.9%, –12.8 to 47.5, control 63.3%, 49.4 to 67.1; $P = 0.002$). However, no significant difference was observed in the Denver study.

To address this apparent lack of concordance between studies we must consider several potential factors:

Method Used to Isolate Cell Populations

Isolation of regulatory and responder cell populations is achieved by two main methods, namely flow cytometric-based cell sorting and immunomagnetic bead isolation. Each method has its own advantages and disadvantages. Flow cytometry-based sorting is considered to be the "gold standard" method for isolation as it provides advantages in terms of the purity of cell populations isolated and well-defined expression levels of CD25. In contrast, the use of immunomagnetic sorting is more convenient and provides more "untouched" cell populations. It has been suggested that *in vitro* suppression assays performed with cells isolated by different methods may yield slightly different results, due in part to the above-mentioned differences in the isolated populations. However, although the London study used immunomagnetic sorting, the Gainesville and Denver studies both used flow-based sorting and it is therefore unlikely that the isolation method used contributed to the apparent discordance between the Denver and London/Gainesville studies.

Patient Group Selected

In contrast to the Denver study, which examined responses only in long-standing T1DM patients, the Gainesville study contained patients with a wide range of disease durations and the London study was based solely on newly diagnosed individuals. It is therefore possible that the inclusion of newly diagnosed patients in the London and Gainesville studies explains the difference between these and the Denver study and that the defect in suppression is only present in individuals close to diagnosis. Future studies in populations with range of T1DM durations will be required to clarify this issue, although the Gainesville study implies that duration has little effect.

Stimulation Conditions

It has previously been demonstrated that the strength of stimulus used to activate the effector T cell population can have a dramatic effect on the suppressive capacity of CD4$^+$ CD25$^+$ T cells.[12] In a key paper by Baecher-Allan and colleagues, it was shown that as T cell signal strength was increased (in terms of the strength of monoclonal anti-CD3 antibody stimulation) the suppressive capacity of CD4$^+$CD25$^+$ T cells was reduced, with suppression ablated at high signal strength.[13] Furthermore, the importance of signal strength in the context of an autoimmune disease has also been suggested by a study examining the suppressive capacity of CD4$^+$CD25$^+$ T cells in individuals with multiple sclerosis (MS) the key finding of which are summarized in FIGURE 2 A.[14] At low signal strength (soluble anti-CD3) CD4$^+$CD25$^+$ T cells from both MS patients and controls show good suppressive function, with no significant difference between the groups. As signal strength is increased, the suppressive capacity of cells from MS patients becomes significantly impaired in comparison to those from controls (plate bound anti-CD3 at 0.1 μg/mL and 0.5 μg/mL). However, at the highest signal strength (plate bound anti-CD3 at 2.5 μg/mL) both the MS patients and controls show impaired suppression, with no difference between the groups. Thus it appears that MS patients become unable to suppress at a lower signal strength than control individuals and thus there is a "window" of stimulation strength that reveals a difference in the regulatory capacity of CD4$^+$CD25$^+$ cells from MS patients and controls.

If a similar defect was present in T1DM patients, that is, a difference in the threshold of stimulation required to break suppression, it is possible that the selection of different signal strengths in the different studies may explain why a difference was noted in some but not other studies. Whereas it is very difficult to compare the signal strengths between studies, it is possible to rank the signal strengths used within a single study. The different signal strengths used within the three published studies and the outcome of the study, in terms of suppression seen in T1DM and control individuals is shown in FIGURE 2 B. Different signal strengths within a single assay are arbitrarily designated as

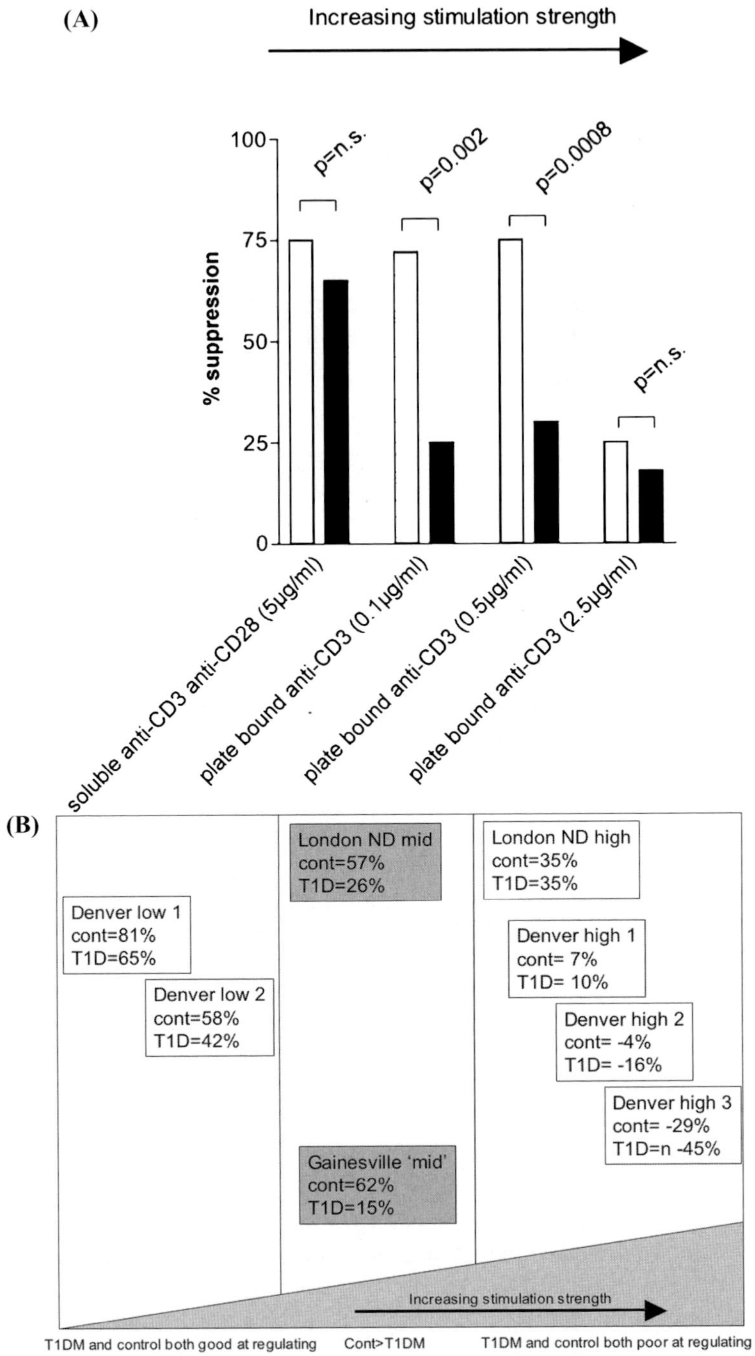
(A)
Increasing stimulation strength
100
75
50
25
0
% suppression
p=n.s.
p=0.002
p=0.0008
p=n.s.
soluble anti-CD3 anti-CD28 (5μg/ml)
plate bound anti-CD3 (0.1μg/ml)
plate bound anti-CD3 (0.5μg/ml)
plate bound anti-CD3 (2.5μg/ml)
(B)
Denver low 1 cont=81% T1D=65%
Denver low 2 cont=58% T1D=42%
London ND mid cont=57% T1D=26%
Gainesville 'mid' cont=62% T1D=15%
London ND high cont=35% T1D=35%
Denver high 1 cont= 7% T1D= 10%
Denver high 2 cont= -4% T1D= -16%
Denver high 3 cont= -29% T1D=n -45%
Increasing stimulation strength
T1DM and control both good at regulating
Cont>T1DM
T1DM and control both poor at regulating

low, medium, or high. In the London study we see that whereas there is a significant difference at medium signal strength (plate bound anti-CD3 at 5 μg/mL) increasing signal strength (high = plate bound anti-CD3 at 10 μg/mL) results in reduced suppressive capacity in both groups with no difference between them. The Denver study used five different signal strengths, two at which both the T1DM patients and controls were equally good at regulating (low 1 and low 2) and three at which both populations show poor regulation (high 1–3). It is important to note that the increment between Denver "low 2" and "high 1" represents a very large increase (50-fold) in anti-CD3 concentration (0.01 μg/mL to 0.5 μg/mL) and the inclusion of an intermediate stimulation strength may have revealed a significant difference between T1DM patients and controls. Although the Gainesville study only reports a single signal strength (and hence is arbitrarily designated as medium), it is noteworthy that this represents an increased signal strength compared to the Denver low 1 signal (soluble anti-CD3 at 5 μg/mL versus soluble anti-CD3 at 2.5 μg/mL, respectively) and may explain why this study found a significant difference between T1DM and control subjects. It is therefore likely that the apparent discordance between the studies is due to the different stimulation conditions used.

CONCLUSIONS AND FUTURE DIRECTIONS

When the data from these four studies are considered together we see considerable concordance. We conclude that whereas there is no significant difference in the frequency of CD4^{+}CD25^{+} T cells in T1DM patients and control subjects, T1DM patients do show defective suppression in this population of cells critical for the maintenance of immunological tolerance. As all the assays were performed in a fully autologous setting, it is as yet impossible to determine whether the defective suppression is due to a difference in the regulatory or responder T cell populations. Further investigations using mixed cultures of responders and regulators from different individuals will be required to address this question. Of particular importance will be investigations in individuals at risk of developing T1DM to determine whether the defective suppression

FIGURE 2. Relationship between signal strength and suppressive capacity of CD4^{+}CD25^{+} T cells in the context of autoimmune disease. (**A**) Summary of CD4^{+}CD25hi regulatory function in MS patients (black bars) and control individuals (open bars) under differing stimulation conditions. Data represents the mean suppression of the proliferative response at a 1:1 ratio responder:regulator cells. All data are derived from Reference 14. (**B**) Summary of relationship between signal strength and regulatory function in T1DM patient and controls. Data represents the mean suppression of the proliferative response at a 1:1 ratio of responder:regulator cells. Signal strengths within each assay are designated as low, medium, or high. Conditions under which a significant difference between T1DM patients and controls was observed are shaded.

contributes to, or is a result of changes in the immune system associated with the development of T1DM. In addition, further studies investigating the phenotype of $CD4^+CD25^+$ T cells in various patient groups using additional markers associated with Treg, for example, the transcription factor FOXP3, may yield useful insight into the role of these cells in the development of T1DM.

ACKNOWLEDGMENTS

The work on $CD4^+CD25^+$ T cells in the laboratory at King's College London is supported by Diabetes UK. Dr. Tree is the recipient of an RD Lawrence Fellowship from Diabetes UK.

REFERENCES

1. ATKINSON, M.A., D.L. KAUFMAN, L. CAMPBELL, *et al.* 1992. Response of peripheral-blood mononuclear cells to glutamate decarboxylase in insulin-dependent diabetes. Lancet **339:** 458–459.
2. HAWKES, C.J., N.C. SCHLOOT, J. MARKS, *et al.* 2000. T-cell lines reactive to an immunodominant epitope of the tyrosine phosphatase-like autoantigen IA-2 in type 1 diabetes. Diabetes **49:** 356–366.
3. ARIF, S., T.I. TREE, T.P. ASTILL, *et al.* 2004. Autoreactive T cell responses show proinflammatory polarization in diabetes but a regulatory phenotype in health. J. Clin. Invest. **113:** 451–463.
4. WALKER, L.S. & A.K. ABBAS. 2002. The enemy within: keeping self-reactive T cells at bay in the periphery. Nat. Rev. Immunol. **2:** 11–19.
5. FRANCOIS BACH, J. 2003. Regulatory T cells under scrutiny. Nat. Rev. Immunol. **3:** 189–198.
6. SHEVACH, E.M. 2002. $CD4^+$ $CD25^+$ suppressor T cells: more questions than answers. Nat. Rev. Immunol. **2:** 389–400.
7. CHATENOUD, L., B. SALOMON & J.A. BLUESTONE. 2001. Suppressor T cells–they're back and critical for regulation of autoimmunity! Immunol. Rev. **182:** 149–163.
8. LINDLEY, S., C.M. DAYAN, A. BISHOP, *et al.* 2005. Defective suppressor function in CD4(+)CD25(+) T-cells from patients with type 1 diabetes. Diabetes **54:** 92–99.
9. PUTNAM, A.L., F. VENDRAME, F. DOTTA & P.A. GOTTLIEB. 2005. $CD4^+$CD25high regulatory T cells in human autoimmune diabetes. J. Autoimmun. **24:** 55–62.
10. BRUSKO, T.M., C.H. WASSERFALL, M.J. CLARE-SALZLER, *et al.* 2005. Functional defects and the influence of age on the frequency of $CD4^+$ $CD25^+$ T-cells in type 1 diabetes. Diabetes **54:** 1407–1414.
11. KUKREJA, A., G. COST, J. MARKER, *et al.* 2002. Multiple immuno-regulatory defects in type-1 diabetes. J. Clin. Invest. **109:** 131–140.
12. BAECHER-ALLAN, C., J.A. BROWN, G.J. FREEMAN & D.A. HAFLER. 2001. $CD4^+$CD25high regulatory cells in human peripheral blood. J. Immunol. **167:** 1245–1253.
13. BAECHER-ALLAN, C., V. VIGLIETTA & D.A. HAFLER. 2002. Inhibition of human CD4(+)CD25(+high) regulatory T cell function. J. Immunol. **169:** 6210–6217.
14. VIGLIETTA, V., C. BAECHER-ALLAN, H.L. WEINER & D.A. HAFLER. 2004. Loss of functional suppression by $CD4^+CD25^+$ regulatory T cells in patients with multiple sclerosis. J. Exp. Med. **199:** 971–979.

HLA Class I Epitope Discovery in Type 1 Diabetes

Independent and Reproducible Identification of Proinsulin Epitopes of CD8 T Cells—Report of the IDS T Cell Workshop Committee

GABRIELLE G.M. PINKSE,[a] CHRISTIAN BOITARD,[b]
TIMOTHY I.M. TREE,[c] MARK PEAKMAN,[c] AND BART O. ROEP[a]

[a]*Department of Immunohematology and Blood Transfusion, Leiden University Medical Center, 2300 RC Leiden, The Netherlands*

[b]*INSERM U561, Université René Descartes, Hôpital Cochin-St. Vincent de Paul, 82 Avenue Denfert Rochereau, 75014 Paris, France*

[c]*Department of Immunobiology, King's College London, School of Medicine, London SE1 9RT, United Kingdom*

ABSTRACT: Islet autoreactive CD8 T cells are plausible candidates for direct beta cell toxicity in type 1 diabetes (T1DM). In 2005, cellular studies in the pathogenesis of this disease have reached a new milestone. Autoreactive CD8 T cells have been defined and several target islet epitopes of these have been discovered and validated simultaneously in three independent studies. The insulin B10–B18 peptide that displays exceptional binding affinity for HLA-A2 has been reported in all three studies, and its recognition shows an association with autoimmune beta cell destruction and T1DM. These studies imply that CD8 T cell-based HLA tetramers and ELISPOT analyses can be useful to monitor T1DM as well as islet transplantation, and may provide useful tools to assess immunological efficacy of immune intervention trials.

KEYWORDS: CD8 T cell; autoimmune disease; cytotoxicity

Type 1 diabetes mellitus (T1DM) is characterized by a T cell-mediated autoimmune destruction of the pancreatic beta cells, resulting in an irreversible loss of insulin production.[1] How lymphocytes target beta cells has been unclear, but it is conceivable that HLA class I-restricted CD8 T cells are responsible for the direct cytolysis of beta cells. Autoreactive cytotoxic T cells can rec-

Address for correspondence: Bart O. Roep, Department of Immunohematology and Blood Transfusion, E3Q, Leiden University Medical Center, PO Box 9600, 2300 RC Leiden, The Netherlands. Voice: 31-71-526-3869; fax: 31-71-521-6751.
e-mail: boroep@lumc.nl

Ann. N.Y. Acad. Sci. 1079: 19–23 (2006). © 2006 New York Academy of Sciences.
doi: 10.1196/annals.1375.003

ognize peptide epitopes displayed on the beta cell surface in the context of HLA class I molecules. These 8–10 amino acid epitopes are primarily derived from endogenous (beta cell) proteins, and are processed by proteasomes that determine the C terminus of the epitopes that are critical for binding to HLA class I. Next, transporters associated with antigen processing (TAP) selectively transfer certain processed peptides from the cytosol into the ER, where they can bind to HLA class I.

Remarkably, little is known of autoreactive CD8 T cells in clinical T1DM. Such T cells have been described against an HLA-A2 binding peptide of GAD65.[2] However, these T cells seem unable to lyse beta cells, and we have preliminary data that this GAD65 peptide is not naturally processed by constitutive proteasomes. This could explain the lack of beta cell lysis, in spite of lysis of GAD65-transfected B cell lines. Second, human cytotoxic T lymphocytes (CTLs) to a peptide with strong HLA-A2 binding affinity from islet amyloid polypeptide (IAPP or amylin) were reported in individuals with recent-onset T1DM.[3]

In 2005, three breakthrough studies have been reported that independently addressed the discovery of beta cell epitopes of CD8 T cells (Hassainya *et al.* [4], Toma *et al.*,[5] and Pinkse *et al.* [6]). All three studies pursued similar experimental designs that included intracellular mechanisms, such as proteolytic breakdown of intracytosolic peptides by the proteasome, translocation by TAP, and binding of peptides into the groove of MHC class I molecules. Finally, T cell responses

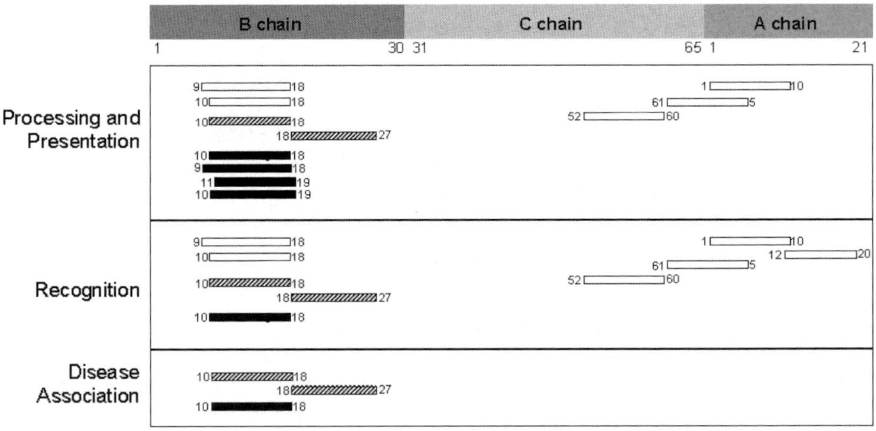

FIGURE 1. Discovery of HLA-A2-restricted peptides of (pro)insulin in three independent studies. Processing and presentation of peptides with high HLA-A2 and TAP affinities and correct proteasome cleavage sites, recognition of HLA-A2-restricted proinsulin epitopes recognized by T cells in humans or a humanized mouse model, and disease association of epitope recognition are summarized. Peptides are presented as open, hatched, or black bars, as defined in Hassainya *et al.*[4] Toma *et al.*[5] and Pinkse *et al.*[6] respectively.

TABLE 1. Overview of generation and recognition of proinsulin epitopes of CD8 T cells

Position	HLA-A2-peptide binding	TAP affinity*	Proteasome cleavage	Notes
B9–B18	H	H	+	Recognized by HHD2 mice
B10–B18	H	H	+	Recognized by type 1 diabetic patients and islet transplant recipients with loss of function
B18–B27	I	I	+	Recognized by type 1 diabetic patients
C52–C60	L	L	+	Recognized by HHD2 mice, sequence difference between mice and human
C61–A5	L	L	+	Recognized by HHD2 mice, sequence difference between mice and human
A1–A10	H	I	+	Epitope generated inefficiently by antigen presenting cells
A12–A20	H	H	−	Recognized by HHD2 mice

*L = low affinity; I = intermediate affinity; H = high affinity

to these HLA class A2-restricted islet epitopes were studied in humans[5,6] or a humanized mouse model.[4] Two of these studies went on to evaluate whether the processed peptides were recognized by human CD8 T cells, and tested for an association with (the pathogenesis) of T1DM.[5,6]

Insulin is an important autoantigen that initiates the immune response leading to autoimmune diabetes in mice. CD4 T cell reactivity to the insulin B chain was frequently detectable in diabetic patients,[7,8] and insulin was suggested to be a major target in T cells in pancreas-draining lymph nodes of long-standing T1DM patients.[9] Since ulin is only expressed in pancreatic beta cells, peptides derived from proinsulin should be a major target for cytotoxic T cells causing beta cell destruction. It was therefore logical to test proinsulin as target of autoreactive CD8 T cells.

All three studies have in common that they identify novel epitopes in T1DM for the class I allele HLA-A2 (0201) that has been shown to confer additional risk to the development of T1DM in patients possessing the high-risk class II alleles HLA-DR3 and HLA-DR4. Indeed, introduction of human HLA-A2 in an animal model of spontaneous autoimmune diabetes leads to an accelerated disease onset.[10] The three studies have independently identified HLA-A2-restricted epitopes of proinsulin (FIG. 1, TABLE 1). All these epitopes can be naturally processed. Each study independently identified the insulin B10–B18 epitope as a candidate target of autoreactive CD8 T cells with extremely high binding affinity for HLA-A2. Preliminary data support recognition of the naturally processed endogenous insulin B10–B18 epitope on the surface of human beta cells. Importantly, this epitope was differentially recognized in T1DM patients both at disease onset and after longer disease duration, but not in T2DM patients or HLA-A2-matched nondiabetic control subjects in ELISPOT studies.[5] Importantly, HLA-$A2^{insB10-B18}$ tetramer studies indicate that insulin B10–B18-specific CD8 T cells are present in the circulation of islet transplant recipients with recurrent autoimmunity, but rarely in those with persistent beta cell function or patients that rejected their islet allograft.[6] One study further identified candidate proinsulin epitopes of HLA-B8 and HLA-A1.[5] The epitopes C52–C60 and C61–A5 identified by Hassainya *et al.* do not necessarily bear relevance to humans in view of sequence differences between murine and human proinsulin, although their potential immunogenicity was demonstrated in HHD2- transgenic mice.[4] Epitope A12–A20 is recognized by HDD2 T cells, but lacks evidence of being naturally processed.

We conclude that cellular studies on the pathogenesis of T1DM have reached a new milestone. Autoreactive CD8 T cells have been defined and several target islet epitopes of these have been discovered and validated. The insulin B10–B18 peptide that displays exceptional binding affinity for HLA-A2 has been identified independently in the three studies. Recognition of this epitope indicates an association with autoimmune beta cell destruction and T1DM. These studies imply that class I HLA tetramers and ELISPOT analyses can be useful to study new-onset T1DM patients as well as type 1 diabetic islet transplant recipients, and may provide useful tools to assess immunological efficacy of immune intervention trials.

REFERENCES

1. ROEP, B.O. 2003. The role of T-cells in the pathogenesis of type 1 diabetes: from cause to cure. Diabetologia **46:** 305–321.
2. PANINA-BORDIGNON, P., R. LANG, P.M. VAN ENDERT, *et al.* 1995. Cytotoxic T cells specific for glutamic acid decarboxylase in autoimmune diabetes. J. Exp. Med. **181:** 1923–1927.
3. PANAGIOTOPOULOS, C., H. QIN, R. TAN & C.B. VERCHERE. 2003. Identification of a beta-cell-specific HLA class I restricted epitope in type 1 diabetes. Diabetes **52:** 2647–2651.
4. HASSAINYA, Y., F. GARCIA-PONS, R. KRATZER, *et al.* 2005. Identification of naturally processed HLA-A2-restricted proinsulin epitopes by reverse immunology. Diabetes **54:** 2053–2059.
5. TOMA, A., S. HADDOUK, J.P. BRIAND, *et al.* 2005. Recognition of a subregion of human proinsulin by class I-restricted T cells in type 1 diabetic patients. Proc. Natl. Acad. Sci. USA **102:** 10581–10586.

6. PINKSE, G.G., O.H. TYSMA, C.A. BERGEN, *et al.* 2005. Autoreactive CD8 T cells associated with β-cell destruction in type 1 diabetes. Proc. Natl. Acad. Sci. USA **102:** 18425–18430.
7. ARIF, S., T.I. TREE, T.P. ASTILL, *et al.* 2004. Autoreactive T cell responses show proinflammatory polarization in diabetes but a regulatory phenotype in health. J. Clin. Invest **113:** 451–463.
8. DURINOVIC-BELLO, I., M. SCHLOSSER, M. RIEDL, *et al.* 2004. Pro- and anti-inflammatory cytokine production by autoimmune T cells against preproinsulin in HLA-DRB1*04, DQ8 Type 1 diabetes. Diabetologia **47:** 439–450.
9. KENT, S.C., Y. CHEN, L. BREGOLI, *et al.* 2005. Expanded T cells from pancreatic lymph nodes of type 1 diabetic subjects recognize an insulin epitope. Nature **435:** 224–228.
10. MARRON, M.P., R.T. GRASER, H.D. CHAPMAN & D.V. SERREZE. 2002. Functional evidence for the mediation of diabetogenic T cell responses by HLA-A2.1 MHC class I molecules through transgenic expression in NOD mice. Proc. Natl. Acad. Sci. USA **99:** 13753–13758.

Genetics of Fulminant Type 1 Diabetes

EIJI KAWASAKI[a] AND KATSUMI EGUCHI[b]

[a]*Department of Metabolism/Diabetes and Clinical Nutrition, Nagasaki University Hospital of Medicine and Dentistry, Nagasaki 852-8501, Japan*

[b]*The First Department of Internal Medicine, Graduate School of Biomedical Sciences, Nagasaki 852-8501, Japan*

ABSTRACT: Fulminant type 1 diabetes exhibits distinct clinical futures from "classic" autoimmune type 1 diabetes. Although the etiology of fulminant type 1 diabetes is not fully elucidated, class II HLA could contribute to the development of fulminant type 1 diabetes. In Japanese patients with "classic" type 1 diabetes, DRB1*0405-DQB1*0401 and DRB1*0901-DQB1*0303 are major susceptible HLA-DR-DQ haplotypes, whereas DRB1*1502-DQB1*0601 and DRB1*1501-DQB1*0602 are protective. In contrast, only DRB1*0405-DQB1*0401, but not DRB1*0901-DQB1*0303, is a susceptible haplotype in fulminant type 1 diabetes. In addition, neither DRB1*1502-DQB1*0601 nor DRB1*1501-DQB1*0602 are protective haplotypes in fulminant type 1 diabetes. In genotypic combination analysis, the homozygotes of DRB1*0405-DQB1*0401 are associated with both fulminant type 1 diabetes and "classic" type 1 diabetes, whereas the homozygotes of DRB1*0901-DQB1*0303 are associated with only "classic" type 1 diabetes. These findings suggest a different contribution of class II HLA in the mechanisms of beta cell damage between fulminant and "classic" type 1 diabetes. To further address the pathogenesis of fulminant type 1 diabetes, HNF-1α gene mutation and mutation of the mitochondrial DNA were analyzed in patients with fulminant type 1 diabetes admitted to our department during the period from 1990 to 2000. Neither mutations of HNF-1α gene nor A-to-G mutation at nucleotide position 3,243 of the mitochondrial tRNA$^{LEU(UUR)}$ gene were identified in these patients. These results suggest that the HNF-1α gene mutation and mutation of the mitochondrial DNA are not likely associated with diabetic patients with fulminant clinical symptoms at disease onset. In this article we will summarize the current findings on the genetics of Japanese patients with fulminant type 1 diabetes.

KEYWORDS: type 1 diabetes; Japanese; fulminant; genetics; HLA

Address for correspondence: Eiji Kawasaki, M.D., Ph.D., Department of Metabolism/Diabetes and Clinical Nutrition, Nagasaki University Hospital of Medicine and Dentistry, 1-7-1 Sakamoto, Nagasaki 852-8501, Japan. Voice: +81-95-849-7550; fax: +81-95-849-7552.
e-mail: eijikawa@nagasaki-u.ac.jp

Ann. N.Y. Acad. Sci. 1079: 24–30 (2006). © 2006 New York Academy of Sciences.
doi: 10.1196/annals.1375.004

INTRODUCTION

Type 1 diabetes is characterized by insulin deficiency from the chronic and progressive autoimmune destruction of islet beta cells. This type of type 1 diabetes is classified as "immune-mediated" (type 1A) diabetes. Another type of type 1 diabetes is a disease with no evidence of an autoimmune disorder at disease onset and classified as "idiopathic" (type 1B) diabetes.[1,2] It is well known that clinical characteristics of type 1 diabetes are heterogenous in terms of age at onset, mode of onset, etc. It has been recently documented as a new subtype of type 1 diabetes in Japan, termed as *fulminant type 1 diabetes* characterized by remarkably abrupt onset and fulminant symptoms, including marked hyperglycemia and severe diabetic ketoacidosis with normal-to-near normal HbA1c levels.[3] Genetic factors are important on the development of type 1 diabetes and more than 20 putative diabetes-predisposing genes have been identified by linkage and association studies.[4] Among them most of the genetic susceptibility for type 1 diabetes is determined by HLA class II genes on chromosome 6q21.[5] Other major disease-associated loci identified so far are the insulin gene on chromosome 11p15,[6] and the CTLA4 locus on 2q33.[7] On the other hand, several disorders other than type 1 diabetes lead to extensive pancreatic islet beta cell destruction. Among them relatively common genetic disorders associated with insulin-dependent diabetes include MODY3 by mutations in the HNF-1α gene[8] and the maternally inherited diabetes mellitus (MIDD) caused by a point mutation in the mitochondrial gene coding for tRNA $^{\text{LEU(UUR)}}$ (especially nucleotide position at 3,243).[9] In this article we will summarize the current findings on the genetics of Japanese patients with fulminant type 1 diabetes.

FULMINANT TYPE 1 DIABETES

TABLE 1 summarizes the clinical features of patients with fulminant type 1 diabetes. Fulminant type 1 diabetes have distinct clinical features from type 1 A diabetes characterized by (*a*) extremely rapid onset, (*b*) male predominance, adult-onset, and frequent flu-like symptoms precede the onset of diabetes occurrence of diabetic ketoacidosis, (*c*) exhausted insulin secretory capacity at onset, (*d*) no anti-islet autoantibodies, (*e*) elevated serum pancreatic enzyme, and (*f*) T cell infiltration of the exocrine pancreas in biopsy specimens. Based on a nationwide survey of fulminant type 1 diabetes in Japan conducted by the Committee on the Study of Fulminant Type 1 Diabetes under the auspices of Japan Diabetes Society, the diagnostic criteria for fulminant type 1 diabetes have been established (TABLE 2).

CLASS II HLA AND FULMINANT TYPE 1 DIABETES

Many studies have shown that the class II HLA loci on chromosome 6q21.3 are most strongly associated with type 1 diabetes risk. The DRB1

TABLE 1. Clinical characteristics of fulminant type 1 diabetes

1. ~20% among Japanese type 1 diabetes with ketosis or ketoacidosis at onset
2. Mostly (>90%) adult onset
3. Remarkably abrupt onset (duration before diagnosis 4 ~ 5 days) with diabetic ketoacidosis
4. Extremely high plasma glucose (average 44 mM) with low level of HbA1c (<8.5%) at onset
5. High frequency of flu-like symptoms preceding the diabetes onset
6. Elevated serum pancreatic enzyme levels
7. Negative for anti-islet autoantibodies
8. No endogenous insulin secretion at onset (urine C-peptide < 10 μg/day)
9. No honeymoon period
10. Typical form of type 1 diabetes associated with pregnancy

and DQB1 genes are the major determinants of HLA-encoded susceptibility to type 1 diabetes. Although disease associations with the DQB1 genes are stronger than with DRB1 gene,[10] it has been shown that both loci are important for determining overall disease risk. HLA-DRB1*0405-DQB1*0401 and DRB1*0901-DQB1*0303 are two major diabetes-susceptible haplotypes in Japanese population. In contrast, DRB1*1501-DQB1*0602 confers strong protection against type 1 diabetes and this protective effect is dominant over susceptibility conferred by HLA-DRB1*0405-DQB1*0401 and DRB1*0901-DQB1*0303.[11] Furthermore, DRB1*1502-DQB1*0601 also protects against type 1 diabetes in Japanese population, but its effect is not as strong as that of DRB1*1501-DQB1*0602 haplotype. Recent studies of the HLA subtype identified associations between fulminant type 1 diabetes and the class II HLA. In contrast to the association of HLA-DR9 with typical type 1A diabetes, HLA-DR4, but not DR9, was associated with fulminant type 1 diabetes. In fulminant type 1 diabetes, the homozygotes of DR4-DQ4 showed highest odds ratio (OR) (OR = 13.3, 95% CI: 3.8–47.0, $P = 2.87 \times 10^{-6}$) (FIG. 1).[12] However, the contribution of class II HLA is distinct in patients with fulminant type 1 diabetes who developed during the pregnancy or immediately after delivery.[13] The patients associated with pregnancy account for 21% of female fulminant type 1 diabetic patients aged 13–49 years. In those patients, homozygotes for

TABLE 2. Diagnostic criteria for fulminant type 1 diabetes (Committee on the Study of Fulminant Type 1 Diabetes, Japan Diabetes Society)

1. Occurrence of diabetic ketosis or ketoacidosis soon after (around 7 days) the onset of hyperglycemic symptoms (elevation of urinary keton or serum keton at onset)

and

2. Plasma glucose > 16.0 mM and HbA1c level < 8.5% at onset

and

3. (1) Urinary C-peptide excretion < 10 μg/day or (2) Fasting serum C-peptide < 0.3 ng/mL and serum C-peptide < 0.5 ng/mL after i.v. glucagon (or after meal)

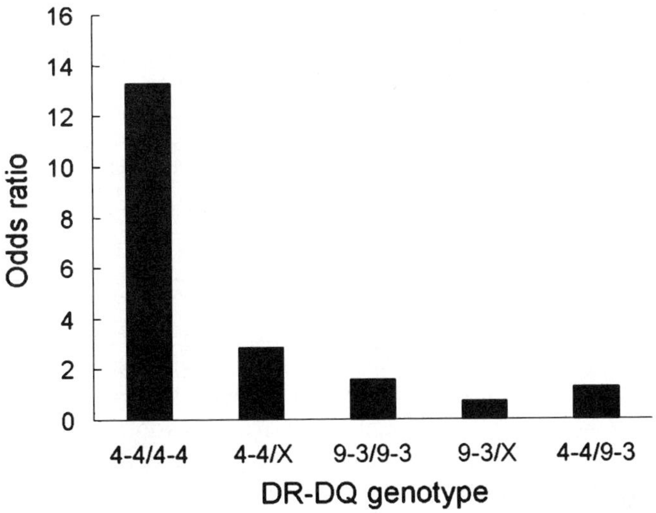

FIGURE 1. OR for the genotypic combination of DR4-DQ4 and DR9-DQ3 in fulminant type 1 diabetes.[12] X, neither DR4-DQ4 nor DR9-DQ3.

DR9-DQ3 is strongly associated with the susceptibility to fulminant type 1 diabetes (OR = 10.0, 95% CI: 2.0–49.0, $P = 0.0007$), even though the clinical phenotypes of these patients are almost the same as those whose onset were not associated with pregnancy. These results suggest that a differential contribution of class II HLA in the mechanisms of beta cell damage between pregnancy-associated and nonpregnancy-associated fulminant type 1 diabetes.

HNF-1α GENE AND MITOCHONDRIAL GENE IN FULMINANT TYPE 1 DIABETES

Several disorders other than type 1 diabetes lead to extensive pancreatic islet beta cell destruction. Among them relatively common genetic disorders associated with insulin-dependent diabetes include MODY3 by mutations in the HNF-1α gene[8] and the MIDD caused by a point mutation in the mitochondrial gene coding for tRNA $^{LEU(UUR)}$ (especially nucleotide position at 3,243).[9] To address the pathogenesis of fulminant type 1 diabetes, HNF-1α gene mutation and mutation of the mitochondrial DNA were analyzed in our patients diagnosed as fulminant type 1 diabetes who were admitted to Nagasaki University Hospital during the period from 1990 to 2000. The protocol was approved by the Institutional Review Board of the Nagasaki University School of Medicine. For the systemic search of the mutation in the HNF-1α gene the 10 exons, flanking introns, and the minimal promotor region were amplified by PCR and analyzed by direct sequencing method on an ABI Prism 377 DNA Sequencer (ABI Perkin-Elmer Corp., Foster City, CA).[14] Furthermore, A-to-G mutation at position 3,243 of the mitochondrial $tRNA^{LEU(UUR)}$ gene was analyzed by PCR–RFLP using *Apa* I restriction enzyme.[9] However, none of the patients with fulminant type 1 diabetes had mutations in the HNF-1α gene. Furthermore, no A-to-G substitution at position 3,243 of the mitochondrial $tRNA^{LEU(UUR)}$ gene was identified in these patients.

DISCUSSION

Fulminant type 1 diabetes is a subtype of type 1 diabetes that accounts for approximately 20% of abrupt onset type 1 diabetes in Japan.[15] It is currently unknown whether or not fulminant type 1 diabetes is a unique disease in Japanese population. Few cases have been reported outside Japan.[16–18] Because greater than 90% of patients develop in adulthood, it might be possible that this subtype has been disregarded among the majority of typical type 1A diabetes in children. The pathogenesis underlying beta cell destruction in fulminant type 1 diabetes is largely unknown. In the original paper published in the *New England Journal of Medicine* in 2000, Imagawa and co-workers described that fulminant type 1 diabetes is a nonautoimmune diabetes.[3] However, there are some evidences that support the fact that fulminant type 1 diabetes is autoimmune related. Tanaka and co-workers reported the evidence of insulitis in an autopsy case of fulminant type 1 diabetes.[19] Furthermore, about 5% of patients with fulminant type 1 diabetes express autoantibodies to GAD65.[15] GAD-reactive or insulin B9–B23-reactive Th1 cells were also identified in peripheral blood lymphocyte from patients with fulminant type 1 diabetes.[20] The strong association of DRB1*0405-DQB1*0401, which has close linkage disequilibrium with class I HLA-A24, with fulminant type 1 diabetes also suggests that immunogenetic predisposition contributes to beta cell destruction in this subtype of type 1 diabetes. The class I HLA-A24 gene has been reported to promote pancreatic beta cell destruction in an additive manner in the patients with type 1 diabetes-susceptible HLA class II genes.[21] These findings suggest that the etiology of fulminant type 1 diabetes might be heterogenous and a part of patients is autoimmune related.

It has been reported that MODY3 caused by the mutations in the HNF-1α gene is characterized by rapid progress to overt diabetes and severe insulin secretory defects to glucose.[22] Furthermore, patients with MIDD caused by a point mutation in the mitochondrial gene coding for $tRNA^{LEU(UUR)}$ often show the insulin-deficient diabetes.[9] We have previously reported that about 7% of Japanese patients with type 1 diabetes who lack anti-islet autoantibodies have the mutations in the HNF-1α gene.[14] These highlight the difficulties in distinguishing between insulin-dependent diabetic patients with MODY3 or MIDD and patients with type 1B diabetes because of the lack of anti-islet autoantibodies in these patients. Because of the severe hyperglycemia and the deficient insulin secretion of patients with MODY3 or MIDD, we hypothesized that some patients classified as having fulminant type 1 diabetes could have MODY3 or MIDD. However, neither mutations of HNF-1α gene nor mitochondrial tRNA$^{LEU(UUR)}$ gene were identified in our patients diagnosed as having fulminant type 1 diabetes. These results suggest that the HNF-1α gene mutation and mutation of the mitochondrial DNA are not likely associated with diabetic patients with fulminant clinical symptoms at disease onset. Further investigations are needed to understand the pathophysiological mechanisms involved in the beta cell destruction in fulminant type 1 diabetes.

ACKNOWLEDGMENTS

This work is supported in part by a grant-in-aid from the Ministry of Education, Culture, Science, Sports and Technology of Japan and from the Japan Diabetes Foundation. Committee members on the Study of Fulminant Type 1 Diabetes are as follows: Chairman: Hideichi Makino (Ehime University School of Medicine), Secretary: Toshiaki Hanafusa (Osaka Medical College), Akihisa Imagawa (Osaka Medical College), Hiromi Iwahashi (Osaka University), Yasuko Uchigata (Tokyo Women's Medical University School of Medicine), Azuma Kanatsuka (Kasori Hospital), Eiji Kawasaki (Nagasaki University Hospital of Medicine and Dentistry), Tetsuro Kobayashi (University of Yamanashi School of Medicine), Akira Shimada (Keio University School of Medicine), Ikki Shimizu (Ehime Prefectural Central Hospital), and Taro Maruyama (Saitama Social Insurance Hospital).

REFERENCES

1. THE EXPERT COMMITTEE ON THE DIAGNOSIS AND CLASSIFICATION OF DIABETES MELLITUS. 1997. Report of the Expert Committee on the Diagnosis and Classification of Diabetes Mellitus. Diabetes Care **20:** 1183–1197.
2. ALBERTI, K.G. & P.Z. ZIMMET. 1998. Definition, diagnosis and classification of diabetes mellitus and its complications. Part 1: diagnosis and classification of diabetes mellitus provisional report of a WHO consultation. Diabet. Med. **15:** 539–553.
3. IMAGAWA, A. *et al.* 2000. A novel subtype of type 1 diabetes mellitus characterized by a rapid onset and an absence of diabetes-related antibodies. Osaka IDDM Study Group. N. Engl. J. Med. **342:** 301–307.
4. KAWASAKI, E., R.G. GILL & G.S. EISENBARTH. 1999. Type 1 diabetes. *In* Endocrine and Organ Specific Autoimmunity. G.S. Eisenbarth, Ed.: 149–182. R.G. Landes. Austin, TX.
5. TODD, J.A., J.I. BELL & H.O. MCDEVITT. 1987. HLA-DQB gene contributes to susceptibility and resistance to insulin-dependent diabetes mellitus. Nature **329:** 599–604.

6. BELL, G.I., S. HORITA & J.H. KARAM. 1984. A polymorphic locus near the human insulin gene is associated with insulin-dependent diabetes mellitus. Diabetes **33:** 176–183.
7. UEDA, H. *et al.* 2003. Association of the T-cell regulatory gene CTLA4 with susceptibility to autoimmune disease. Nature **423:** 506–511.
8. YAMAGATA, K. *et al.* 1996. Mutations in the hepatocyte nuclear factor-1 α gene in maturity-onset diabetes of the young. Nature **384:** 455–458.
9. KADOWAKI, T. *et al.* 1994. A subtype of diabetes mellitus associated with a mutation of mitochondrial DNA. N. Engl. J. Med. **330:** 962–968.
10. SHE, J. 1996. Susceptibility to type I diabetes: HLA-DQ and DR revisited. Immunol. Today **17:** 323–329.
11. ABIRU, N., E. KAWASAKI & K. EGUCHI. 2002. Current knowledge of Japanese type 1 diabetic syndrome. Diabetes Metab. Res. Rev. **18:** 357–366.
12. IMAGAWA, A. *et al.* 2005. Different contribution of class II HLA in fulminant and typical autoimmune type 1 diabetes mellitus. Diabetologia **48:** 294–300.
13. SHIMIZU, I. *et al.* 2005. Clinical and immunogenetic characteristics of fulminant type 1 diabetes associated with pregnancy. J. Clin. Endocrinol. Metab. **91:** 471–476.
14. KAWASAKI, E. *et al.* 2000. Identification and functional analysis of mutations in the hepatocyte nuclear factor-1 α gene in anti-islet autoantibody-negative Japanese patients with type 1 diabetes. J. Clin. Endocrinol. Metab. **85:** 331–335.
15. IMAGAWA, A. *et al.* 2003. Fulminant type 1 diabetes: a nationwide survey in Japan. Diabetes Care **26:** 2345–2352.
16. JUNG, T.S. *et al.* 2004. A Korean patient with fulminant autoantibody-negative type 1 diabetes. Diabetes Care **27:** 3023–3024.
17. TANIYAMA, M. *et al.* 2004. A Filipino patient with fulminant type 1 diabetes. Diabetes Care **27:** 842–843.
18. VREUGDENHIL, G.R. *et al.* 2000. Acute onset of type I diabetes mellitus after severe echovirus 9 infection: putative pathogenic pathways. Clin. Infect. Dis. **31:** 1025–1031.
19. TANAKA, S., T. KOBAYASHI & T. MOMOTSU. 2000. A novel subtype of type 1 diabetes mellitus. N. Engl. J. Med. **342:** 1835–1837.
20. KOTANI, R. *et al.* 2004. T lymphocyte response against pancreatic beta cell antigens in fulminant type 1 diabetes. Diabetologia **47:** 1285–1291.
21. NAKANISHI, K. *et al.* 1993. Association of HLA-A24 with complete β-cell destruction in IDDM. Diabetes **42:** 1086–1098.
22. LEHTO, M. *et al.* 1997. Characterization of the MODY3 phenotype. Early-onset diabetes caused by an insulin secretion defect. J. Clin. Invest. **99:** 582–591.

Why Is Type 1 Diabetes Uncommon in Asia?

YONGSOO PARK

Division of Endocrinology and Metabolism, Department of Internal Medicine, Hanyang University Hospital, Hanyang University College of Medicine, 471-020 Seoul, Korea

Department of Bioengineering, Hanyang University College of Engineering, 471-020 Seoul, Korea

Abstract: T1D (type 1 diabetes) incidence rates are extremely low in Asian populations. The prevalences of islet-specific autoantibodies are reported to be low compared with Caucasians. Although the clinical and immunologic characteristics of T1D in Asians appear to be different from those of Caucasians, if we apply correct patient definition and standardized methods, the typical T1D patients are very similar, in the immunologic as well as genetic perspectives. Although the association of individual allele seems to be different between populations, if we compare the identical DR-DQ haplotypes, the association and transmission to diabetic offspring were similar for Asians and Caucasians. The high-risk HLA genotypes/haplotypes were found to be independent determinants of diabetes in the first-degree relatives of individuals with T1D, particularly in the presence of autoantibodies. A different genetic susceptibility including a low frequency of high-risk HLA alleles could explain the lower prevalence of islet-specific autoantibodies and the low incidence of T1D, or different genetic and environmental interactions might be involved in the etiology of T1D. It is certain that DR-DQ linkage disequilibrium (LD) is an important factor explaining the difference in T1D incidence in different countries. LD between highly susceptible DRB1 alleles and protective DQB1 alleles, and *vice versa*, is the major contributing factor to the low incidence of T1D in Asians. We also suggested that different genetic/environmental interactions might operate in the etiology of T1D between Caucasians and Asians. It would be of great help for primary prevention to investigate to what degree genetic determinants influence the well-known regional differences in incidences, since we can identify environmental risk factors that may either initiate the autoimmune process or promote already ongoing β cell damage in different countries. For this, population-based epidemiological studies are necessary to identify risk determinants that may be useful for primary prevention strategies.

Address for correspondence: Yongsoo Park, M.D., Department of Internal Medicine, Hanyang University Hospital, 249-1 Kyomun-dong, Kuri, Kyunggi-do, 471-020, Korea. Voice: 82-31-560-2239; fax: 82-31-553-7369.

e-mail: parkys@hanyang.ac.kr

Ann. N.Y. Acad. Sci. 1079: 31–40 (2006).
doi: 10.1196/annals.1375.005

KEYWORDS: type 1 diabetes; incidence; genetic determinants; environmental etiologies

Is Type 1 Diabetes (T1D) Uncommon in Asia?

Immune-mediated T1D is an etiologic subtype of diabetes caused by autoimmune destruction of the insulin-secreting β cells of the islets of Langerhans. Unlike T2D, a more common form of diabetes with onset mostly, but not exclusively in adults, T1D is among the most prevalent life-threatening disorders affecting children around the world. The incidence of T1D in different ethnic groups is extremely variable, suggesting the involvement of genetic as well as environmental elements. The incidence rate of T1D occurring below the age of 15 years has been registered in many parts of the world, owing to the activities of the WHO-DIAMOND collaborative studies.[1] In Caucasian populations, T1D incidence rates are high with rates in excess of 20 cases/year/100,000 individuals, while Asian countries have extremely low T1D incidence rates with the rate less than 1 case/year/100,000 individuals. A mail survey to investigate the T1D incidence has been conducted in all hospitals with more than 20 beds in Seoul, Korea since the year 1986.[2,3] All T1D patients had been registered thereafter. The annual incidence rates did not show significant temporal variation ranging from 0.6 to 2.2 cases per 100,000. Additional T1D incidence data in Japan with a high degree of ascertainment have demonstrated that the incidence is similar with no temporal variation.[4] From these, we can indicate that T1D is much less frequent in Asia than in countries with a predominantly Caucasian population.

The average ascertainment level of TID in Asian countries is low, and incorrect patient definition might lead to a false conclusion on the demographic characteristics of T1D in Asia. There is a difference in the relative proportion of T1D by age of onset in Asia and Europe.[5] The percentage of T2D in young diabetic subjects in Asians is higher than in Caucasoid population. In accordance with the view that development of T1D involves heterogeneous mechanisms, different clinical courses of β cell destruction have been reported in Asian T1D patients. The most prevalent clinical manifestation is abrupt onset with severe clinical symptoms, very high blood glucose levels and ketonemia at diagnosis, which shares similar clinical features with that seen in Caucasian populations. Another subtype of T1D in the Asian population is a slow-onset form. The eventual clinical features of these patients include ketosis proneness, unstable blood glucose levels, and extremely diminished 24-h urinary C-peptide excretion rate. The majority of Asian patients with T2D have been reported to be a non-obese type with low insulin secretion. It is also true that the clinical distinction between T1D and T2D has been difficult to determine in some of the Asian population. In our Seoul T1D genetic consortium, we would like to monitor every single development of T1D prospectively.[6] Having sera as well as DNA, we could define the patient more correctly and we may be able to get an access to the etiology of T1D. We have the hypothesis that the high-risk haplotypes/genotypes are independent determinants of diabetes in the first-degree relatives, particularly in the presence of islet-specific antibodies. Concordant siblings or T1D patients and multiple autoantibody (+) siblings appeared to share the same 2 HLA DR-DQ haplotypes. We are following up every single case prospectively whether he or she has autoantibodies.

Is T1D in Asia also Caused by Autoimmunity?

T1D is now perceived as an autoimmune disease characterized by selective destruction of pancreatic β cells. In the Asian populations, it has been known that the clinical and immunologic characteristics of T1D are quite different from those of Caucasians. Besides the low incidence rate of T1D in Asia, the prevalences of islet cell cytoplasmic antibody (ICA) in Asian T1D patients had been reported to be extremely low compared with those of the Caucasians.[7] However, not only is the detection of the islet-specific autoantibodies in a conventional way rather complicated and time-consuming, but incorrect patient definition might lead to false conclusion on the immunologic characteristics of T1D in Asia.[8] Previous studies have shown a low prevalence of ICA (14–16%) in recent-onset Japanese patients with T1D, suggesting that the autoimmune component may not be so important in the pathogenesis of T1D in Japanese.[7] However, a series of recent well-standardized study on the prevalence of ICA in Asians with T1D demonstrated that more than 80% of recent-onset patients had ICA.[8,9]

During the past decade investigators have identified, cloned, and expressed a series of islet autoantigens, including GAD65 and IA-2 and applied as an alternative to ICA. We also applied a new radioligand-binding assay in T1D patients, whose age at onset was less than 15 years and the prevalences of IA-2 autoantibodies, anti-GAD65, and ICA in recent-onset patients (duration < 1 year) reached those of Caucasian levels.[9] In contrast, in a subset of these patients with long standing diabetes (duration > 3 years), the prevalence of IA-2 autoantibodies, anti-GAD65, and ICA were decreased to 22%, 49%, and 25%, respectively. The overall prevalence of islet-specific autoantibodies in this childhood-onset T1D in Korea was comparable to Caucasians, especially among those in recent-onset cases (duration less than 1 year). In our Korean patients, IA-2 autoantibodies as well as anti-GAD65 were significantly associated with the presence of ICA, especially in those with onset age < 15 years. Although there should be some other T1D related with insulin deficiency, the major part of T1D with onset age less than 15 is mainly caused by autoimmunity.

Is T1D in Asia also Determined by the Genetic Susceptibility?

T1D is much less frequent in Asia than in countries with a predominantly Caucasian population.[3,4] To investigate whether the genetic determinants influence the development of T1D in these low incidence countries, Ikegami *et al*. studied siblings of T1D probands with age at onset under 20 years.[10] The ratio of the risk for siblings of T1D patients and the population prevalence (λs), often used to assess the degree of familial clustering of a disease is more than 200, a much higher value than that in Caucasian populations. Familial clustering of a disease does not necessarily indicate a genetic component, since it may be caused by sharing of the same environment among family members. If a genetic factor is responsible for the high λs value for T1D with low population prevalence in Asians, then susceptibility alleles whose frequencies are very low in the general population may be segregating in T1D families.

Is HLA also Important in Asia?

HLA Association in Asians

The HLA class II alleles on chromosome 6p21 are the most highly related to T1D susceptibility.[11–13] Affected siblings-pairs (ASPs) with T1D share HLA alleles more often than expected. Multiple candidate genes in the HLA together with strong linkage disequilibrium (LD) in the HLA make it difficult to pinpoint the locus responsible for T1D susceptibility. To overcome this, we have used simultaneous analysis of multiple candidate gene polymorphisms in the same patients. Even in Asians, both the DR and DQ alleles are the ones to have the highest association with T1D.[6,8,11] In Korean T1D cases, HLA DR3 and DR9 were increased. DR4 as a group was not significantly increased in diabetic patients compared to controls. Among the DR4 subtypes, DRB1*0401 and DRB1*0405 had increased frequencies in patients. Two DR4 subtypes (0403 and 0406) had lower frequencies in patients. As expected, DR15 confers strong protection. DR12 was also strongly protective. When the HLA DQB1 alleles were identified in the T1D patients, the only DQB1*0201 allele had significantly higher frequencies in patients, while three DQB1 alleles (0301, 0601, 0602) had significantly lower frequencies in patients compared to controls. Five haplotypes (DRB1*03-DQB1*0201, DRB1*0401-DQB1*0302, DRB1*0405-DQB1*0302, DRB1*0407-DQB1*0302, and DRB1*0901-DQB1*0303) had significantly increased frequencies in diabetic patients. Four other haplotypes (DRB1*15-DQB1*0601, DRB1*15-DQB1*0602, DRB1*08-DQB1*0601, and DRB1*10-DQB1*05) had significantly lower frequencies in patients.[11]

HLA Genotypic and Haplotypic Associations

It has been proposed that the contribution of the HLA DQ molecule to overall disease susceptibility may be genotype dependent. We analyzed the association of DQ8 (DQA1*0301-DQB1*0302) and DQ4 (DQA1*0301-DQB1*0401) haplotypes in Asian patients with T1D.[14] Although the prevalence of the DR4-DQ8 haplotype did not differ in patients versus controls, the HLA DR3/4-DQ8 genotype had an increased risk indicating a synergistic effect. When DR3/4 diabetic patients are compared to all other DR4 positive patients, a significant association of DQ8 with the DR3/4 genotype was found. In contrast, a significant association of DQ4 with DR4/X (X: other than 1, 3, 4) was found. High-risk DR4 subtypes (DRB1*0401, *0402, *0405) were predominant in DR4/X, whereas protective DR4 subtypes (DRB1*0403, *0406) were observed mainly in the DR3/4 genotype. The association of DR4 haplotypes with diabetes varies depending on the haplotype borne on the homologous chromosome. This might contribute not only to the synergistic effect of DR3/4, but also to the susceptibility influence of DQ4 haplotypes confined to DR4/X.

Common Transmission of HLA Haplotypes Across Ethnicity

It has been suggested that HLA alleles of Asian patients associated with T1D differ from those of Caucasians. It is apparent that population frequencies of DR and DQ alleles and haplotypes vary dramatically between ethnic groups. Because of this, some highly "diabetogenic" DR or DQ alleles, which are relatively uncommon in a population may be mistakenly considered neutral in population association studies. Only haplotype analyses can reveal the effect of DR and DQ alleles simultaneously. Although the nature of association for a particular allele may be very different in various ethnic groups, the effect of a given allele (or a haplotype) on T1D susceptibility is probably consistent in all populations. In our transracial study, for all parental haplotypes, which were identical at DRB1 and DQB1, the association with T1D and the transmission of the haplotypes from nondiabetic parents to diabetic offspring was similar for Korean and Caucasian families.[15] Thus, the influence of class II susceptibility and resistance alleles appears to transcend ethnic and geographic diversity of T1D incidence.

Other Intra-HLA Susceptibility Genes

It is known that more than one genetic locus even within the HLA is important for disease risk. The highest risk genotype for T1D consists of individuals heterozygous for DR3- and DR4-associated haplotypes. This HLA DR3/4 genotype can only explain some 20% or 12% of the total genetic contribution in Caucasians, assuming a 30% or 50% concordance rate in monozygotic twins, respectively.[13,16] In Asians, the contribution of this genotype to overall susceptibility of T1D appeared to be less than that in Caucasians.[6,8] Moreover, the population frequency of this genotype in Caucasians is still 10–20 times higher than the prevalence of T1D associated with this genotype. DRB1 subtyping might influence the risk of T1D in this high-risk DQ population, though it is assumed to account for only 10% of additional familial aggregation. This implies that additional protective risk genes (HLA or non-HLA) and/or environmental factors influence susceptibility to the disease, especially in Asians. We found independent susceptibility of D6S273 and D6S2223 microsatellite markers in DQ8/DQ2 heterozygous individuals from the Caucasian Diabetes Autoimmunity Study in the Young (DAISY) repository.[17] In our Koreans, MIC-A and tumor necrosis factor-α (TNF-α) microsatellites were also associated with T1D independently.[6,18]

Are Susceptible Genes Similar Everywhere?

T1D is one of the first disorders with a complex genetic basis that researchers have begun to unravel. More than 20 years ago, the HLA region was found to contain a major locus that influences predisposition to T1D, and a decade ago a locus with a smaller effect was identified in the insulin gene region. With the advent of numerous microsatellite markers suitable for genome screening, additional 20 loci that influence susceptibility to T1D have been reported.[8,19] Some of the new loci appear to predispose people to T1D independently of HLA and may be important factors in families with T1D who lack strong HLA susceptibility. Other loci may interact to cause susceptibility, and specific combinations may be diabetogenic. Some highly "diabetogenic" genes, which are relatively uncommon in a population may be mistakenly considered neutral in population association studies. Because of these interactions, the effect of some susceptibility genes, whose influence is evident in one population, becomes obscure in other population. Notwithstanding, although isolating the actual predisposing genes in T1D is more difficult than isolating those involved in single-locus genetic disorders, the fact that the genes can be identified with the use of a reasonable number of multiethnic families is very encouraging for future research on other genetically complex disorders.

One of the confirmed T1D susceptibility loci is *IDDM12* located on chromosome 2q33. However, there are still inconsistencies between different studies. Transmission disequilibrium test (TDT) revealed highly significant deviation of transmission for alleles at the (AT)n microsatellite marker and the A/G polymorphism within the *CTLA4* gene in the data sets with Mediterranean origins (Italian, Spanish, French, and Mexican Americans).[20] In contrast to a negative result in Japanese and Chinese, a positive result was also observed in a small Korean data set.[21] Recent large-scale studies performed in Caucasians indicated CTLA4 gene to be responsible for T1D as well as autoimmune thyroid disease (ATD) susceptibility. We studied the association of CTLA4 polymorphism with T1D, ATD, and T1D patients with ATD in a large genetically distinct Korean cohort. The +6230 G>A polymorphism of CTLA4 was significantly associated with Graves' disease patients and T1D patients with ATD, but not with T1D without ATD (unpublished observation). Given the high prevalence of ATD in patients with T1D, we may suggest that ATD may be etiologically and genetically distinct from T1D and T1D patients should be separately classified according to the ATD phenotype in genetic studies as well as in clinical trials.

We reported highly significant evidence for association between T1D and multiple single nucleotide polymorphisms (SNPs) from 180 kb of genomic DNA within the *IDDM5* interval in a large multiethnic family.[22] We also performed fine mapping using a high density of SNPs in our Korean population.[23] We found several SNPs associated with T1D. Importantly, M55V polymorphism is one of the highest associations. Although there have been inconsistent reports, mostly from the Caucasians, we confirmed the susceptibility influence of M55V polymorphism in our Korean case–control studies, not only in T1D patients[23] but also in Graves' disease patients (unpublished observation). This susceptibility influence was also confirmed in the Japanese population.[24] A single amino acid substitution (M55V) of SUMO4 encoding a small ubiquitin-like modifier type 4 protein was found to be strongly associated with T1D. SUMO4 was shown to be able to conjugate to IkBa and negatively regulate NF-κB transcriptional activity. The M55V substitution results in a considerable increase of NF-κB transcriptional activity and about twofold higher expression of NF-κB-dependent genes. These findings suggest a novel pathway implicated in T1D pathogenesis.

Concannon *et al.* reported the results of a genome screen for linkage with T1D and analyzed the data by multipoint linkage methods.[19] An initial panel of 212 ASPs were genotyped for 438 markers spanning all autosomes, and additional 467 ASPs were used for follow-up genotyping. Other than the well-established linkage with the HLA region at 6p21.3, they found only 1 region, located on 1q. Being ascribed to a weak effect of the disease genes, genetic heterogeniety or random variation, these sorts of differences will give us big obstacle for the confirmation and fine mapping of susceptibility intervals and identification of etiologic mutations. If oligogenicity rather than polygenicity applies to human T1D, studies of large multiplex families from genetically and culturally homogeneous populations are likely to improve the prospects of identifying susceptibility genes by genetic linkage studies followed by positional cloning.

From these, it may be evident that susceptible genes are working everywhere, although their contribution might vary across geographical regions or ethnicity. However, different genetic make-up, LD pattern, or varying interaction with other genes may influence differentially which diseases are popular in one population and which genes are important in susceptibility. Comorbidities are also important in determining susceptibility.

Why Is T1D so Uncommon in Asia?

The frequencies of T1D-associated HLA antigens are correlated with the worldwide diabetes incidences, which differ by ethnicity as well as geographic regions. Dorman *et al.* plotted the association of the frequency of DQB1 non-ASP with T1D incidences.[25] At that time Japan and Korea were the exceptions. Because they ignored the contribution of DRB1 alleles, that plot counts as one of oversimplified view. The Sardinians and the Scandinavian population have the highest T1D incidence in the world (17.6–28.6/100,000 per year). The high frequencies of DRB1*0301, DRB1*0401, the 0301/0302, and 0301/0201 DQ dimers correlate with the high incidence of T1D in Scandinavians, while the high frequency of DRB1*0301 is consistent with the high disease incidence in Sardinians. In contrast, the Asian populations, such as Japanese and Koreans, have a very low incidence. The absence of the DR3 haplotype also correlates with the low incidence of T1D in Japanese. The contribution of DR3/4 to T1D susceptibility appears less important in Korea than in Caucasoid population. Instead, other rare genotypes are important in accordance with the prevalent haplotypes in the general population. Among the DR genotypes, DR3/9, DR9/9, and DR3/X (X: other than 3, 4) were susceptible genotypes. In Asians, more moderate risk haplotypes rather than highly susceptible DR3 and DR4 haplotypes are prevalent and there are less chances of the DQ0201/0302 dimers to be formed. Therefore, it becomes evident that T1D is uncommon in Asia considering the frequency of DRB1-DQB1 genotypes in the general population. Moreover, LD between highly susceptible DRB1 alleles and protective DQB1 alleles, and *vice versa*, is also the major contributing factor to the low incidence of T1D in Japanese, Korean, and Chinese. We analyzed the association of the different DR4 subtypes with susceptible DQ8 (DQA1*0301-DQB1*0302) and neutral DQ4 (DQA1*0301-DQB1*0401) haplotypes in Asian general population. In Asians, DQ8 is usually combined with protective DR4 subtypes (DRB1*0403, *0406), while DQ4 is in LD with susceptible DRB1*0405. High-risk DR4 subtypes (DRB1*0401, *0402, *0405) were predominant in DR4/X, whereas protective DR4 subtypes (DRB1*0403, *0406) were observed mainly in the DR3/4 genotype. The low incidence rate in the Asian population may be explained by the counterbalancing effect of the DRB1 and DQB1 alleles in the general population.

However, the genetic contribution does not explain the whole portion of T1D incidence variability across population. In genetically rather similar populations, such as in Estonia and Finland, up to sixfold variation in incidence rates have been found. In addition, in the genetically very homogenous Swedish population, significant and consistent incidence variability is present pointing to the importance of nongenetic risk factors. This suggestion is also supported by the finding that the incidence is increasing with time in many countries that have population-based registries. Korea has the lowest documented incidence of T1D in the world, and prevalences of islet-specific autoantibodies are reported to be low compared with Caucasians. A different genetic susceptibility including a low frequency of high-risk HLA alleles could explain the lower prevalence of islet-specific autoantibodies to GAD and islet cells cytoplasm (ICA) and the low incidence of T1D, or different genetic and environmental interactions that might be involved in the etiology of T1D. Although Asians may be genetically protected against T1D compared with the Caucasians, it is unknown to what degree genetic determinants influence the well-known regional differences in incidence. We suggested that different genetic–environmental interactions do operate in the etiology of T1D between Caucasians and Asians.

ACKNOWLEDGMENTS

This work was supported by the grants from Korea Science and Engineering Foundation (R01-2001-00177 and R01-2005-10075) and a grant from the Korea Health 21 R and D Project, Ministry of Health and Welfare, Republic of Korea (A05-0463-B50704-05N1-00030B).

REFERENCES

1. WHO DIAMOND PROJECT GROUP. 1990. WHO multinational project for childhood diabetes. Diabetes Care **13:** 1062–1068.
2. KO, K. *et al.* 1994. The incidence of IDDM in Seoul from 1985 to 1988. Diabetes Care **17:** 1473–1475.
3. PARK, Y. *et al.* 1996. Molecular epidemiology of insulin-dependent diabetes mellitus (IDDM) in Korea. Diabetes Res. Clin. Pract. **34:** S55–S59.
4. TAJIMA, N. *et al.* 1985. A comparison of the epidemiology of youth-onset insulin-dependent diabetes mellitus between Japan and the United States. Diabetes Care **11:** 17–23.
5. KUZUYA T. *et al.* 2002. Report of the committee on the classification and diagnostic criteria of diabetes mellitus. Diabetes Res. Clin. Pract. **55:** 65–85.
6. PARK, Y. 2004. Prediction of the risk of type 1 diabetes from polymorphisms in candidate genes. Diabetes Res. Clin. Pract. **66**(Suppl):S19–S25.
7. NOTSU, K. *et al.* 1983. A population survey of pancreatic islet cell antibodies and antithyroid antibodies. Tohoku J. Exp. Med. **141:** 261–263.
8. PARK, Y. & G.S. EISENBARTH. 2001. Genetic susceptibility factors of type 1 diabetes in Asians and their functional evaluation. Diabetes Metab. Res. Rev. **17:** 2–11.
9. PARK, Y. *et al.* Evaluation of the efficacy of multiple autoantibody screening in Korean patients with IDDM. Acta Diabetologica **37:** 213–217.
10. IKEGAMI, H. & T. OGIHARA. 1996. Genetics of insulin-dependent diabetes mellitus. Endocr. J. **43:** 605–613.
11. PARK, Y. *et al.* 1998. Combination of HLA DR and DQ molecules determine the susceptibility to insulin-dependent diabetes mellitus in Koreans. Hum. Immunol. **59:** 794–801.
12. TODD, J. *et al.* 1987. HLA-DQB gene contributes to susceptibility and resistance to insulin-dependent diabetes mellitus. Nature **329:** 599–604.
13. RISCH, N. 1987. Assessing the role of HLA-liked and unlinked determinants of disease. Am. J. Hum. Genet. **40:** 1–14.
14. PARK, Y. *et al.* 2001. Transracial evidence for the influence of the homologous HLA DR-DQ haplotype on transmission of HLA DR4 haplotypes to diabetic children. Tissue Antigens **57:** 185–191.

15. PARK, Y. *et al.* 2000. Common susceptibility and transmission pattern of HLA DRB1-DQB1 haplotypes to Korean and Caucasian patients with type 1 diabetes. J. Clin. Endocrinol. Metab. **85:** 4538–4542.
16. NOBLE, J. *et al.* 1996. The role of HLA class II genes in insulin-dependent diabetes mellitus: molecular analysis of 180 Caucasians, multiplex families. Am. J. Hum. Genet. **59:** 1134–1148.
17. PARK, Y. *et al.* 1999. D6S2223 alleles associated with risk of IDDM in DR3-DQ2/DR4-DQ8 heterozygotes. Diabetes **48:** A183.
18. PARK, Y. *et al.* 2001. MICA polymorphism is associated with type 1 diabetes in Korean Population. Diabetes Care **24:** 33–38.
19. CONCANNON, P. *et al.* 1998. A second-generation screen of the human genome for susceptibility to insulin-dependent diabetes mellitus. Nat. Genet. **19:** 292–296.
20. MARRON, M. *et al.* 1997. Insulin-dependent diabetes mellitus (IDDM) is associated with CTLA4 polymorphisms in multiple ethnic groups. Hum. Mol. Genet. **8:** 1275–1282.
21. MARRON, M. *et al.* 2000. Genetic and physical fine-mapping of a type 1 diabetes susceptibility gene (IDDM12) to a 100-kb phagemid artificial chromosome clone containing D2S72-CTLA4-D2S105 on chromosome 2q33. Diabetes **49:** 492–499.
22. GUO, D. *et al.* 2004. A new IkBa modifier, SUMO-L, is associated with type 1 diabetes. Nat. Genet. **36:** 837–841.
23. PARK, Y. *et al.* 2005. Assessing the validity of the association between the SUMO4 M55V variant and risk of type 1 diabetes. Nat. Genet. **37:** 112.
24. NOSO, S. *et al.* 2005. Genetic heterogeneity in association of the SUMO4 M55V variant with susceptibility to type 1 diabetes. Diabetes **54:** 3582–3586.
25. DORMAN, J. *et al.* 1990. Worldwide differences in the incidence of type I diabetes are associated with amino acid variation at position 57 of the HLA-DQ beta chain. Proc. Natl. Acad. Sci. USA **87:** 7370–7374.

Association of *SUMO4*, as a Candidate Gene for *IDDM5*, with Susceptibility to Type 1 Diabetes in Asian Populations

SHINSUKE NOSO,[a] HIROSHI IKEGAMI,[a,b] TOMOMI FUJISAWA,[a] YUMIKO KAWABATA,[a,b] KATSUAKI ASANO,[a] YOSHIHISA HIROMINE,[a] SHIGETAKA SUGIHARA,[c] INKYU LEE,[d] EIJI KAWASAKI,[e] TAKUYA AWATA,[f] AND TOSHIO OGIHARA[a]

[a]*Department of Geriatric Medicine, Osaka University Graduate School of Medicine, Osaka 565-0871, Japan*

[b]*Department of Endocrinology, Diabetes and Metabolism, Kinki University School of Medicine, Osaka 589-8511, Japan*

[c]*Department of Pediatrics, Tokyo Women's Medical University Daini Hospital, Tokyo 116-8567, Japan*

[d]*Department of Internal Medicine, Kyungpook National University Hospital, School of Medicine, Kyungpook National University, Daegu 700-721, Korea*

[e]*Department of Metabolism/Diabetes and Clinical Nutrition, Nagasaki University Hospital of Medicine and Dentistry, Nagasaki 852-8501, Japan*

[f]*Division of Endocrinology and Diabetes, Department of Medicine, Saitama Medical School, Saitama 350-0495, Japan*

ABSTRACT: Recent study demonstrated that M55V variant in *SUMO4* at *IDDM5* was associated with susceptibility to type 1 diabetes. Subsequent studies, however, showed inconsistency in the association. To clarify the population-wide effect on the association of *SUMO4* with type 1 diabetes, we have performed meta-analysis including our own data in Asian populations, which confirmed a highly significant association in Asian populations (summary odds ratio [OR]: 1.29, $P = 7.0 \times 10^{-6}$), but indicated significant heterogeneity in the genetic effect of the *SUMO4* gene on type 1 diabetes among diverse ethnic groups. These observations indicated the association of *SUMO4* with type 1 diabetes in Asian populations.

KEYWORDS: type 1 diabetes; *IDDM5*; *SUMO4*; genetic heterogeneity; Asian populations

Address for correspondence: Dr. Hiroshi Ikegami, Department of Endocrinology, Diabetes and Metabolism, Kinki University School of Medicine, 377-2 Ohno-higashi, Sayama-shi, Osaka 589-8511, Japan. Voice: +81-72-366-0221; ext.: 3123 fax: +81-72-366-2095.
e-mail: ikegami@med.kindai.ac.jp.

Ann. N.Y. Acad. Sci. 1079: 41–46 (2006). © 2006 New York Academy of Sciences.
doi: 10.1196/annals.1375.006

INTRODUCTION

Type 1 diabetes is an autoimmune disease caused by the destruction of insulin-producing beta cells of the pancreas by lymphocyte infiltration, leading to an absolute loss of endogenous insulin secretion and a requirement of exogenous insulin therapy to survive. To identify the susceptibility gene(s) for common multifactorial diseases, such as type 1 diabetes, two major approaches were often adopted: candidate gene approach based on biochemical knowledge of the gene products and positional cloning based on linkage analysis. Identification of susceptibility genes for type 1 diabetes, however, largely depended on the candidate gene approach so far as is observed for *HLA* class II, *INS-VNTR*, *CTLA4*, and *PTPN22*. Identification of methionine to valine substitution at codon 55 (M55V) of a novel susceptibility gene, *SUMO4*, as a causal variant for *IDDM5* locus on chromosome 6 was the first instance for type 1 diabetes gene identified by positional cloning approach.[1] In the present article, we compared the contribution of the *SUMO4* variant to susceptibility to type 1 diabetes between Caucasian and Asian populations.

POSITIONAL CLONING OF THE SUSCEPTIBILITY GENE FOR *IDDM5*

An association between type 1 diabetes and multiple single nucleotide polymorphisms (SNPs) in 197 kb of genomic DNA in the *IDDM5* interval was recently reported by Guo and colleagues (A, FIG. 1).[1] Almost simultaneously,

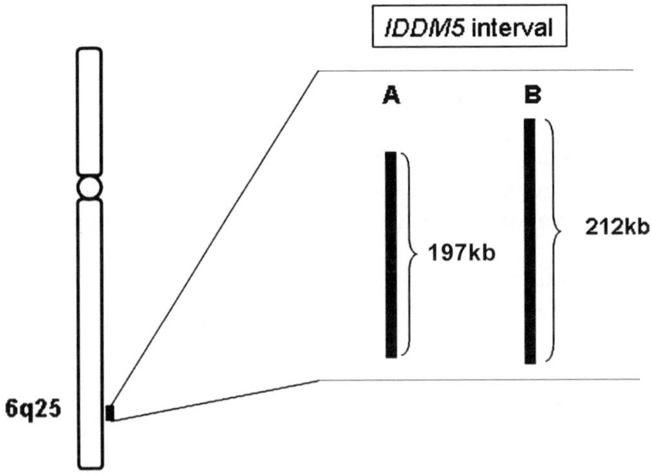

FIGURE 1. *IDDM5* locus was recently narrowed to an approximately 200-kb interval on chromosome 6q25 by two independent groups (**A** and **B**).

Owerbach *et al.*[2] have also mapped the *IDDM5* locus to a near-identical 212-kb interval in the region (B, FIG. 1). Guo and colleagues have cloned a novel gene belonging to small ubiquitin-like modifier family, designated as *SUMO4*, in the *IDDM5* interval, and exonic SNP leading to methionine to valine substitution at codon 55 located in evolutionally conserved domain showed significant association with susceptibility to type 1 diabetes in diverse ethnic groups with functional evidence.

Subsequent studies, however, showed inconsistency in the association of the *SUMO4* gene with type 1 diabetes. The original report by Guo *et al.* with subjects from diverse ethnic groups and the subsequent study by Park *et al.*[3] in Korean subjects showed that possession of the G allele was significantly associated with increased risk for type 1 diabetes, whereas studies in Caucasian subjects of European descent showed no association[4,5] or even an association of the A allele with the disease.[6] Of note is the positive association in studies with subjects from Asian populations in contrast to the lack of association in subjects of European descent[4,5] and a tendency for an opposite association in British subjects.[6]

VALIDATION OF THE ASSOCIATION OF *SUMO4* WITH TYPE 1 DIABETES IN ASIAN POPULATIONS

To clarify the contribution of the M55V polymorphism of the *SUMO4* gene to type 1 diabetes susceptibility, we have studied 541 type 1 diabetic patients and 768 control subjects in Asian populations.[7] The Japanese case and control subjects were recruited from three geographical areas in Japan: Osaka, Nagasaki, and Saitama. Subjects were independently genotyped in these three panels. Similar allele and genotype frequencies were observed in each geographical area (I^2: 0.0%, Mantel–Haenszel test, TABLE 1), suggesting homogeneity of the Japanese data in present study. In total, the frequency of subjects with the G allele was significantly higher in cases than controls (odds ratio [or] [95% CI]: 1.43 [1.12–1.81], $P = 4.0 \times 10^{-3}$, χ^2 test, TABLE 1). A similar tendency was observed in Korean subjects (0.58 versus 0.44, OR: 1.75 [0.94–3.24]). In the combined data from Japanese and Korean subjects, the G allele was significantly associated with type 1 diabetes (OR: 1.46 [1.17–1.83], $P = 0.00083$, Mantel–Haenszel test).

MARKED HETEROGENEITY IN THE ASSOCIATION AMONG DIVERSE ETHNIC GROUPS: META-ANALYSIS

To test whether the M55V variant of the *SUMO4* gene has a population-wide effect on its association with type 1 diabetes, we performed a meta-analysis of published studies with our own data.[7] From 7 articles detected

TABLE 1. Association of M55V polymorphism of *SUMO4* gene in Japanese population

	Panel 1 (Osaka)		Panel 2 (Nagasaki)		Panel 3 (Saitama)		Total				
	T1DM $n = 206$ (%)	Control $n = 226$ (%)	T1DM $n = 150$ (%)	Control $n = 116$ (%)	T1DM $n = 116$ (%)	Control $n = 299$ (%)	T1DM $n = 472$ (%)	Control $n = 641$ (%)	I^2(%)	OR (95% CI)	p
GG	14(7)	20(9)	14(9)	13(11)	15(13)	31(10)	43(9)	64(10)			
GA	106(51)	91(40)	73(49)	48(41)	55(47)	117(39)	234(50)	256(40)			
AA	86(42)	115(51)	63(42)	55(47)	46(40)	151(51)	195(41)	321(50)			0.005
G	134(33)	131(29)	101(34)	74(32)	85(37)	179(30)	320(34)	384(30)			
A	278(67)	321(71)	199(66)	158(68)	147(63)	419(70)	624(66)	898(70)	0.0	1.2 (1.0–1.4)	<0.05
GG+GA	120(58)	111(49)	87(58)	61(53)	70(60)	148(49)	277(59)	320(50)			
AA	86(42)	115(51)	63(42)	55(47)	46(40)	151(51)	195(41)	321(50)	0.0	1.4 (1.1–1.8)	4.0×10^{-3}

OR: odds ratio, CI: confidential interval, χ^2 test, I^2 was calculated with Mantel–Haenszel test.

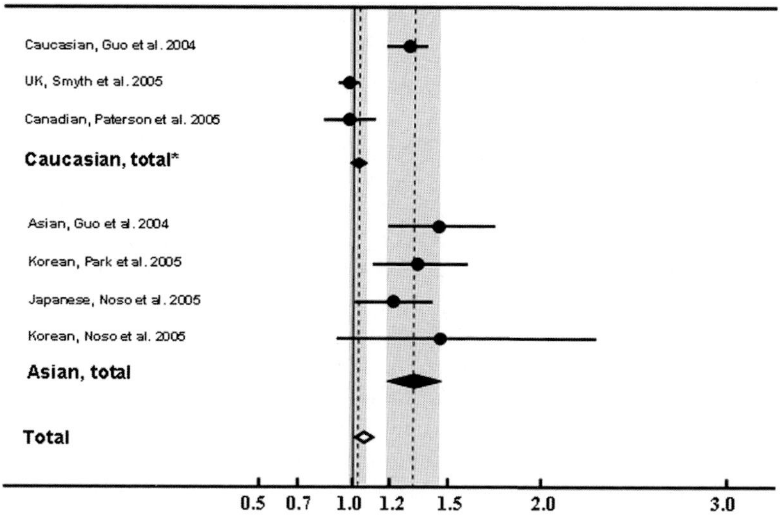

FIGURE 2. Estimates of OR for type 1 diabetes according to M55V (A163G) variant of *SUMO4* gene in Caucasian and Asian populations. Values more than 1 imply an increased OR for type 1 diabetes associated with the G allele. The 95% CI are expressed by bars (for each group) and ♦ (for combined studies). Broken vertical lines represent the summary OR of combined studies for Asian populations. The data from case–control and TDT studies were integrated as described in previous study (Kazeem G.R. & M. Farrall M. 2005. Integrating case–control and TDT studies. *Ann Hum. Genet.* **69**(Pt. 3): 329–335).

by PubMed search, 6 sets of data were available. Two sets of data were excluded from the meta-analysis because some of the subjects from the Human Biological Data Interchange and the Warren repository overlapped with those in another large-scale association study. Korean subjects of case–control study from the original report, which may be overlapped with the data published by Park *et al.*, were also excluded from meta-analysis. Meta-analysis of all Asian data from previous studies and our own study (1126 cases and 1675 controls for case–control studies and 129 families for transmission disequilibrium test [TDT] studies) showed a significant association of the G allele with type 1 diabetes (OR [95%CI]: 1.29 [1.15–1.44], $P = 7.0 \times 10^{-6}$) with very homogenous data (*P* value for heterogeneity: 0.29, NS, FIG. 2). In contrast, the summary OR for European subjects (4053 cases and 5273 controls for case–control studies and 2810 families for TDT studies) was 1.02 (0.98–1.07) (*P* value for heterogeneity within European subjects: 4.0×10^{-8}), with no overlap in the 95% CI with that of Asian data. As a result, when both data were combined, the summary OR was reduced to 1.05 (1.01–1.09) ($P = 0.0087$), although significant heterogeneity (*P* value for heterogeneity: 1.0×10^{-11}) across these data sets was also indicated.

CONCLUSION

Asian specific association of the *SUMO4* gene with type 1 diabetes was demonstrated. Although further assessment in Caucasian and other populations is needed to confirm population-wide contribution of *SUMO4* gene on the development of type 1 diabetes, these results suggest that the heterogeneity of the genetic effect between ethnicities could cause the discrepancy of association between the studies. Careful investigations should be required to conclude the contribution of susceptibility gene(s) to multifactorial diseases with inconsistent results.

ACKNOWLEDGMENTS

We thank M. Moritani and Y. Tsukamoto for their technical assistance and Yoshihiko Kawaguchi for his invaluable suggestions on statistical analysis. This work was supported by a Grant-in-Aid for Scientific Research from the Ministry of Education, Science, Sports, Culture, and Technology, Japan.

REFERENCES

1. Guo, D., M. Li, Y. Zhang, *et al.* 2004. A functional variant of SUMO4, a new I kappa B alpha modifier, is associated with type 1 diabetes. Nat. Genet. **36:** 837–841.
2. Owerbach, D., L. Pina & K.H. Gabbay 2004. A 212-kb region on chromosome 6q25 containing the TAB2 gene is associated with susceptibility to type 1 diabetes. Diabetes **53:** 1890–1893.
3. Park, Y., S. Park, J. Kang, *et al.* 2005. Assessing the validity of the association between the SUMO4 M55V variant and risk of type 1 diabetes. Nat. Genet. **37:** 112.
4. Smyth, D.J., J.M. Howson, C.E. Lowe, *et al.* 2005. Assessing the validity of the association between the SUMO4 M55V variant and risk of type 1 diabetes. Nat. Genet. **37:** 110–111.
5. Qu, H., B. Bharaj, X.Q. Liu, *et al.* 2005. Assessing the validity of the association between the SUMO4 M55V variant and risk of type 1 diabetes. Nat. Genet. **37:** 111–112.
6. Bohren, K.M., V. Nadkarni, J.H. Song, *et al.* 2004. A M55V polymorphism in a novel SUMO gene (SUMO-4) differentially activates heat shock transcription factors and is associated with susceptibility to type I diabetes mellitus. J. Biol. Chem. **279:** 27233–27238.
7. Noso, S., H. Ikegami, T. Fujisawa, *et al.* 2005. Genetic heterogeneity in association of the SUMO4 M55V variant with susceptibility to type 1 diabetes. Diabetes **54:** 3582–3586.

The Gene for Human IL-21 and Genetic Susceptibility to Type 1 Diabetes in the Japanese

KATSUAKI ASANO,[a] HIROSHI IKEGAMI,[a,b] TOMOMI FUJISAWA,[a] YUMIKO KAWABATA,[a,b] SHINSUKE NOSO,[a] YOSHIHISA HIROMINE,[a] AND TOSHIO OGIHARA[a]

[a]*Department of Geriatric Medicine, Osaka University Graduate School of Medicine, Suita, Osaka 565-0871, Japan*

[b]*Department of Endocrinology, Diabetes and Metabolism, Kinki University School of Medicine, Sayama, Osaka 589-8511, Japan*

ABSTRACT: Type 1 diabetes is under polygenic control both in humans and the NOD mouse. Recently a possible role of IL-21 in the pathogenesis of type 1 diabetes was demonstrated in the NOD mouse. Furthermore, the murine IL-21 gene is mapped to the *Idd3* interval, making the human IL-21 gene (*IL21*) a functional as well as positional candidate for susceptibility. We therefore screened sequence variants of *IL21* and studied the association with type 1 diabetes. Preliminary data showed no association of *IL21* polymorphisms with the disease, suggesting that *IL21* plays little role in susceptibility to type 1 diabetes in Japanese.

KEYWORDS: type 1 diabetes; interleukin-21; genetics; autoimmune disease

INTRODUCTION

Type 1 diabetes, an organ-specific autoimmune disease, is increasing in many countries and, therefore, better strategies for prediction and prevention of the disease are clinically warranted. Genetic susceptibility and environmental factors are known to be involved in the development of type 1 diabetes, and a number of studies have demonstrated that, in addition to human leukocyte antigen (HLA), non-HLA genes are important in the susceptibility to type 1 diabetes.[1] Several non-HLA loci have been reported to be linked to or associated with type 1 diabetes, but for most of these loci, responsible genes are yet to be determined, except for insulin and CTLA4 genes for *IDDM2*

Address for correspondence: Dr. Hiroshi Ikegami, Department of Endocrinology, Diabetes and Metabolism, Kinki University School of Medicine, 377-2 Ohno-higashi, Sayama, Osaka 589-8511, Japan. Voice: +81-72-366-0221; ext.: 3123; fax: +81-72-366-2095.
e-mail: ikegami@med.kindai.ac.jp

Ann. N.Y. Acad. Sci. 1079: 47–50 (2006). © 2006 New York Academy of Sciences.
doi: 10.1196/annals.1375.007

and *IDDM12*, respectively. Elucidation of susceptibility genes will not only be useful to identify individuals at high risk for future development of type 1 diabetes, but would also facilitate our understanding of the pathogenesis of the disease, leading to establishment of novel strategies for prevention and cure of the disease.

A recent study in non-obese diabetic (NOD) mice, an animal model for type 1 diabetes, indicated that lymphopenia and its compensatory homeostatic expansion drive autoimmunity against beta cells through increased responses to a cytokine interleukin-21 (IL-21).[2] As IL-21 was found to have pleiotropic effects on immune regulation, alteration in function and regulation of IL-21 would affect the autoimmune process leading to beta cell destruction. *IL21* encoding human IL-21 is therefore considered as a functional candidate for susceptibility gene to type 1 diabetes.

As in the case of humans, type 1 diabetes in the NOD mouse is under polygenic control, with the strongest component linked to the major histocompatibility complex (MHC). Among multiple non-MHC loci, *Idd3* is one of the strongest susceptibility loci, and has been mapped to an 780-kb interval, including *Il21*, a gene for murine IL-21.[3] Given that several susceptibility genes are shared between humans and NOD mouse, as is evidenced by the MHC genes (*IDDM1* and *Idd1*),[4] genes for *CTLA4* (*IDDM12* and *Idd5.1*),[5] and *SLC11A1* (*IDDM13* and *Idd5.2*),[6] it is possible to consider *IL21*, the human ortholog of murine *Il21,* as a positional candidate gene for type 1 diabetes.

Taken together, *IL21* is a functional as well as a positional candidate gene for type 1 diabetes in humans, which prompted us to investigate a possible involvement of *IL21* in genetic susceptibility to the disease. In this article, we screened for sequence variants in *IL21* and studied the association with type 1 diabetes.

METHODS

For screening sequence variants, a total of greater than 20 patients with type 1 diabetes and control subjects were studied. Genomic DNA was extracted from peripheral leukocytes. The human IL-21 gene is composed of 5 exons with a length of 8.38 kb. Primers were designed to cover all the 5 exons and exon–intron junctions. Sequencing was performed using ABI 3100 capillary sequencer (Applied Biosystems, Tokyo, Japan) with ABI PRISM®BigDye™Terminators v3.1 Cycle Sequencing Kit (Applied Biosystems) and analyzed using ABI PRISM®3730 Genetic Analyzer (Applied Biosystems).

For the association study, three single nucleotide polymorphisms (SNPs) were genotyped by PCR–RFLP methods in a total of more than 150 Japanese subjects.

RESULTS

In a total of approximately 4000-bp interval sequenced, only one SNP was identified with low minor allele frequency, suggesting that sequence variants are rare in exons and exon–intron junctions of *IL21*. We therefore searched NCBI genome database and selected additional three SNPs located in introns 2 and 3, and in the 3′-downstream of *IL21*, and studied the association of these SNPs with type 1 diabetes.

Preliminary data suggested that none of the SNPs was associated with type 1 diabetes.

DISCUSSION

In the present study, no difference was observed in the distribution of SNPs between patients with type 1 diabetes and control subjects, suggesting that *IL21* plays little, if any, role in susceptibility to type 1 diabetes in Japanese. Since the results are still preliminary, further studies with larger number of subjects are required to elucidate a contribution of *IL21* in genetic susceptibility to type 1 diabetes.

IL-21 is one of the newest members of the common γ-chain family of cytokines, whose biological functions have recently been clarified. These functions include augmentation of the proliferation of T cells, driving the differentiation of B cells into memory cells, and activation of natural killer cells,[7] which collectively are expected to affect the autoimmune process. In particular, a recent study in the NOD mouse pointed to a crucial role of IL-21 in compensatory expansion of lymphocytes. Since lymphopenia is often associated with viral infections, which are known to trigger type 1 diabetes, it is possible that alteration in *IL21* affects T cell turnover and modifies autoimmune process, as observed in the NOD mouse.[2] Therefore, a putative polymorphism of *IL21* that affects dynamics or function of IL-21, could play a role in conferring susceptibility to type 1 diabetes. Provided that such a polymorphism as well as its biological effect is elucidated, the information will make prevention and intervention of type 1 diabetes more feasible by modifying IL-21 action, as in the case of NOD mice.

ACKNOWLEDGMENTS

We thank M. Moritani and Y. Tsukamoto for their skillful technical assistance. This work was supported by a Grant-in-Aid for Scientific Research from the Ministry of Education, Science, Sports, Culture, and Technology, Japan.

REFERENCES

1. IKEGAMI, H. & T. OGIHARA. 1996. Genetics of insulin-dependent diabetes mellitus. Endocr. J. **43:** 605–613.
2. KING, C., A. ILIC, K. KOELSCH, *et al.* 2004. Homeostatic expansion of T cells during immune insufficiency generates autoimmunity. Cell **117:** 265–277.
3. LYONS, P.A., N. ARMITAGE, F. ARGENTINA, *et al.* 2000. Congenic mapping of the type 1 diabetes locus, *Idd3*, to a 780-kb region of mouse chromosome 3: identification of a candidate segment of ancestral DNA by haplotype mapping. Genome Res. **10:** 446–453.
4. KAWABATA, Y., H. IKEGAMI, Y. KAWAGUCHI, *et al.* 2002. Asian-specific HLA haplotypes reveal heterogeneity of the contribution of HLA-DR and -DQ haplotypes to susceptibility to type 1 diabetes. Diabetes **51:** 545–551.
5. UEDA, H., J.M. HOWSON, L. ESPOSITO, *et al.* 2003. Association of the T-cell regulatory gene *CTLA4* with susceptibility to autoimmune disease. Nature **423:** 506–511.
6. NISHINO, M., H. IKEGAMI, T. FUJISAWA, *et al.* 2005. Functional polymorphism in Z-DNA-forming motif of promoter of *SLC11A1* gene and type 1 diabetes in Japanese subjects: association study and meta-analysis. Metabolism **54:** 628–633.
7. LEONARD, W.J. & R. SPOLSKI. 2005. Interleukin-21: a modulator of lymphoid proliferation, apoptosis and differentiation. Nat. Rev. Immunol. **5:** 688–698.

Genetics of Type 1 Diabetes: Similarities and Differences between Asian and Caucasian Populations

HIROSHI IKEGAMI,[a,b] TOMOMI FUJISAWA,[a] YUMIKO KAWABATA,[a,b] SHINSUKE NOSO,[a] AND TOSHIO OGIHARA[a]

[a]*Department of Geriatric Medicine, Osaka University Graduate School of Medicine, Suita, Osaka 565-0871, Japan*

[b]*Department of Endocrinology, Metabolism and Diabetes, Kinki University School of Medicine, Osaka-sayama, Osaka 589-8511, Japan*

ABSTRACT: Transracial studies are a powerful tool for genetic association studies of multifactorial diseases, such as type 1 diabetes. We therefore studied the association of candidate genes, *HLA, INS, CTLA4, PTPN22,* and *SUMO4*, with type 1 diabetes in Asian populations in comparison with Caucasian populations. Class II HLA was strongly associated with type 1 diabetes in both Asian and Caucasian populations, but alleles associated with type 1 diabetes are different among different ethnic groups due to difference in allele distribution in general populations. *INS* was associated with type 1 diabetes in both Japanese and Caucasian populations, but frequency of disease-associated haplotype was markedly higher in Japanese than in Caucasian populations. *CTLA4* association was reported for both type 1 diabetes and autoimmune thyroid diseases (AITD) in Caucasian populations, but the association with type 1 diabetes was concentrated in a subset of patients with AITD in Japanese. A variant (R620W) of *PTPN22* was consistently associated with type 1 diabetes in Caucasian populations, but the variant was absent in Asian populations including Japanese. M55V variant of *SUMO4* was significantly associated with type 1 diabetes in Asians, but genetic heterogeneity between Asian and Caucasian populations was suggested. These data indicate the importance of transracial studies with a large number of samples in each ethnic group in genetic dissection of type 1 diabetes.

KEYWORDS: type 1 diabetes; genetics; autoimmune disease; HLA; *INS*; *CTLA4*; *PTPN22*; *SUMO4*

Address for correspondence: H. Ikegami, Department of Endocrinology, Metabolism and Diabetes, Kinki University School of Medicine, 377-2 Ohno-higashi, Osaka-sayama, Osaka. 589-8511, Japan. e-mail: ikegami@med.kindai.ac.jp

Ann. N.Y. Acad. Sci. 1079: 51–59 (2006). © 2006 New York Academy of Sciences.
doi: 10.1196/annals.1375.008

INTRODUCTION

Identification of genes predisposing to common, multifactorial diseases, such as diabetes and hypertension, is important in establishing effective methods for prediction, prevention, and intervention in diseases. Fine mapping and identification of susceptibility genes for multifactorial diseases is, however, still a formidable challenge because of infrequent recombination (linkage disequilibrium) in a small interval where susceptibility genes have been genetically mapped.[1] One way to overcome this problem is to study different ethnic groups where different combinations of alleles at nearby loci, termed *haplotypes*, segregate. Such transracial studies have been prove to be a powerful tool for identification of disease-causing variants in multifactorial diseases, as was demonstrated by the fine mapping and identification of *IDDM1*, a major susceptibility gene for type 1 diabetes in the HLA region.[2,3]

Type 1 diabetes mellitus is caused by a complex interaction of genetic and environmental factors. Genetic factor consists of multiple susceptibility genes with a major locus encoded by HLA region on chromosome 6p21.[4–6] Class II *DQ* and *DR* genes have been consistently reported to be associated with type 1 diabetes in multiple ethnic groups.[7,8] In addition to HLA, several non-HLA loci have been shown to contribute to the disease susceptibility.[4–6] Despite a large number of loci mapped to the genome, only a limited number of genes have been identified as genes responsible for susceptibility conferred by these loci. Among these are the insulin gene (*INS*) for *IDDM2*,[9] *CTLA4* for *IDDM12*,[10] *SUMO4* for *IDDM5*,[11] and *PTPN22* encoding lymphoid tyrosine phosphatase (LYP).[12] Most of these genes, however, were identified in Caucasian populations, and it is yet to be clarified whether or not the effect of these genes on type 1 diabetes susceptibility is universal over different ethnic groups. We therefore studied the contribution of these genes to susceptibility to type 1 diabetes in Asian populations (Japanese and Koreans) in comparison with Caucasian populations.

Familiar Clustering of Type 1 Diabetes

In Caucasian populations, type 1 diabetes clusters in families as is evidenced by the higher lifetime risk in siblings of type 1 diabetic probands than in general populations (6% versus 0.4%, λs 15) (FIG. 1).[13] In Asian countries, however, the incidences of type 1 diabetes are much lower than those in Caucasian countries,[14] making it difficult to study familiar clustering of the disease because of a limited number of multiplex families with type 1 diabetes. We previously performed a nationwide study on multiplex families with type 1 diabetes, and found that 3.8% frequency of type 1 diabetes in siblings of diabetic probands (FIG. 1),[15] which is similar to that in Caucasian populations. Studies using different data sources also suggested much higher frequencies (1.3–3.3%) of type

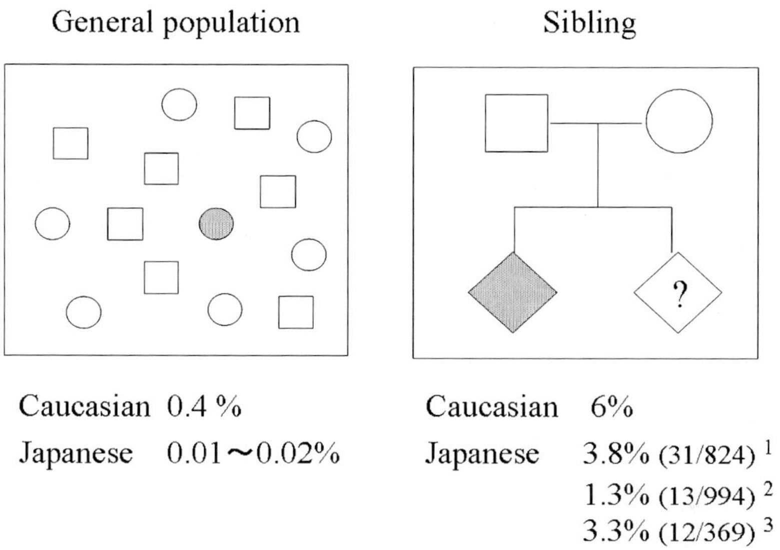

FIGURE 1. Frequencies of type 1 diabetes in siblings of probands with type 1 diabetes as compared with prevalence of type 1 diabetes in general population.
[1]Ikegami H et al. Endocrine J 43:605, 1996.[2] Based on survey on family history of type 1 diabetes at summer camps for childhood diabetes in 1998. [3]Based on report from the committee on immunogenetics of type 1 diabetes of Japan Diabetes Society, 1987. Frequency was estimated from the number of patients with type 1 diabetes in siblings of probands with type 1 diabetes divided by the number of families studied (the number of siblings was not available). Based on average number (approximately 2) of children in each family in Japan in 1987, the frequency may not have been overestimated as compared with the frequency calculated from the number of patients divided by the number of siblings.

1 diabetes in siblings of diabetic probands in Japan (FIG. 1), indicating that type 1 diabetes clusters in families even in low incidence countries like Japan.

Importance of Large-Scale Studies with Sufficient Power

To identify disease-causing variants with a modest effect, as in the case of non-HLA genes for type 1 diabetes, a large number of samples from cases and controls are required. This is clearly illustrated by recent large-scale studies with sufficient statistical power on genetic susceptibility to type 1 diabetes in Caucasian populations.[10] No such study, however, has been performed in Asians because of the very low incidence (less than one-tenth of that in Caucasians) of type 1 diabetes in most Asian countries.[14] To overcome this, a nationwide effort to accumulate a large number of samples from cases and controls for genetic studies of type 1 diabetes is necessary in each population. We therefore started such an effort several years ago to establish a multicenter collaborative study group. Seven leading groups in the field of genetics of type 1 diabetes in Japan agreed to collaborate and the Japanese Study Group on Type 1 Diabetes Genetics was established in 2003. To date, samples from up to greater than 800 patients with type 1 diabetes and greater than 800 control subjects were accumulated, making it possible to perform a large-scale case–control association studies in Japanese population. Given the very low frequency (less than one-tenth of that in Caucasians) of type 1 diabetes in Japan, the time and effort taken to collect this number of patients with type 1 diabetes may correspond to greater than 8000 patients in Caucasian populations.

HLA (IDDM1): A Major Susceptibility Gene

HLA-*DRB1* and *DQB1* have been consistently reported to be associated with type 1 diabetes. Substantial differences, however, in alleles and haplotypes conferring susceptibility to type 1 diabetes have been reported among different ethnic groups. In Caucasian populations, DR3 (*DRB1*0301-DQB1*0201*) and DR4 (*DRB1*0401-DQB1*0302*) haplotypes are positively associated with type 1 diabetes, whereas DR4 (*DRB1*0405-DQB1*0401*) and DR9 (*DRB1*0901-DQB1*0303*) haplotypes are associated with the disease in Japanese and most east Asian populations.[8] The reason for the differences in haplotypes associated with type 1 diabetes in Japanese and Caucasian populations is due to the difference in available haplotypes in each population. Disease-associated DR3 and DR4 haplotypes in Caucasians are very rare in Japanese, and therefore the contribution of these haplotypes to type 1 diabetes susceptibility is unknown in Japanese (TABLE 1). The same is true for Asian-specific DR4 and DR9 haplotypes in that these haplotypes are almost absent in Caucasian populations and therefore their effect on susceptibility to type 1 diabetes is unknown in Caucasians (TABLE 1). Thus, the difference in haplotypes associated with type 1 diabetes between Japanese and Caucasian populations can be explained by the presence or absence of haplotypes in each population. In fact, a DR2 haplotype (*DRB1*1501-DQB1*0602*), which is present in both Japanese and Caucasian

TABLE 1. Difference in Class II HLA haplotypes associated with type 1 diabetes in Japanese and Caucasian populations

	Japanese		Caucasian	
DRB1-DQB1 Haplotype	Type 1 diabetes susceptibility	HF*	Type 1 diabetes susceptibility	HF
*DRB1*0405-DQB1*0401*	susceptible	present	unknown	rare
*DRB1*0901-DQB1*0303*	susceptible	present	unknown	rare
*DRB1*0301-DQB1*0201*	unknown	rare	susceptible	present
*DRB1*0401-DQB1*0302*	unknown	rare	susceptible	present
*DRB1*1501-DQB1*0602*	protective	present	protective	present

*HF: haplotype frequency.

populations, is negatively associated with type 1 diabetes in both populations (Table 1), further confirming that differential association of HLA haplotypes with type 1 diabetes among different ethnic groups is due to the difference in the presence or absence of haplotypes in each population.

INS (IDDM2): β *Cell Specificity*

Insulin is specifically expressed in β cells of the pancreas, and therefore is a candidate gene for type 1 diabetes determining β cell specificity of the disease. In fact, accumulating lines of evidence in both humans and animal models suggested that insulin is an autoantigen in type 1 diabetes.[16] In addition, insulin gene region has been repeatedly reported to be associated with type 1 diabetes in Caucasian populations.[9,17,18] Allelic variation in the variable number of tandem repeats (VNTR) located 5' upstream region of *INS* has been implicated to be responsible for the disease susceptibility.[17,18] Class I haplotype with shorter VNTR confers susceptibility, while class III haplotype with longer VNTR provides dominant protection. In Japanese, however, frequency of disease-associated class I haplotype was markedly high (>90%) in general population,[19] making it difficult to assess the effect of the insulin gene polymorphism on susceptibility to type 1 diabetes. To overcome this, we performed a meta-analysis of a previously published data and our own data, and the results indicated that class I haplotype is significantly associated with type 1 diabetes in Japanese.[19] This was further confirmed by a recent study with a large number of samples in the collaborative study group,[20]indicating that *INS*-VNTR is associated with type 1 diabetes in both Japanese and Caucasian populations. Recent studies showed that the insulin gene is transcribed not only in pancreatic β cells, but also in the thymus, and transcription levels correlate with allelic variation at the *INS*-VNTR.[21,22] Disease-protective class III haplotype was reported to be associated with two- to threefold higher *INS* mRNA levels in the human thymus than disease-susceptible class I haplotype.[21,22] Higher levels of *INS* expression in the thymus with class III haplotype is thought to facilitate immune tolerance induction through negative selection of insulin-specific T lymphocytes, proving a plausible explanation for the dominant protective effect of class III VNTR.

CTLA4 (IDDM12): A Negative Regulator

CTLA4 polymorphism has been reported to be associated with susceptibility to autoimmune thyroid disease (AITD), but its effect on type 1 diabetes was controversial. A recent large-scale study on the association of *CTLA4* with autoimmune diseases confirmed that *CTLA4* is significantly associated with AITD (odds ratio [OR]: 1.4–1.5), but also with type 1 diabetes (OR: 1.1).[10]

We studied the association of *CTLA4* with type 1 diabetes in Japanese using a large number of samples from the collaborative study group.[23] *CTLA4* was significantly associated with AITD, but not with type 1 diabetes. When type 1 diabetic patients were divided into two groups, those with and without AITD, *CTLA4* was significantly associated with type 1 diabetes with AITD, but not without AITD, suggesting that association of *CTLA4* with type 1 diabetes is concentrated in a subset of patients complicated with AITD.

PTPN22 Encoding Lymphoid Tyrosine Phosphatase (LYP)

An arginine-to-tryptophan substitution at codon 620 (R620W) of *PTPN22* was consistently reported to be associated with type 1 diabetes as well as other autoimmune diseases, such as rheumatoid arthritis, systemic lupus erythematosis (SLE), and Graves' disease, in Caucasian populations.[12,24] To clarify the contribution of the variant to type 1 diabetes in Asian populations, a large number of Japanese samples ($n > 1500$) in the collaborative study group as well as Korean samples ($n > 150$) were genotyped, but none had the variant, indicating that the variant is absent in Asian populations.[25] By resequencing of *PTPN22* in Japanese samples for additional single nucleotide polymorphisms (SNPs), five novel SNPs were identified and the –1123 G>C promotor SNP was found to be associated with type 1 diabetes in both Japanese and Korean populations.[25] These data suggested that *PTPN22* contribute to susceptibility to type 1 diabetes, but that disease-associated SNPs may be different between Japanese and Caucasian populations. Preliminary studies on both R620W and the –1123 G>C SNP in Caucasian samples from BDA Warren Repository suggested that the –1123 G>C SNP may be more strongly associated with type 1 diabetes than R620W SNP.[25] Further studies on the association of the newly identified SNP in the promotor region in Caucasian population will clarify whether or not the SNP is primarily associated with type 1 diabetes.

SUMO4 (IDDM5)

A methionine-to-valine substitution at codon 55 (M55V) of *SUMO4* was reported as the causative variant of *IDDM5* on chromosome 6q25 by two groups.[11,26] Subsequent studies, however, showed inconsistency in the association of *SUMO4* with type 1 diabetes.[27–30] To clarify the contribution of *SUMO4* to susceptibility to type 1 diabetes, we sequenced >2000-bp interval of the chromosome 6q25, including the whole *SUMO4* gene, in Japanese.[31] One novel SNP in the promotor region and another in 3'-untranslated region were identified in addition to the M55V variant. These three SNPs were in strong linkage disequilibrium, and three major haplotypes were estimated for these three SNPs. The M55V variant was significantly associated with type 1 diabetes in Japanese and Korean populations.[31] Meta-analysis of published

TABLE 2. Reasons for apparent differences in susceptibility haplotypes and alleles for type 1 diabetes between Japanese and Caucasian populations

		Association		
Gene	Variant	Caucasian	Japanese	Reasons for apparent difference
HLA	Class II haplotype	yes	yes	Available haplotypes[1]
INS	Class I VNTR	yes	yes	Frequency of haplotypes[2]
CTLA4	+6230G>A	yes	restricted	Clinical subtypes[3]
PTPN22	R620W	yes	unknown	Available alleles[4]
SUMO4	M55V	no	yes	Genetic heterogeneity

[1] Haplotypes confer susceptibility in Caucasians are absent in Japanese, and *vice versa*.
[2] Frequency of disease-associated allele is markedly high in Japanese general population.
[3] Association is concentrated in a subtype of diabetes complicated with AITD in Japanese. Re-evaluation in Caucasians needed relative to subtypes with and without AITD.
[4] Disease-associated R620W variant in Caucasians is absent in Asians. Another SNP in the promotor region is associated with type 1 diabetes in Japanese. Re-evaluation in Caucasians needed for this SNP in comparison with R620W to identify the primary SNP-associated with the disease.

studies and our own data confirmed a highly significant association of the M55V variant with type 1 diabetes in Asian populations (summary OR: 1.29, $P = 7.0 \times 10^{-6}$), but not in Caucasian populations,[31] indicating heterogeneity in the genetic effect of *SUMO4* on type 1 diabetes among diverse ethnic groups.

CONCLUSIONS

Similarities and differences in the association of candidate genes for type 1 diabetes were observed between Caucasian and Asian populations. Reasons for observed differences between Caucasian and Asian populations can be summarized as follows (TABLE 2): consistent association, but difference in disease-associated alleles (*HLA*); consistent association, but marked difference in frequencies of disease-associated alleles (*INS*); association concentrated in a subset of patients in Japanese (*CTLA4*); absence of disease-associated allele in Asians (R620W variant of *PTPN22*); and consistent association only in Asians, but not in Caucasians (M55V variant of *SUMO4*). A large number of samples in each ethnic group and comparative studies among different ethnic groups will contribute to genetic dissection of type 1 diabetes and identification of disease-causing variants.

ACKNOWLEDGMENTS

We thank members of the Japanese Study Group of Type 1 Diabetes Genetics: Takuya Awata (Saitama Medical School), Eiji Kawasaki (Nagasaki University), Tetsuro Kobayashi (University of Yamanashi), Taro Maruyama (Saitama Social

Insurance Hospital), Koji Nakanishi (Toranomon Hospital), Akira Shimada (Keio University). This work was supported by a grant-in-aid for Scientific Research from the Ministry of Education, Science, Sports, Culture, and Technology, Japan.

REFERENCES

1. WANG, W.Y.S., B.J. BARRATT, D.G. CLAYTON, *et al.* 2005. Genome-wide association studies: theoretical issues and practical concerns. Nat. Rev. Genet. **6:** 109–118.
2. TODD, J.A., C. MIJOVIC, J. FLETCHER, *et al.* 1989. Identification of susceptibility loci for insulin-dependent diabetes by trans-racial gene mapping. Nature **338:** 587–589.
3. JENKINS, D., C. MIJOVIC, J. FLETCHER, *et al.* 1990. Identification of susceptibility loci for type 1 (insulin-dependent) diabetes by trans-racial gene mapping. Diabetologia **33:** 387–395.
4. DAVIES, J.L., Y. KAWAGUCHI, S.T. BENNETT, *et al.* 1994. A genome-wide search for human type 1 diabetes susceptibility genes. Nature **371:** 130–136.
5. COX, N.J., B. WAPELHORST, V.A. MORRISON, *et al.* 2001 Seven regions of the genome show evidence of linkage to type 1 diabetes in a consensus analysis of 7657 multiplex families. Am. J. Hum. Genet. **69:** 820–830.
6. CONCANNON, P., H.A. ERLICH, C. JULIER, *et al.* 2005. Type 1 diabetes: evidence for susceptibility loci from four genome-wide linkage scans in 1435 multiplex families. Diabetes **54:** 2995–3001.
7. THOMSON, G., W. ROBINSON, M. KUHNER, *et al.* 1988. Genetic heterogeneity, mode of inheritance, and risk estimates for a joint study of Caucasians with insulin-dependent diabetes mellitus. Am. J. Hum. Genet. **43:** 799–816.
8. KAWABATA, Y., H. IKEGAMI, Y. KAWAGUCHI, *et al.* 2002. Asian-specific HLA haplotypes reveal heterogeneity of the contribution of HLA-DR and -DQ haplotypes to susceptibility to type 1 diabetes. Diabetes **51:** 545–551.
9. JULIER, C., R.N. HYER, J. DAVIES, *et al.* 1991. Insulin-IGF2 region on chromosome 11p encodes a gene implicated in HLA-DR4-dependent diabetes susceptibility. Nature **354:** 155–159.
10. UEDA, H., J.M.M. HOWSON, L. ESPOSITO, *et al.* 2003. Association of the T-cell regulatory gene CTLA4 with susceptibility to autoimmune disease. Nature **423:** 506–511.
11. GUO, D., M. LI, Y. ZHANG, *et al.* 2004. A functional variant of SUMO4, a new I kappa B alpha modifier, is associated with type 1 diabetes. Nat. Genet. **36:** 837–841.
12. MELONI, G.F., P. LUCARELLI, M. PELLECCHIA, *et al.* 2004. A functional variant of lymphoid tyrosine phosphatase is associated with type 1 diabetes. Nat. Genet. **36:** 337–338.
13. RISH, N. 1987. Assessing the role of HLA-linked and unlinked determinants of disease. Am. J. Hum. Genet. **40:** 1–14.
14. KARVONEN, M., M. VIIK-KAJANDER, E. MOLTCHANOVA, *et al.* 2000. Incidence of childhood type 1 diabetes worldwide. Diabetes Mondiale (DiaMond) Project Group. Diabetes Care **23:** 1516–1526.
15. IKEGAMI, H. & T. OGIHARA. 1996. Genetics of insulin-dependent diabetes mellitus. Endocrine J. **43:** 605–613.

16. Nakayama, M., N. Abiru, H. Miriyama, *et al.* 2005. Prime role for an insulin epitope in the development of type 1 diabetes in NOD mice. Nature **435:** 220–223.
17. Lucassen, A.M., C. Julier, J.-P. Beressi, *et al.* 1993. Susceptibility to insulin dependent diabetes mellitus maps to a 4.1kb segment of DNA spanning the insulin gene and associated with VNTR. Nat. Genet. **4:** 305–310.
18. Bennett, S.T., A.M. Lucassen, S.C.L. Gough, *et al.* 1995. Susceptibility to human type 1 diabetes at IDDM2 is determined by tandem repeat variation at the insulin gene minisatellite locus. Nat. Genet. **9:** 284–292.
19. Kawaguchi, Y., H. Ikegami, G.-Q. Shen, *et al.* 1997. Insulin gene region contributes to genetic susceptibility to, but may not to low incidence of, insulin-dependent diabetes mellitus in Japanese. Biochem. Biophys. Res. Commun. **233:** 283–287.
20. Awata, T. *et al.* manuscript in preparation.
21. Vafiadia, P., S.T. Bennett, J.A. Todd, *et al.* 1997. Insulin expression in human thymus is modulated by INS VNTR alleles at the IDDM2 locus. Nat. Genet. **15:** 289–292.
22. Pugliese, A., M. Zeller, A. Fernandez, *et al.* 1997. The insulin gene is transcribed in the human thymus and transcription levels correlate with allelic variation at the INS VNTR-IDDM2 susceptibility locus for type 1 diabetes. Nat .Genet. **15:** 293–296.
23. Ikegami, H., T. Awata, E. Kawasaki, *et al.* 2006. The association of CTLA4 polymorphism with type 1 diabetes is concentrated in patients complicated with autoimmune thyroid disease: a multi-center collaborative study in Japan. J. Clin. Endocrino Metab. **91:** 1087–1092.
24. Bottini, N., L. Musumeci, A. Alonso, *et al.* 2004. A functional variant of lymphoid tyrosine phosphatase is associated with type 1 diabetes. Nat. Genet. **36:** 337–338.
25. Kawasaki, E., T. Awata, H. Ikegami, *et al.* 2006. Systematic search for single nucleotide polymorphisms in a lymphoid tyrosine phosphatase (PTPN22) gene: Association between promoter polymorphism and type 1 diabetes in Asian populations. Am. J. Med. Genet. **140:** 586–593.
26. Owerbach, D., L. Pina & K.H. Gabbay. 2004. A 212-kb region on chromosome 6q25 containing the TAB2 gene is associated with susceptibility to type 1 diabetes. Diabetes **53:** 1890–1893.
27. Bohren, K.M., V. Nadkarni, J.H. Song, *et al.* 2004. A M55V polymorphism in a novel SUMO gene (SUMO-4) differentially activates heat shock transcription factors and is associated with susceptibility to type 1 diabetes mellitus. J. Biol. Chem. **279:** 27233–27238.
28. Smyth, D.J., J.M.M. Howson, C.E. Lowe, *et al.* 2005. Assessing the validity of the association between the SUMO4 M55V variant and risk of type 1 diabetes. Nat. Genet. **37:** 110–111.
29. Qu, H., B. Bharaj, X.-Q. Liu, *et al.* 2005. Assessing the validity of the association between the SUMO4 M55V variant and risk of type 1 diabetes. Nat. Genet. **37:** 111–112.
30. Park, Y., S. Park, J. Kang, *et al.* 2005. Assessing the validity of the association between the SUMO4 M55V variant and risk of type 1 diabetes. Nat. Genet. **37:** 112.
31. Noso, S., H. Ikegami, T. Fujisawa, *et al.* 2005. Genetic heterogeneity in association of SUMO4 M55V variant with susceptibility to type 1 diabetes. Diabetes. **54:** 3582–3586.

Immunopathological and Genetic Features in Slowly Progressive Insulin-Dependent Diabetes Mellitus and Latent Autoimmune Diabetes in Adults

TETSURO KOBAYASHI,[a] SHOICHIRO TANAKA,[a] NORIKAZU HARII,[a] KAORU AIDA,[a] HIROKI SHIMURA,[a] MASAYUKI OHMORI,[a] MASAHIRO KANESIGE,[a] AKIRA SHIMADA,[b] AND TARO MARUYAMA[c]

[a]*Third Department of Internal Medical, University of Yamanashi, School of Medicine, Tamaho, Yamanashi 409-3898, Japan*

[b]*Department of Internal Medicine, Keio University, School of Medicine, Tokyo 160-8582, Japan*

[c]*Department of Internal Medicine, Saitama Social Insurance Hospital, Saitama 330-0074, Japan*

ABSTRACT: In 1982 we proposed the presence of a subtype of type 1 diabetes [slowly progressive insulin-dependent diabetes mellitus (SPIDDM)], which was characterized by persistently positive islet cell antibody, late age of onset, noninsulin-dependent diabetes, and slowly progressive beta cell failure. Since then many studies demonstrated that this subtype of type 1 diabetes is prevalent in many ethnic groups and was later called the latent autoimmune diabetes in adults (LADA). Recent epidemiological studies reported that about 10% of patients with apparent type 2 diabetes have at least one autoantibodies against islet-specific antigen with high potential to progress to insulin-dependent state. Between SPIDDM and LADA some differences are reported in terms of some genetic predispositions including HLA class II and class I genes, vitamin D receptor gene, and CTLA4 genes. Common features in SPIDDM and LADA including preserved beta cells at the onset of diabetes and weak T cell response to residual beta cells suggest that these subtypes of type 1 diabetes are suitable candidates for prevention treatment for further progression of beta cell failure.

KEYWORDS: slowly progressive IDDM; SPIDDM; LADA; GAD antibody; IA-2 antibody; insulin autoantibody; prevention; insulin; HLA; CTLA4; INS-VNTR; neuro D; vit D

Address for correspondence: Tetsuro Kobayashi, M.D., Ph.D.,Third Department of Internal Medicine, School of Medicine, University of Yamanashi, Tamaho, Yamanashi 409-3898, Japan. Voice: +81-55-273-9602; fax: +81-55-273-9685.
e-mail: tetsurou@yamanashi.ac.jp

Ann. N.Y. Acad. Sci. 1079: 60–66 (2006).
doi: 10.1196/annals.1375.009

INTRODUCTION

There is a current need to assess the environmental and genetic factors, which contribute to progressive betacell failure in slowly progressive insulin-dependent diabetes mellitus (SPIDDM).[1–6] This is because the number of patients with SPIDDM is higher than classic childhood type 1 diabetes: According to nationwide survey of Japan Diabetes Society about 10% of patients with apparent type 2 diabetes have at least one pancreatic autoantibody including islet cell antibody (ICA), glutamic acid decarboxylase autoantibody (GADAb), IA-2 autoantibody (IA-2Ab), and insulin autoantibody (IAA) and most of them will progress to an insulin-dependent state in several years. The patients with SPIDDM are candidates for intervention to prevent progressive beta cell failure. Why are patients with SPIDDM a suitable target for intervention? In SPIDDM patients endogenous insulin secretion is preserved enough to keep stable glycemic control at the time of onset and the rate of decline of beta cell function occurs over a long time. T cell response to islet cell antigen is weaker than those in acute-onset insulin-dependent (type 1) diabetes mellitus (AIDDM).[7] Environmental and genetic risk factors that will be described below are weak and are sharply contrasted with those in classical AIDDM. Clinical and genetic characterization of SPIDDM comparing some features in latent autoimmune diabetes in adults (LADA)[8] will provide strong insights for prevention of those syndromes (FIG.1).

Definition and Nomenclature of SPIDDM

In 1982, based on a 2-year prospective observation on ICA-positive patients with noninsulin-dependent diabetes (NIDDM), we have suggested that there might be a distinct subtype of type 1 diabetes called SPIDDM. The clinical phenotypes are characterized by (*a*) persistently positive ICA with low titer, (*b*) late age of onset, and (*c*) slowly progressive beta cell failure to insulin-dependent stage.[1] Since then many rigorous efforts have been made to characterize the features of SPIDDM in terms of the genetic, immunological, and clinical aspects.

We have extended our study to include a larger number of patients on their beta cell response to oral glucose test (OGTT) and their changes in level of ICA in patients with SPIDDM based on both prospective and retrospective examinations in Japanese populations.[2,4] In addition to the distinct characteristics from those in patients with AIDDM as mentioned above, we can identify some characteristic findings of SPIDDM: First, serum C-peptide response to OGTT as represented by the sum value of C-peptide at 0, 30, 60, 90, and 120 min during OGTT: sigma C-peptide (normal range: 22–41 ng/mL) was shown to be the most sensitive and specific marker of residual beta cell function.[4] This was because fasting C-peptide level varied day by day and glucagon-stimulation test was weak for C-peptide elicitation and therefore is a less sensitive measure

	SPIDDM	LADA
I. Genetic Factors	HLA-class II (DR4)	HLA-class II (DR4/DR3)
	No association with class I HLA (HLA-A24)	
	No association with CTLA4, INS-VNTR genes	CTLA4, INS-VNTR, IL-10 promoter genes
	No association with Neuro D, Vit D Receptor genes	MICA 5.0/5.1 genes
II. Factors for progression	Sulfonylureas	
	GADAb titer (Cutoff 180 WHO u/ml)	GADAb titer, Age
	Initial beta cell function	
	Epitopes of autoantibodies (GADAb: E4, IA-2Ab)	Epitopes of autoantibodies (GADAb: E1, IA-2Ab)
III. T cell response and Insulitis	Weak T cell response	Weak T cell response
	Less predominant insulitis	

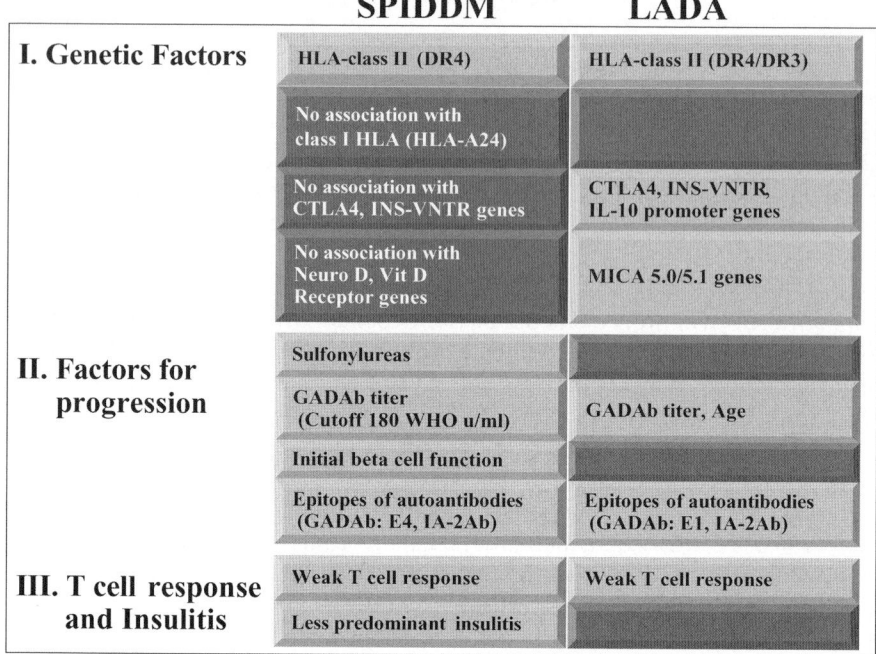

FIGURE 1. Genetic factors and other risk factors, which contribute or not contribute to slowly progressive beta cell dysfunction in SPIDDM and LADA. Blanked board denotes an absence of reports.

for assessing residual beta cell function in SPIDDM. Sigma C-peptide value in SPIDDM patients decreased progressively and most of the patients lapsed to ketosis-prone stage when sigma C-peptide level decreased to less than 4 ng/mL.[4] Second, SPIDDM occurs more frequently in males than females, however, AIDDM occurs more frequently in females than males,[2] and a decline in serum C-peptide values occurs more steeply in male patients than those in female patients.[5] Third, a family history of type 2 NIDDM in SPIDDM patients was more prevalent than that in AIDDM,[2] suggesting that some genetic and/or environmental factors other than HLA are related with progression of beta cell failure in SPIDDM.[9]

LADA is defined as islet antibody-positive NIDDM with slowly progressive beta cell failure and late age (>40 years) of onset.[8,10] However, young onset cases are reported and called latent autoimmune diabetes in children (LADC)[11] or latent autoimmune diabetes in the young (LADY).[12] It, therefore, would be more suitable to change the term *latent* to *slowly progressive* and change the term *LADA* to *slowly progressive IDDM or slowly progressive form of type 1 diabetes* following a WHO recommendation,[13] where the nomenclature must clearly describe the clinical course of the syndrome.

Genetic Factors of SPIDDM

Japanese AIDDM relates with two kinds of diabetogenic haplotypes in homozygous or heterozygous manner (HLA-DRB1*0901-DQB1*0303 / HLA-DRB1*0901-DQB1*0303 or HLA-DRB1*0405-DQB1*0401 / HLA-DRB1*0901-DQB1*0303) while SPIDDM relates only with single diabetogenic haplotype (HLA-DRB1*0405-DQB1*0401 or DRB1*0901-DQB1*0303).[2,14] In addition, AIDDM is closely associated with class I HLA; HLA-A24 (A*2401), which contributes to complete destruction of beta cells and the age of onset in AIDDM[15–17] while patients with SPIDDM lack an association with these diabetogenic haplotypes.[2] The neuroD / beta 2 gene and vitamin D receptor gene are also lacking in the patients with SPIDDM while patients with AIDDM usually have those genes.[18,19] Most patients with SPIDDM do not have an association with CTLA4 or INS-VNTR polymorphisms,[21] while those polymorphisms are found frequently in patient with LADA in Caucasian population.[21,22] These results suggest that genetic predisposition in SPIDDM is less predominant in terms of number of diabetogenic haplotypes of HLA class II and class I genes and other diabetogenic predispositions when compared with LADA and AIDDM. These differences of genetic factors between SPIDDM and LADA do not always mean that those two syndromes are etiologically different, because the clinical phenotype of AIDDM is the same among Caucasian population, even if the variation of genetic factors in AIDDM (mainly HLA genes) are reported differently among the same Caucasian population.[23]

Other Risk Factors for Beta Cell Dysfunction and Implications for Prevention of SPIDDM

In addition to the genetic predispositions, other factors will be related with the rate of decline of progressive beta cell dysfunction. Our previous study demonstrated that sulfonylurea (SU) treatment, duration of ICA, and initial body weight were identified as independent risk factors.[24] We have conducted an intervention trial using early insulin injections instead of SU.[25] Our prevention trial demonstrated that early insulin treatment instead of SU could prevent or slow down the progression of beta cell failure in SPIDDM patients with negative conversion of ICA.[25] Results of multiple randomized clinical trial to prevent the slowly progressive beta cell dysfunction in SPIDDM completed in 2005 will present more clear evidence of the beneficial effects of the early insulin intervention treatment (submitted).

GADAb Epitopes in SPIDDM

Immunological epitope of GADAb in SPIDDM is unique and the epitope resides on N-terminal region of GAD65 molecules (AA 1-83).[26] This epitope was not detected in AIDDM in any other populations, and we named this specific GADAb epitope as E4. In LADA cases Hampe *et al.*[27] reported the presence of epitope on the N-terminal region of GAD65 molecules in accordance with our report.

CONCLUSIONS

Are SPIDDM and LADA the same? Before answering this initial question, we should recognize that various number of cases with islet autoantibody-positive "type 2 diabetes" and slowly progressive betacell dysfunction are reported in many ethnic groups and are called using other terms besides SPIDDM or LADA (slow-onset IDDM, type 1 1/2 diabetes, slowly progressive adult-onset type 1 diabetes, slowly progressive adult-onset type 1 diabetes, etc.).[28] It should also be recognized that a high proportion (around 10%) of patients with apparent type 2 diabetes has islet autoantibodies.

The following issues remain unclear. (*A*) Are there any specific gene(s) related with the syndrome named SPIDDM or LADA? (*B*) Do any etiological mechanism(s) other than T cell-mediated mechanisms relate to beta cell dysfunction? To resolve these issues a whole genome analysis on SPIDDM cases using multiple single nucleotide polymorphisms will be helpful. It may contribute not only to understanding the etiological mechanisms of type 1 diabetes but to provide new insights for prevention of type 1 diabetes.

REFERENCES

1. Kobayashi, T. *et al.* 1982. Islet-cell antibodies in insulin-dependent and non-insulin-dependent diabetics in Japan: their prevalence and clinical significance. *In* Clinico-genetic Genesis of Diabetes Mellitus (International Congress Series 597). G., Mimura S. Baba, Y. Goto, & J. Köbberling, Eds.: 150–160. Excerpta Medica Amesterdam.
2. Kobayashi, T., K. Tamemoto, K. Nakanishi, *et al.* 1993. Immunogenetic and clinical characterization of slowly progressive IDDM. Diabetes Care **16:** 780–788.
3. Kobayashi, T. 1994. Subtype of insulin-dependent diabetes mellitus (IDDM) in Japan: slowly progressive IDDM–the clinical characteristics and pathogenesis of the syndrome [review]. Diabetes Res. Clin. Pract. **24** (Suppl): S95–S99.
4. Kobayashi, T., T. Itoh, K. Kosaka, *et al.* 1987. Time course of islet cell antibodies and beta-cell function in non-insulin-dependent stage of type I diabetes. Diabetes **36:** 510–517.
5. Kobayashi, T., K. Nakanishi, T. Sugimoto, *et al.* 1989. Maleness as risk factor for slowly progressive IDDM. Diabetes Care **12:** 7–11.
6. Kobayashi, T., K. Nakanishi, M. Okubo, *et al.* 1996. GAD antibodies seldom disappear in slowly progressive IDDM. Diabetes Care **19:** 1031.

7. SHIMADA, A., Y. IMAZU, S. MORINAGA, *et al.* 1999. T-cell insulitis found in anti-GAD65+ diabetes with residual beta-cell function. A case report. Diabetes Care **22:** 615–617.
8. TUOMI, T., L.C. GROOP, P.Z. ZIMMET, *et al.* 1993. Antibodies to glutamic acid decarboxylase reveal latent autoimmune diabetes mellitus in adults with a non-insulin-dependent onset of diabetes. Diabetes **42:** 359–362.
9. KAJIO, H., T. KOBAYASHI, K. NAKANISHI, *et al.* 1995. Relationship between insulin-dependent diabetes mellitus (IDDM) and non-insulin-dependent diabetes mellitus: beta-cell function, islet cell antibody, and haptoglobin in parents of IDDM patients. Metabolism **44:** 869–875.
10. FOURLANOS, S., F. DOTTA, C.J. GREENBAUM, *et al.* 2005. Latent autoimmune diabetes in adults (LADA) should be less latent. Diabetologia **48:** 2206–2212.
11. LOHMANN, T., U. NIETZSCHMANN & W. KIESS. 2000. "Lady-like": is there a latent autoimmune diabetes in the young? Diabetes Care **23:** 1707–1708.
12. AYCAN, Z., M. BERBEROGLU, P. ADIYAMAN, *et al.* 2004. Latent autoimmune diabetes mellitus in children (LADC) with autoimmune thyroiditis and celiac disease. J. Pediatr. Endocrinol. Metab. **17:** 1565–1569.
13. ALBERTI, K.G. & P.Z. ZIMMET. 1998. Definition, diagnosis and classification of diabetes mellitus and its complications. Part 1: diagnosis and classification of diabetes mellitus provisional report of a WHO consultation. Diabet. Med. **15:** 539–553.
14. MURAO, S., H. MAKINO, Y. KAINO, *et al.* 2004. Differences in the contribution of HLA-DR and -DQ haplotypes to susceptibility to adult- and childhood-onset type 1 diabetes in Japanese patients. Diabetes **53:** 2684–2690.
15. NAKANISHI, K., T. KOBAYASHI, T. MURASE, *et al.* 1993. Association of HLA-A24 with complete beta-cell destruction in IDDM. Diabetes **42:** 1086–1093.
16. NAKANISHI, K., T. KOBAYASHI, T. MURASE, *et al.* 1999. Human leukocyte antigen-A24 and -DQA1*0301 in Japanese insulin-dependent diabetes mellitus: independent contributions to susceptibility to the disease and additive contributions to acceleration of beta-cell destruction. J. Clin. Endocrinol. Metab. **84:** 3721–3725.
17. AWATA, T., R. HAGURA, T. URAKAMI & Y. KANAZAWA. 1995. Age-dependent HLA genetic heterogeneity of IDDM in Japanese patients. Diabetologia **38:** 748–749.
18. YAMADA, S., Y. MOTOHASHI, T. YANAGAWA, *et al.* 2001. NeuroD/beta2 gene G–>A polymorphism may affect onset pattern of type 1 diabetes in Japanese. Diabetes Care **24:** 1438–1441.
19. MOTOHASHI, Y., S. YAMADA, T. YANAGAWA, *et al.* 2003. Vitamin D receptor gene polymorphism affects onset pattern of type 1 diabetes. J. Clin. Endocrinol. Metab. **88:** 3137–3140.
20. ABE, T., Y. YAMAGUCHI, H. TAKINO, *et al.* 2001. CTLA4 gene polymorphism contributes to the mode of onset of diabetes with antiglutamic acid decarboxylase antibody in Japanese patients: genetic analysis of diabetic patients with antiglutamic acid decarboxylase antibody. Diabet. Med. **18:** 726–731.
21. CAPUTO, M., G.E. CERRONE, A.P. LOPEZ, *et al.* 2005. Cytotoxic T lymphocyte antigen 4 heterozygous codon 49 A/G dimorphism is associated to latent autoimmune diabetes in adults (LADA). Autoimmunity **38:** 277–281.
22. CERRONE, G.E., M. CAPUTO, A.P. LOPEZ, *et al.* 2004. Variable number of tandem repeats of the insulin gene determines susceptibility to latent autoimmune diabetes in adults. Mol. Diagn. **8:** 43–49.
23. RONNINGEN, K.S., N. KEIDING, A. GREEN. 2001. EURODIAB ACE Study Group. Europe and Diabetes: Correlations between the incidence of childhood-onset

type I diabetes in Europe and HLA genotypes. Diabetologia **44**(Suppl 3): B51–B59.

24. Kobayashi, T., S. Sawano, T. Sugimoto, *et al.* 1984. Risk factors of slowly progressive insulin-dependent (type I) diabetes mellitus. J. Steroid Biochem. **20:** 1488.
25. Kobayashi, T., K. Nakanishi, T. Murase & K. Kosaka. 1996. Small doses of subcutaneous-insulin as a strategy for preventing slowly progressive beta-cell failure in islet cell antibody-positive patients with clinical features of NIDDM. Diabetes **45:** 622–626.
26. Kobayashi, T., S. Tanaka, M. Okubo, *et al.* 2003. Unique epitopes of glutamic acid decarboxylase autoantibodies in slowly progressive type 1 diabetes. J Clin Endocrinol Metab. **88:** 4768–4775.
27. Hampe, C.S., I. Kockum, M. Landin-Olsson, *et al.* 2002. GAD65 antibody epitope patterns of type 1.5 diabetic patients are consistent with slow-onset autoimmune diabetes [letter]. Diabetes Care **25:** 1481–1482.
28. Stenstrom, G., A. Gottsater, E. Bakhtadze, *et al.* 2005. Latent autoimmune diabetes in adults: definition, prevalence, beta-cell function, and treatment. Diabetes **54**(Suppl 2): S68–S72.

Genes Influencing Innate and Acquired Immunity in Type 1 Diabetes and Latent Autoimmune Diabetes in Adults

CARANI B. SANJEEVI

Department of Molecular Medicine, Karolinska Hospital Campus, Karolinska Institute, S-17176 Stockholm, Sweden

ABSTRACT: **DQ8 and DQ2 are associated with susceptibility to and DQ6 with protection from type 1 diabetes mellitus (T1DM). A set of polymorphic genes, called MHC class I chain-related genes (MIC-A) in HLA class I region interact with NK cells. In Italians, MICA allele 5 increases T1DM risk by 6.1. Together with HLA-DQ8 and DQ2 the risk increases severalfold. HLA class I genes, also identified as susceptibility genes for T1DM, interact with polymorphic killer immunoglobulin-like receptors (KIR) on NK cells. HLA-DQ8 and DQ2 and MICA-5 in Swedish and other populations also show positive association with disease. Studies on KIR in Latvian patients with T1DM also suggest a role for KIR in the etiology of T1DM. The results from MICA and KIR studies suggest that polymorphism of these genes of the innate immune system identify possible defects in the first line of antiviral defense in the etiology of T1DM. Screening for these genes could be important in the prediction strategies for T1DM.**

KEYWORDS: **T1DM; KIR; MICA; HLA-DR; LADA**

INTRODUCTION

The autoimmune destruction of the pancreatic islet beta cells that results in type 1 diabetes mellitus (T1DM) are thought to be due to an attack by lymphocytes from the patient's own immune system. T1DM is common in Finland and Sardinia. The incidence increases approximately 20% every 10 years. Environmental factors play a major role in the etiology of the disease. This is evident from studies on monozygotic twins where only 33% to 50% concordance is observed.[1] Currently studies aimed at preventing T1DM have largely been performed in relatives of individuals with T1DM and not in general population. However 90% of the patients with T1DM do not have a close relative

Address for correspondence: Dr. C.B. Sanjeevi, Karolinska Institute, Department of Molecular Medicine, Karolinska Hospital Campus, CMM L5:01, S-17176, Stockholm, Sweden. Voice: +46-8-51776254; fax: +46-8-51776179.
e-mail: Sanjeevi.Carani@ki.se

Ann. N.Y. Acad. Sci. 1079: 67–80 (2006).
doi: 10.1196/annals.1375.010

with the disease and therefore improved prediction in the general population is necessary before we can design prevention trials on a public health scale.

In Swedish children with T1DM, 89% of the newly diagnosed patients can be accounted for by the high-risk susceptibility alleles HLA-DQ8 and DQ2 located in the major histocompatibility complex (MHC) region in the short arm of chromosome 6.[2–6] The remaining 11% develop T1DM without the high-risk HLA. Several DQ6 subtypes are present. One such subtype called DQ6 (DQB1*0604) is associated with susceptibility to T1DM. Structural and functional studies on susceptibility DQ6 (DQB1*0604) and protective DQ6 (DQB1*0602) show that critical differences between the susceptible and protective HLA-DQ6 lie in two key residues (residue 57 DQβ and residue 70 DQβ). Residue 70 interacts with the T cell receptor and residue 57 interacts with peptide and forms important residue of P9 pocket.[7–9] Polymorphic substitution at 57β might have a major impact on peptide binding and substitution at 70β could have significant effect on T cell interactions. The protective effect of DQ6 (B*0602), identified to be due to changes at Asp (D) β57 and Gly (G) β70 were evaluated in T1DM patients and controls. The combination of D57/G70-D57/G70 gave absolute protection suggesting the important role these two residues play in protection from T1DM.[10]

Immunological and Genetic Markers in Prediction Studies

The major autoantigens in T1DM are insulin, glutamic acid decarboxylase-isoform 65 (GAD65), and protein tyrosine phosphatase (ICA512 or IA-2).[11] Antibodies to insulin (IAA), GAD65 (GAD65-Ab), and ICA512 or IA-2 are markers for the disease. Their presence in the serum denotes the underlying β cell autoimmunity. They develop well before the signs of clinical diabetes and their presence in the sera of nondiabetic individuals may indicate impending diabetes development. Therefore these markers along with the high-risk genetic markers (e.g., HLA DR and DQ genes) have been used to predict T1DM. The high-risk genetic markers used in prediction studies include the presence of HLA-DQ8 and DQ2. These prediction studies do not take into account the 11% of individuals who may develop T1DM but do not carry the high-risk HLA. The development of T1DM in these 11% of patients suggests that additional genes play a crucial role in conferring protection from or susceptibility to T1DM. Therefore these additional genetic markers associated with susceptibility need to be identified.

Slowly Progressive Form of T1DM or Latent Autoimmune Diabetes in Adults (LADA)

The term *LADA* was coined to describe patients who appeared to have a slowly progressive form of autoimmune or T1DM, managed initially with diet and oral hypoglycemic agents before requiring insulin. LADA, has been known for more than two decades. In 1979 Irvine *et al.*[12] showed that islet cell antibodies (ICAs) can predict secondary failure of oral hypoglycemic agent therapy in type 2 diabetes mellitus (T2DM) patients. In 1986 Groop *et al.* showed[13] that islet cell antibodies identify latent T1DM in patients aged 35–75 years at diagnosis.

The recognition of LADA was facilitated by the development of robust islet autoantibody assays, in particular for GAD.[14] However, earlier studies[15,16] had identified T1DM relatives with high titer GADAb, accounting for ICA detected by immunofluorescence staining, who had a lower risk of progression to diabetes. The diagnosis of LADA is currently based on three criteria: (*a*) adult age at onset of diabetes, (*b*) the presence of circulating islet autoantibodies, and (*c*) lack of a requirement for insulin for at least 6 months after diagnosis. Islet autoantibodies are markers of β cell autoimmunity that distinguish LADA from T2DM. The period of insulin independence (a minimum period of 6 months) after diagnosis distinguishes LADA from classic T1DM. The Immunology of Diabetes Society (IDS) has proposed that an age of 30 years be used as a cut off when using the age criteria until more data are available from longitudinal studies. It is still unclear whether LADA is under the control of distinct genetic markers or is only the consequence of the action of protective environmental factors on a genetic background predisposing for autoimmune diabetes.

LADA, like classic T1DM, is associated with HLA class II genes. In 1986 Ludvigsson *et al.* demonstrated that T1DM is a genetically heterogeneous disease and that HLA-DR3 is associated with a more slowly progressive form of insulin-dependent diabetes.[17] In Finnish LADA patients, Tuomi *et al.* found the frequency of DQB1*0302 to be significantly higher in GAD65 antibody-positive patients than in healthy controls.[18] In a large LADA cohort (age 25–65 years, $n = 236$) from the United Kingdom Prospective Diabetes Study (UKPDS), the frequencies of HLA DR3 (28%), DR4 (27%), HLA DR3/4 (22%) were similar to each other and declined with age at diagnosis.[19] The frequency of the risk HLA genotype DR3-DQ2 in LADA patients is reported increased[17] or unchanged,[20] possibly reflecting the selection or ethnicity of subjects.

MICA and T1DM

The family of MIC (MHC class I chain-related) genes were identified on the short arm of chromosome 6 within the MHC class I region. Since then this group of genes (MICA and MICB) has been widely studied.[21–23] The MICA gene is very polymorphic. Sequence analysis reveals trinucleotide repeat (GCT) microsatellite polymorphism on exon 5 encoding for the transmembrane region of the MICA protein. The MICA protein lacks β2 microglobulin and does not present any peptides.

MICA molecules are not expressed constitutively. It has been shown that the expression of MICA is stress induced, for example, after heat shock,[24] viral infection,[25] bacterial infection,[26] or oxidative stress.[27] MICA gene products interact with $\gamma\delta$ T cells expressing variable region Vγ1. These are CD8 negative $\gamma\delta$ T cells that have been conceptualized to interact with self-antigen instead of foreign peptide or nonpeptide antigens. As these $\gamma\delta$ T cells recognize MICA, MICA may be involved in immune surveillance of stressed epithelial cells. MICA interacts with an activating receptor, NKG2D, expressed at the surface of most circulating $\alpha\beta$ CD8 T cells, $\gamma\delta$ T cells, and natural killer (NK) cells in humans.[22,28–30] Engagement of NKG2D by MICA triggers NK cells and costimulates some $\gamma\delta$ T cells and antigen-specific $\alpha\beta$ CD8 T cells. In CD8 $\alpha\beta$ T cells, NKG2D/MIC engagement delivers a costimulatory signal that complements T cell receptor (TCR)-mediated Ag recognition on target cells (TABLE 1).[25]

The TM region polymorphism of MICA gene has been shown to be associated with several autoimmune disorders including psoriasis, ankylosing, spondylitis,[22] autoimmune Addison's disease,[31] and juvenile rheumatoid arthritis.[32] Previous studies done in different populations have also reported MICA allele associations with T1DM. In the Chinese population, MICA9 is positively associated,[33] whereas in Japanese[34] and Koreans[35] MICA4 is positively and MICA6 is negatively associated with T1DM. In Latvians[36] and Asian Indians[37] MICA5 is positively associated.

Effect of MICA on Age at Onset of T1DM

The risk for T1DM with positively associated DQ2-DQ8 and negatively associated DQ6 is decreasing with increasing age.[7,38] In Swedish patients diagnosed between the age of 0–35 years, those aged 20 years or less (younger onset group) and those aged above 20 years (older onset group) were compared to see if MICA association shows similar age effect. The risk associated with MICA5, was higher in younger onset group compared to the older onset group. MICA6 was negatively associated with the disease in the younger onset group but not in the older onset group. MICA6 has previously been shown to be negatively associated with the disease in Japanese and Koreans.[34,35,39–41]

MICA and LADA

MICA polymorphism has been studied in LADA in Italian, Swedish, Indian, Latvian patients with T1DM.[36,37,39,40] In an Italian study MICA5 was associated with younger onset T1DM ($<$25 years; odds ratio [OR] $=$12.5) independent of high risk DQ2/DQ8. The odds ratio of simultaneous presence of MICA5 and DQ2/DQ8 was 172. Also, MICA5.1 was associated with adult-onset T1DM ($>$25 years; OR $=$ 3.4) and LADA (OR $=$7.0) independent of

DR3-DQ2/DR4-DQ8 and a combination of MICA5.1 and DR3-DQ2/DR4-DQ8 conferred an increased risk for adult-onset T1DM (OR = 18.2) and LADA (OR = 34.4).

This distinction in association of allele 5 with T1DM and allele 5.1 with LADA was the first to be reported. It is not clear whether this distinction can be used as a marker for diagnosis of LADA and in the prediction studies in newborns.[39]

Viral Etiology of T1DM: Is MICA Involved?

Polymorphism of MICA and HLA and infection with Coxsackie B virus (CBV) has been associated with T1DM.[42] In Swedish patients with T1DM, especially in the Linköping region of Sweden, CBV increased in DR3-MICA5.1 positive patients versus DR3-MICA5.1 negative patients and in DR3-DR4-MICA5.1 positive patients versus DR3-DR4-MICA5.1 negative patients ($P <$ 0.02 for both). This suggests that MICA5.1 has an influence on immune response against CBV 3 or 5 infection in patients from Linköping. When the patients from the whole of Sweden were divided based on the presence or absence of DR3, DR4, or DR3-DR4 (heterozygous); MICA5, -5.1, or -6; and DR3- MICA5.1, DR4-MICA5.1, or DR3-DR4-MICA5.1, no difference in the frequency of CBV antibodies was observed in any of the three groups. It is difficult to say how association of CBV-IgM to MICA5.1 could be relevant in pathogenesis of T1DM.[43] There is evidence that early innate immune response (via NK cells) against CBV4 may directly be responsible for the development of diabetes in mice.[44] MICA is one of the activating factors for NK cells.[45,46] Induction of MICA expression after viral infection (CMV) has been shown.[25] It needs to be tested if MICA expression can be induced by CBV infection, particularly in the β cells. Induced expression of MICA after CBV infection might be important in the pathogenesis of T1DM through NKG2D bearing NK cells and also αβ T cells.

MICA as a Marker for Newborn Screening

The Diabetes Autoimmunity Study in the Young (DAISY) is a newborn screening and follow-up study in the state of Colorado, United States. Here children are followed up from birth to define the incidence of beta cell autoimmunity by age, race/ethnicity, HLA genotype, family history of T1DM, and environmental factors.[47] In this study material, homozygosity of MICA 5.1/5.1 is associated with early activation of autoimmunity of DR3/4-DQ2/8 DAISY relatives.[46] This suggests that MICA may be, important in early events of autoimmunity that is, events before acute onset of the disease.

KIR and T1DM

NK cells of the innate immune system are important in antiviral and antitumor immunity. Like CD4$^+$ cells they have the capacity to directly lyse target cells. This may occur either as a result of direct recognition of the target cell by activating receptors expressed by NK cells or antibody-dependent cellular cytotoxicity mediated through antibody binding. Human NK cells express multiple receptors that interact with HLA class I molecules. In the absence of antigen receptors it was not known how NK cells discriminate healthy cells from transformed or virus-infected ones. NK cell function is regulated by the interaction of MHC class I molecules with inhibitory cell surface receptors. This mechanism is believed to protect healthy cells from lysis by autologous NK cells, while rendering cells for which class I expression is compromised by infection or transformation susceptible to NK cell-mediated lysis.[48–50]

It has been observed that expression of MHC class I molecules by target cells is inversely correlated with susceptibility to NK cell-mediated lysis. The best-studied groups of human NK cell receptors that interact with HLA class I molecules are termed *killer cell immunoglobulin-like receptors* (KIR). KIRs form a family of highly homologous immune receptors that regulate the response of NK cells and some T cells. These receptors were first identified by their ability to impart some specificity on NK cytolysis.[51] The discovery of KIRs has also imparted an additional function of the MHC class I molecules. Thus, it is likely that KIRs play significant role in the control of immune response and susceptibility to some immune-mediated diseases. NK cells need to discriminate between healthy and infected or transformed cells, corresponding with the observed phenotypic dominance of KIR-mediated inhibition over activation. Diversity at the locus may be a result of selection pressures, in a manner autologous to that proposed for HLA locus. Thus, disease resistance conferred by KIR locus is likely to vary in a haplotypic manner depending on disease type.[49]

KIR genes are a family of genes clustered on the long arm of chromosome 19 (q13.4). The KIR region is polymorphic. A significant feature of KIR locus is that content and number of genes vary between haplotypes.[49] Variation at the KIR gene complex is a function of both—allelic polymorphism at several KIR genes and variability in the number of genes present on any given haplotype. However, the genes 2DL4, 3DP1, 3DL2, and 3DL3 are present on virtually all haplotypes and therefore have been named framework loci.[52] All the other genes exist only as fractions of the total haplotypic pool.

The genes encoding KIR receptors share similar structure, being composed of 9 exons and 8 introns. KIR receptors are divided into two functional groups, based on sequence differences in the transmembrane and cytoplasmic regions. One of these groups has "long" cytoplasmic tails, for example KIR2DL or KIR3DL (2D or 3D refers to the number of IG-like domains in the receptor, "L" refers to "long" cytoplasmic tail). These KIR receptors have inhibitory

TABLE 1. Association of MICA alleles with T1DM in different populations

MICA allele/genotype	Population studied	Association	Reference
5 and 5.1	HBDI T1DM families	Positive	73
5	Latvians, Asian Indians	Positive	36, 37, 74
Italians			
4	Japanese, Koreans, Spanish	Positive	34, 35, 75
Basques			
9	Chinese	Positive	33
6	Japanese, Koreans	Negative	34, 35
4/5.1 and 9/9	Brazilians	Positive	76

function. Activation of these receptors leads to the inhibition of NK cell activation. The other group of KIR receptors, for example, KIR2DS and KIR3DS ("S" refers to short) have shorter cytoplasmic domains. These KIRs have activating function. The genes for KIR, HLA are on different chromosomes, so that ligands and receptors segregate independently in human pedigrees.

Based on the genes present, haplotypes have been divided into two primary sets termed A and B haplotypes, which differ in the number of genes encoding for stimulatory receptors. Haplotype A contains only one gene encoding for a stimulatory receptor—2DS4, but haplotype B may contain various combinations of 2DS1, 2DS2, 2DS3, 2DS5, 3DS1, and 2DS4. The frequencies of A and B haplotypes are roughly similar in Caucasians, but vary in different ethnic groups.[53,54] KIR-A haplotypes differ only at the allelic level, but not in gene content, as opposed to B haplotype, which has a much greater variety of subtypes both varying at the allelic level and gene content.

KIRs and TCRs have overlapping binding sites and therefore cannot bind to the same HLA/peptide complex.[55,56] This may generate some control over T cell activity, since TCRs and KIRs would act as competitors for HLA binding (see TABLE 2). Although interactions with KIRs have been showed to be independent of peptide presented on HLA class I,[57] some studies indicate that specificity of binding does indeed depend on the peptide presented through HLA class I molecules.[57,58] It has been suggested that inhibiting and activating receptors of the same specificity for HLA may respond differentially depending on bound peptides. These distinct binding affinities of activating KIRs compared to inhibiting ones may contribute to dominance of inhibition. For example, KIR 2DL2 has a higher affinity for HLA Cw3 than 2DS2, due to a single amino acid substitution.[55,59]

Studies of KIR genes in different immune-mediated diseases are limited. Few studies have looked at the importance of these genes in HIV-infected individuals, rheumatoid arthritis and psoriatic arthritis, pre-eclampsia, transplantation, as well as diabetes mellitus and celiac disease. There was no difference in the KIR gene repertoire in pre-eclampsia and normotensive controls.[60] Case–control analysis found no association of the five KIR genotype categories, the A or B KIR haplotypes, also transmission disequilibrium test found no

TABLE 2. KIR genes, ligand, and function

KIR gene	HLA class I ligand	Function
2DL1	Cw (Asn77 and Lys80)	inhibitory
2DL2	Cw (Ser77 and Asn80)	inhibitory
2DL3	Cw (Ser 77 and Asn80)	inhibitory
2DS1	Cw (Asn 77 and Lys80)	stimulating
2DS2	Cw (Ser 77 and Asn80)	stimulating
2DS3	unknown	stimulating
2DS4	unknown	stimulating
2DS5	unknown	stimulating
2DL4	probably HLA-G	inhibitory, stimulating, or both (framework locus)
2DL5	unknown	likely inhibitory
3DL1	HLA-B (Bw4)	inhibitory, allele 3DS1-stim
3DL2	HLA-A alleles	inhibitory (framework locus)
3DL3	unknown	unknown (framework locus)

association of the A and B KIR haplotypes with celiac disease.[61] Martin *et al.* reported that subjects with activating KIR2DS1 and/or KIR2DS2 genes are susceptible to developing psoriatic arthritis, but only when HLA ligands for their homologous inhibitory receptors, KIR2DL1 and KIR2DL2/3, are missing.[62]

In studies of KIR genes in Latvian patients with T1DM, KIR2DL2 and KIR2DS2 were positively associated with disease. The combined risk of KIR2DL2 with HLA-DR3 (OR = 73.4) or DR4 (OR = 66.8), or DR3 and DR4 (OR = 88.3), was higher than MICA4 and KIR2DL2 (OR = 26.7). This indicates that these KIR genes, probably together with their ligands, are important in the pathogenesis of T1DM in the Latvian population. When the KIR genotypes were studied, the presence of KIR2DL2 (homozygous or as single copy) was associated with susceptibility and its absence was associated with protection in T1DM. This might indicate the particular importance of this gene for the disease in Latvian population.[63]

Inhibitory KIR receptors, such as those represented by 2DL2, if present on NK cells and other immune cells, would probably prevent them from killing an infected or transformed target cell that expresses a sufficient amount of HLA class I molecules, because engagement of these inhibitory receptors would suppress the activating signal necessary to trigger cell killing. If the target cell does express other ligands, such as a MICA, that can override the inhibitory signal from the KIR-HLA class I interaction by binding with NKG2D, the pathogenic process mediated by the target cell can continue. But if an infected or transformed cell downregulates its class I molecules, which is usually the case, the inhibitory receptors would not have ligands; thus, KIR-expressing cells would be activated and would proceed to kill the target cell.

One such hypothesis might be initial direct recognition of pancreatic beta cells, with downregulated MHC class I due to infection, by NK cells, which could lead to direct lysis of β cells, release of autoantigens, and triggering of T cells.[64] In the case of infected or transformed cell, which is expressing sufficient amount of HLA class I, NK cells, as well as other cells expressing KIR receptors, will probably not kill the cell, because of the lack of activating signal resulting from engagement of inhibitory receptors. This would cause survival of affected cell and the pathogenic process can continue, in case if this cell does not express other ligands, like MICA molecule, engagement of which by NKG2D can override inhibitory signal from KIR/HLA class I interaction. Yet another hypothesis is that recognition of HLA class I molecules by activating KIRs on NK and T cells may affect the immune response due to the secretion of IFN-γ.[65] Van der Slik *et al.*[64] in their study of KIR genes in T1DM hypothesized that activating KIRs may enhance rapid induction of T cell-mediated immune responses in the presence of specific HLA class I ligand. Costimulation of T cells by engagement of KIR receptors may contribute to initiation of T1DM by activation of T cell subsets, which interact weakly with low amounts of self peptide.

Toll-Like Receptors and T1DM

Toll-like receptors (TLRs) are a part of innate immune defense that recognize conserved patterns on micro-organisms. Eleven different TLRs have been identified so far. TLR signaling following recognition of distinct pathogen pattern can also influence the production of proinflammatory cytokines and chemokines by dendritic cells and macrophages.[66] These recognize molecular patterns, such as RNA (TLR3, TLR7, and TLR8),[67,68] DNA (TLR9),[69] or lipopolysaccharide (TLR4).[70] The pattern of cytokine production following TLR ligation depends on the type of TLR, which results in a specifically optimized pathogen–host balance and may occasionally result in autoimmune disease.[71] Thus TLR signaling represents a key component of the innate immune response to microbial infection.

According to the recent paper from Rolf Zinkernagel's group,[66] immunization with lymphocytic choriomeningitis virus (LCMV) glycoprotein (GP)-derived peptide did not induce autoimmune diabetes in mice expressing LCMV-GP as a transgene under the control of rat insulin promoter. This is inspite of the fact that there were large numbers of autoreactive cytotoxic T cells. Only subsequent treatment with TLR ligands elicited overt autoimmune disease. In another study, viral mimicry induced the development of diabetes in 'C57BL/6-rat insulin promotor-B7.1 mice.' This suggests a combination of direct recognition of this virus-like stimulus by pancreatic islets occurs through the expression of TLR3.[72] These studies suggest a role of TLR3 in the etiopathogenesis of T1DM.

In conclusion, MICA, KIR, and may be TLRs (based on evidence from mouse model) together or separately play important role in the etiology of T1DM. More studies are needed to understand the interaction of these molecules that might lead to the development of T1DM.

ACKNOWLEDGMENTS

I sincerely acknowledge the support of Swedish Medical Research Council (for research grant and fellowship grant to CBS), Swedish Diabetes Association, Children's Diabetes Fund of Sweden (Barndiabetesfonden), Karolinska Institute, and Karolinska Hospital. I thank my former graduate students Peter Hjlemstrom, Mehran Ghaderi, Aija Shtauvere-Bremeus, Liene Nikitina-Zake, Giovanni Gambelunghe, and Manu Gupta and my visiting guest researchers Alok Kanungo, Madhuri Balaji, A.G.Unnikrishnan, Nikhil Tandon, Valeria Tica for their help.

REFERENCES

1. Deschamps, I., C. Boitard, J. Hors, *et al.* 1992. Life table analysis of the risk of type 1 (insulin-dependent) diabetes mellitus in siblings according to islet cell antibodies and HLA markers. An 8-year prospective study. Diabetologia **35:** 951–957.
2. Sanjeevi, C.B., T.P. Lybrand, M. Landin-Olsson, *et al.* 1994. Analysis of antibody markers, DRB1, DRB5, DQA1 and DQB1 genes and modeling of DR2 molecules in DR2 positive patients with type 1 diabetes. Tissue Antigens **44:** 110–119.
3. Sanjeevi, C.B., T.P. Lybrand, C. DeWeese, *et al.* 1995. Polymorphic amino acids variations in HLA-DQ are associated with systematic physical property changes and occurrence of insulin-dependent diabetes mellitus. Diabetes **44:** 125–131.
4. Sanjeevi, C.B., M. Landin-Olsson, I. Kockum, *et al.* 1995. Effects of the second haplotype on the association with childhood insulin-dependent diabetes mellitus. Tissue Antigens **45:** 148–152.
5. Sanjeevi, C.B., P. Höök, M. Landin-Olsson, *et al.* 1996. Analysis of DR4 subtypes and their molecular properties in a population based study of Swedish childhood diabetes. Tissue Antigens **47:** 275–283.
6. Kockum, I., C.B. Sanjeevi, S. Eastman, *et al.* 1999. Complex interaction between HLA DR and DQ in conferring risk for childhood type 1 diabetes. Eur. J. Immunogenet. **26:** 361–372.
7. Graham, J., I. Kockum, C.B. Sanjeevi, *et al.* 1999. Negative association between type 1 diabetes and HLA DQB1*0602- DQA1*0102 is attenuated with age at onset. Swedish Childhood Diabetes Study Group. Eur. J. Immunogenet. **26:** 117–128.
8. Sanjeevi, C.B., C. Dewessee, T.P. Lybrand, *et al.* 1997. Analysis of critical residues of DQ6 molecules associated with insulin-dependent diabetes. Tissue Antigens **50:** 61–65.
9. Sanjeevi, C.B., W.A. Hagopian, M. Landin-Olsson, *et al.* 1998. Association between autoantibody markers and subtypes of DR4 and DR4-DQ in Swedish children with insulin-dependent diabetes reveals closer association of tyrosine

pyrophosphatase autoimmunity with DR4 than DQ8. Tissue Antigens **51:** 281–286.
10. SANJEEVI, C.B. 2000. DQ6 mediated protection in human insulin-dependent diabetes mellitus. Hum. Immunol. **61:** 148–153.
11. HAGOPIAN, W.A., C.B. SANJEEVI, I. KOCKUM, *et al.* 1995. Glutamate decarboxylase-, insulin- and islet cell-antibodies, and HLA typing to detect diabetes in a general population-based study of Swedish children. J. Clin. Invest. **95:** 1505–1511.
12. IRVINE, W.J. *et al.* 1979. The value of islet cell antibody in predicting secondary failure of oral hypoglycaemic agent therapy in diabetes mellitus. J. Clin. Lab. Immunol. **2:** 23–26.
13. GROOP, L.C. *et al.* 1986. Islet cell antibodies identify latent type 1 diabetes in patients aged 35-75 years at diagnosis. Diabetes **35:** 237–241.
14. HAGOPIAN, W.A., A.E. KARLSEN, A. GOTTSATER, *et al.* 1993. Quantitative assay using recombinant human islet glutamic acid decarboxylase (GAD65) shows that 64K autoantibody positivity at onset predicts diabetes type. J. Clin. Invest. **91:** 368–374.
15. GENOVESE, S., E. BONIFACIO, J.M. MCNALLY, *et al.* 1992. Distinct cytoplasmic islet cell antibodies with different risks for type 1 (insulin-dependent) diabetes mellitus. Diabetologia **35:** 385–388.
16. GIANANI, R., A. PUGLIESE, S. BONNER-WEIR, *et al.* 1992. Prognostically significant heterogeneity of cytoplasmic islet cell antibodies in relatives of patients with type I diabetes. Diabetes **41:** 347–353.
17. LUDVIGSSON, J.U. *et al.* 1986. HLA-DR 3 is associated with a more slowly progressive form of type 1 (insulin-dependent) diabetes. Diabetologia **29:** 207–210.
18. TUOMI, T. *et al.* 1999. Clinical and genetic characteristics of type 2 diabetes with and without GAD antibodies. Diabetes **48:** 150–157.
19. HORTON, V., I. STRATTON, G.F. BOTTAZZO, *et al.* 1999. Genetic heterogeneity of autoimmune diabetes: age of presentation in adults is influenced by HLA DRB1 and DQB1 genotypes (UKPDS 43). UK Prospective Diabetes Study (UKPDS) Group. Diabetologia **42:** 608–616.
20. SANJEEVI, C.B., G. GAMBELUNGHE, A. FALORNI, *et al.* 2002. Genetics of latent autoimmune diabetes in adults. Ann. N. Y. Acad. Sci. **958:** 107–111.
21. BAHRAM, S., M. BRESNAHAN, D.E. GERAGHTY & T. SPIES. 1994. A second lineage of mammalian major histocompatibility complex class I genes. Proc. Natl. Acad. Sci. USA **91:** 6259–6263.
22. BAHRAM, S. 2000. MIC genes: from genetics to biology. Adv. Immunol. **76:** 1–60.
23. OTA, M. *et al.* 1997. Trinucleotide repeat polymorphism within exon 5 of the MICA gene (MHC class I chain-related gene A): allele frequency data in the nine population groups Japanese, Northern Han, Hui, Uygur, Kazakhstan, Iranian, Saudi Arabian, Greek and Italian. Tissue Antigens **49:** 448–454.
24. GROH, V., S. BAHRAM, S. BAUER, *et al.* 1996. Cell stress regulated human major histocompatibility complex class I gene expressed in gastrointestinal epithelium. Proc. Natl. Acad. Sci. USA **93:** 12445–12450.
25. GROH, V., R. RHINEHART, J. RANDOLPH-HABECKER, *et al.* 2001. Costimulation of CD8alphabeta T cells by NKG2D via engagement by MIC induced on virus-infected cells. Nat. Immunol. **2:** 255–260.
26. TIENG, V., C. LE BOUGUENEC, L. DU MERLE, *et al.* 2002. Binding of Escherichia coli adhesin AfaE to CD55 triggers cell-surface expression of the MHC class I-related molecule MICA. Proc. Natl. Acad. Sci. USA **99:** 2977–2982.

27. YAMAMOTO, K., Y. FUJIYAMA, A. ANDOH, *et al.* 2001. Oxidative stress increases MICA and MICB gene expression in the human colon carcinoma cell line (CaCo-2). Biochim. Biophys. Acta **1526:** 10–12.
28. WU, J. *et al.* 1999. An activating immunoreceptor complex formed by NKG2D and DAP10. Science **285:** 730–732.
29. SALIH, H.R., H.G. RAMMENSEE & A. STEINLE. 2002. Cutting edge: down-regulation of MICA on human tumors by proteolytic shedding. J. Immunol. **169:** 4098–4102.
30. GROH, V., J. WU, C. YEE & T. SPIES. 2002. Tumour-derived soluble MIC ligands impair expression of NKG2D and T-cell activation. Nature **419:** 734–738.
31. GAMBELUNGHE, G., A. FALORNI, M. GHADERI, *et al.* 1999. Microsatellite polymorphism of the MHC class I chain related (MIC-A and MIC-B) genes marks the risk for autoimmune Addison's disease. J. Clin. Endocrinol. Metab. **84:** 3701–3707.
32. NIKITINA ZAKE, L., I. CIMDINA, I. RUMBA, *et al.* 2002. Major histocompatibility complex class I chain related (MIC) A gene, TNFa microsatellite alleles and TNFB alleles in juvenile idiopathic arthritis patients from Latvia. Hum. Immunol. **63:** 418–423.
33. LEE, Y.J., F.Y. HUANG, C.H. WANG, *et al.* 2000. Polymorphism in the transmembrane region of the MICA gene and type 1 diabetes. J. Pediatr. Endocrinol. Metab. **13:** 489–496.
34. KAWABATA, Y., H. IKEGAMI, Y. KAWAGUCHI, *et al.* 2000. Age-related association of MHC class I chain-related gene A (MICA) with type 1 (insulin-dependent) diabetes mellitus. Hum. Immunol. **61:** 624–629.
35. PARK, Y., H. LEE, C.B. SANJEEVI & G.S. EISENBARTH. 2001. MICA polymorphism is associated with type 1 diabetes in the Korean population. Diabetes Care **24:** 33–38.
36. SHTAUVERE-BRAMEUS, A., M. GHADERI, I. RUMBA & C.B. SANJEEVI. 2002. Microsatellite allele 5 of MHC class I chain-related gene a increases the risk for insulin-dependent diabetes mellitus in Latvians. Ann. N. Y. Acad. Sci. **958:** 349–352.
37. SANJEEVI, C.B., A. KANUNGO, L. BERZINA, *et al.* 2002. Samal. MHC class I chain related gene A (MICA) alleles distinguishes malnutrition modulated diabetes (MMDM), insulin-dependent diabetes patients (IDDM) and non-insulin dependent diabetes mellitus (NIDDM) patients from Eastern India. Ann. N. Y. Acad. Sci. **958:** 341–344.
38. LOHMANN, T., J. SESSLER, H.J. VERLOHREN, *et al.* 1997. Distinct genetic and immunological features in patients with onset of IDDM before and after age 40. Diabetes Care **20:** 524–529.
39. GUPTA, M., L. NIKITINA-ZAKE, M. ZARGHAMI, *et al.* 2003. Association between the transmembrane region polymorphism of MHC class I chain related Gene-A and type 1 diabetes mellitus in Sweden. Hum. Immunol. **64:** 553–561.
40. GAMBELUNGHE, G., M. GHADERI, C. TORTOIOLI, *et al.* 2001. Two distinct MICA gene markers discriminate major autoimmune diabetes types. J. Clin. Endocrinol. Metab. **86:** 3754–3760.
41. TÖRN, C., M. GUPTA, L. NIKITINA ZAKE, *et al.* 2003. Heterozygosity for MICA5.0/MICA5.1 and HLA-DR3-DQ2/DR4-DQ8 are independent genetic risk factors for latent autoimmune diabetes in adults. Hum. Immunol. **64:** 902–909.
42. VREUGDENHIL, G.R., A. GELUK, T.H. OTTENHOFF, *et al.* 1998. Molecular mimicry in diabetes mellitus: the homologous domain in coxsackie B virus protein 2C

and islet autoantigen GAD65 is highly conserved in the coxsackie B-like enteroviruses and binds to the diabetes associated HLA-DR3 molecule. Diabetologia **41:** 40.

43. Gupta, M., L.N. Zake, M. Landin-Olsson, *et al.* 2003. Coxsackie virus V antibodies are increased in HLA DR3-MICA5.1 positive type 1 diabetes (T1DM) patients in Linköping region in Sweden. Hum. Immunol. **64:** 874–879.
44. Flodstrom, M., A. Maday, D. Balakrishna, *et al.* 2002. Target cell defense prevents the development of diabetes after viral infection. Nat. Immunol. **3:** 373–382.
45. Bauer, S., V. Groh, J. Wu, *et al.* 1999. Activation of NK cells and T cells by NKG2D, a receptor for stress-inducible MICA. Science **285:** 727–729.
46. Ide, A., S.R. Babu, D.T. Robles, *et al.* 2005. Homozygosity for premature stop codon of the MHC class I chain-related gene A (MIC-A) is associated with early activation of islet auto immunity of DR3/4-DQZ/8 high risk DAISY relatives. J. Clin. Immunol. **25:** 303–308.
47. Rewers, M., J.M. Norris, G.S. Eisenbarth, *et al.* 1996. Beta-cell autoantibodies in infants and toddlers without IDDM relatives: diabetes autoimmunity study in the young (DAISY). J. Autoimmun. **9:** 405–410.
48. Trowsdale, J. 2001. Genetic and functional relationships between MHC and NK receptor genes. Immunity **15:** 363–374.
49. Parham, P. 2005. MHC class I molecules and KIRS in human history, health and survival. Nat. Rev. Immunol. **5:** 201–214.
50. Rajagopalan, S. & E.O. Long. 2005. Understanding how combinations of HLA and KIR genes influence disease. J. Exp. Med. **201:** 1025–1029.
51. Harel-Bellan, A. *et al.* 1986. Natural killer susceptibility of human cells may be regulated by genes in the HLA region on chromosome 6. Proc. Natl. Acad. Sci. USA **83:** 5688–5692.
52. Wilson, M.J. *et al.* 2000. Plasticity in the organization and sequences of human KIR/ILTgene families. Proc. Natl. Acad. Sci. USA **97:** 4778–4783.
53. Rajalingam, R. *et al.* 2002. Distinctive KIR and HLA diversity in a panel of north Indian Hindus. Immunogenetics **53:** 1009–1019.
54. Yawata, M. *et al.* 2002. Predominance of group A KIR haplotypes in Japanese associated with diverse NK cell repertoires of KIR expression. Immunogenetics **54:** 543–550.
55. Boyington, J.C. *et al.* 2000. Crystal structure of an NK cell immunoglobulin-like receptor in complex with its class I MHC ligand. Nature **405:** 537–543.
56. Mandelboim, O. *et al.* 1996. Protection from lysis by natural killer cells of group 1 and 2 specificity is mediated by residue 80 in human histocompatibility leukocyte antigen C alleles and also occurs with empty major histocompatibility complex molecules. J. Exp. Med. **184:** 913–922.
57. Peruzzi, M. *et al.* 1996. A p70 killer cell inhibitory receptor specific for several HLA-B allotypes discriminates among peptides bound to HLA-B*2705. J. Exp. Med. **184:** 1585–1590.
58. Rajagopalan, S. & E.O. Long. 1997. The direct binding of a p58 killer cell inhibitory receptor to human histocompatibility leukocyte antigen (HLA)-Cw4 exhibits peptide selectivity. J. Exp. Med. **185:** 1523–1528.
59. Boyington, J.C. & P.D. Sun. 2002. A structural perspective on MHC class I recognition by killer cell immunoglobulin-like receptors. Mol. Immunol. **38:** 1007–1021.

60. WITT, C.S. *et al.* 2002. Alleles of the KIR2DL4 receptor and their lack of association with preeclampsia. Eur. J. Immunol. **32:** 18–29.
61. MOODIE, S.J. *et al.* 2002. Analysis of candidate genes on chromosome 19 in coeliac disease: an association study of the KIR and LILR gene clusters. Eur. J. Immunogenet. **29:** 287–291.
62. MARTIN, M.P. *et al.* 2002. Cutting edge: susceptibility to psoriatic arthritis: influence of activating killer Ig-like receptor genes in the absence of specific HLA-C alleles. J. Immunol. **169:** 2818–2822.
63. NIKITINA-ZAKE, L., R. RAJALINGHAM, I. RUMBA & C.B. SANJEEVI. 2004. Killer-cell immunoglobulin-like receptor genes in Latvian patients with type 1 diabetes mellitus and healthy controls. Ann. N. Y. Acad. Sci. **1037:** 161–169.
64. VAN DER SLIK, A.R. *et al.* 2003. KIR in type 1 diabetes: disparate distribution of activating and inhibitory natural killer cell receptors in patients versus HLA-matched control subjects. Diabetes **52:** 2639–2642.
65. YEN, J.H. *et al.* 2001. Major histocompatibility complex class I-recognizing receptors are disease risk genes in rheumatoid arthritis. J. Exp. Med. **193:** 1159–1167.
66. LANG, K.S., RECHER, M., T. JUNT, *et al.* 2005. Toll-like receptor engagement converts T-cell autoreactivity into overt autoimmune disease. Nat. Med., **11:** 138–145.
67. ALEXOPOLOU, L., A.C. HOLT, R. MEDZHITOV & R.A. FLAVELL. 2001. Recognition of double-stranded RNA and activation of NF-kB by Toll-like receptor3. Nature **413:** 732–738.
68. HEIL, F. *et al.* 2004. Species-specific recognition of single-stranded RNA via toll-like receptor 7 and 8. Science **303:** 1526–1529.
69. HEMMI, H. *et al.* 2000. A toll-like receptor recognizes bacterial DNA. Nature **408:** 740–745.
70. POLTORAK, A. *et al.* 1998. Defective LPS signaling in C3H/HeJ and C57BL/10ScCr mice: mutations in Tlr4 gene. Science **282:** 2085–2088.
71. MEAGHER, C. *et al.* 2003. Cytokines and chemokines in the pathogenesis of type 1 diabetes. Adv. Exp. Med. Biol. **520:** 133–158.
72. WEN, L., J. PENG, Z. LI & S.F. WONG. 2004. The effect of innate immunity on autoimmune diabetes and expression of TLR on pancreatic islets. J. Immunol. **172:** 3173–3180.
73. ZAKE, L.N., M. GHADERI, Y.S. PARK, *et al.* 2002. MHC class I chain-related gene alleles 5 and 5.1 are transmitted more frequently to type 1 diabetes offspring in HBDI families. Ann. N. Y. Acad. Sci. **958:** 309–311.
74. GAMBELUNGHE, G., M. GHADERI, A. COSENTINO, *et al.* 2000. Association of MHC Class I chain-related A (MIC-A) gene polymorphism with type I diabetes. Diabetologia **43:** 507–514.
75. BILBAO, R., A. MARTIN-PAGOLA & B. CALVO. 2001. Contribution of MICA polymorphism to type I diabetes in Basques. Diabetes Metab. Res. Rev. **17**(Suppl 1):27.
76. TICA, V., L. NIKITINA-ZAKE, E. DONADI & C.B. SANJEEVI. 2003. MIC-A genotypes 4/5.1 and 9/9 are positively associated with type 1 diabetes mellitus in Brazilian population. Ann. N. Y. Acad. Sci. **1005:** 310–313.

Progression of Autoimmune Diabetes

Slowly Progressive Insulin-Dependent Diabetes Mellitus or Latent Autoimmune Diabetes of Adult

HURIYA BEYAN, THOMAS OLA, R. DAVID, AND G. LESLIE

Institute of Cell and Molecular Science, Queen Mary College, University of London, London E1 2AT, UK

ABSTRACT: Autoimmune diabetes is due to destruction of insulin-secreting beta islet cells by an immune-mediated process, which is induced and promoted by the interaction of genetic and environmental factors. This form of diabetes is one of a group of autoimmune diseases that affect about 10% of the population in the developed world. The detection of diabetes-associated autoantibodies, including glutamic acid decarboxylase antibodies (GADA), islet cell antibodies (ICA), and insulinoma-associated (IA-2) autoantibodies is widely held to reflect an underlying autoimmune pathology but the clinical features associated with the presence of these diabetes-associated autoantibodies is highly variable ranging from lack of symptoms with normal glucose tolerance to catastrophic and potentially fatal diabetic ketoacidosis. It is the purpose of this article to establish the range of metabolic features associated with diabetes-associated autoimmune changes and discuss how this metabolic spectrum itself reflects a spectrum of immune and clinical changes that cast light on the nature of autoimmune diabetes.

KEYWORDS: autoimmune diabetes; glutamic acid decarboxylase antibodies; islet cell antibodies; insulinoma-associated antigen-2; ketoacidosis

DEFINING AN AUTOIMMUNE DISEASE

From the outset we should make it clear that we refer to "autoimmune diabetes" when we mean diabetes associated with specific autoantibodies. These diabetes-associated autoantibodies include glutamic acid decarboxylase antibodies (GADA), islet cell antibodies (ICA), insulinoma-associated (IA-2)

Address for correspondence: Prof. David Leslie, Institute of Cell and Molecular Science, Centre for Diabetes & Metabolic Medicine, Bart's and The London, Queen Mary's School of Medicine & Dentistry, 4 Newark Street, Nondon, E1 2AT. Voice: +44 (0)20 7882 2482 or +44 (0)20 7601 7446; fax: +44 (0) 20 7882 2186 or +44 (0) 20 7601 7449.
e-mail: r.d.g.leslie@qmul.ac.uk

**Ann. N.Y. Acad. Sci. 1079: 81–89 (2006). © 2006 New York Academy of Sciences.
doi: 10.1196/annals.1375.011**

autoantibodies, and autoantibodies to insulin (IAA).[1] But the detection of autoantibodies in the peripheral blood is a far cry from affirming that autoimmune diabetes is due to an autoimmune destructive process. If we are to accept that type 1 diabetes mellitus (T1DM) is an autoimmune disease then we must acknowledge that the evidence is incomplete. Rose and Bona[2] defined autoimmune diseases as those that show: (*a*) defined autoantigens and autoantibodies; (*b*) that passive transfer of T lymphocytes (specific or nonspecific) can lead to disease development; and (*c*) that immunomodulation of subjects with the disease can ameliorate symptoms. We know that the first of these is true and that diabetes-associated autoantibodies can predict T1DM with a degree of certainty. However, transfer of disease is ethically unacceptable though a single case has been described of apparent and accidental transfer of T1DM following a bone marrow transplant from a diabetic donor to a nondiabetic recipient.[3] Further, there was rapid destruction of apparently normal islet insulin secretory cells when part of a pancreas was transplanted into diabetic identical co-twins from their nondiabetic twins indicating that the destructive process must be outside the islet, insulin secretory cell specific, and retain its cytotoxic memory since the diabetic twins had been diabetic for at least 12 years.[4] The immune system is the most likely candidate for such an extra islet effect. Finally, we are currently unable to immunomodulate T1DM consistently and to achieve significant clinical benefit. There is some evidence that the disease process can be modified by immunotherapy, thus, subjects with newly diagnosed T1DM given cyclosporine, a modifier of T cell activation, are more likely to show a transient improvement in metabolic control in the first 2 years postdiagnosis.[5] But a word of caution, diabetes associated with congenital rubella, a virus, can each cause tissue-specific destruction, inflammation, associated HLA susceptibility and protection, as well as show islet tissue autoantibodies—so none of these features can be held to specifically denote an autoimmune disease.[6] Only the result of the cyclosporine trial in T1DM provides strong, but not definitive, support for so-called autoimmune diabetes actually being an autoimmune disease. With this caveat we can explore the features of autoimmune diabetes.

ONE END OF THE AUTOIMMUNE SPECTRUM

Classical T1DM clinically presents most often in childhood and is characterized by an absolute need for insulin therapy to survive (insulin-dependent). Children can present moribund with potentially fatal ketoacidosis but increasingly they present with a moderately severe illness including classical symptoms of weight loss, thirst, and polyuria due to hyperglycemia resulting from insulin deficiency. The disease is thought to be due to the interaction of genetic and environmental factors inducing an immune-mediated destructive attack on the insulin secretory cells.[7] The nature of the environmental factors causing T1DM is unclear. Genetic susceptibility is mediated largely by histocompatability (HLA) alleles that include HLA DR3, DQB1*0201 and DR4, DQB1*0302, while there is a reduced frequency of other alleles suggesting that they are associated with disease protection, for example, HLA DR2, DQB1*0602.[8–10] The proportion of HLA heterozygotes (HLA DR3, DQB1*0201 and DR4, DQB1*0302) declines with age at diagnosis, as does the contribution of gene protection.[9,10] While about 80–90% of patients with childhood-onset T1DM have these HLA susceptibility alleles, it is not clear whether those individuals without HLA genetic susceptibility alleles have a different type of diabetes. It is certainly possible to develop autoimmune diabetes with diabetes-associated autoantibodies and not have the usual HLA risk alleles. Diabetes-associated autoantibodies include GADA, ICA, IA-2 autoantibodies, and IAA.[5] These autoantibodies are found in about 80% of children with T1DM at diagnosis so if we maintain a strict definition of autoimmune diabetes as those cases with both diabetes and diabetes-associated autoantibodies, then we can recognize that not all children presenting with insulin-dependent diabetes can be strictly defined as having autoimmune diabetes.

INSULIN-DEPENDENT DIABETES NEED NOT BE AUTOIMMUNE

If we accept that not all children presenting with insulin-dependent diabetes can be strictly defined as having autoimmune diabetes then we can also accept that there may be several different causes for insulin-dependent diabetes in children, which are not autoimmune. There are at least three conditions in which the insulin secretory cells fail to produce much, if any, insulin due either to immaturity, destruction, or dysfunction. In Wolframs syndrome, an autosomal recessive defect of developmental genes, the insulin secretory cells fail to mature, though levels of insulin secretion can vary substantially between individuals; it occurs in association with diabetes insipidus, optic atrophy, and high-tone deafness (also called DIDMOAD syndrome). Acute and chronic pancreatitis can be complicated by damage to the islet insulin secretory cells whether induced by viruses, alcohol, or gall stones. A form of diabetes (type 1b diabetes), rare in most of the world but relatively common in Japan, affects young adults and is characterized by the severity of its presentation, marked insulin deficiency, rapid onset with evidence of a short prodrome, insulitis, and raised serum alkaline phosphatase, all consistent with a viral infection though supportive evidence is lacking.[11] Finally, inherited defects of the islet potassium ion channels involved in insulin secretion can compromise insulin secretion and present as neonatal diabetes with little or no insulin secretion. Remarkably, these individuals with Kir6.2 mutations, despite being insulin dependent, can discontinue insulin and be controlled using high-dose sulphonylurea tablets. Sulphonylureas increase insulin secretion from the pancreatic beta cell by closing ATP-sensitive potassium (K_{ATP}) channels, depolarizing the beta cell plasma membrane, and increasing intracellular calcium concentration. It follows that sulphonylureas are of value when there is insulin secretory deficiency but not when insulin resistance has a major impact as is the case in forms of type 2 diabetes but also in neonatal diabetes when there is a potassium channel mutation.[12] Functional studies show that the severity of the clinical phenotype is reflected in the functional changes seen in the mutated channel.

AUTOIMMUNE DIABETES NEED NOT BE INSULIN DEPENDENT

Autoimmune diabetes may also present in adults (adult-onset T1DM) and may not require insulin treatment initially. The latter group of patients are only identified as having autoimmune diabetes when their blood is checked for diabetes-associated autoantibodies. Since their autoimmunity is clinically latent, this form of diabetes has been classified as latent autoimmune diabetes of adults (LADA).[13,14]

Noninsulin requiring autoimmune diabetes or LADA is typically diagnosed when the patient is between 30 and 70 years of age, with positive detection of diabetes-associated autoantibodies and remains noninsulin requiring for at least 6 months postdiagnosis,[13,14] though the definition is semantic and can vary in terms of the age at diagnosis and the duration of noninsulin-requiring diabetes. The epidemiology of LADA is influenced by geography, genetic susceptibility, environmental factors, gender, and age at diagnosis. In northern Europe and North America, about 5–10% of newly diagnosed noninsulin-requiring diabetes patients have LADA, according to the mode of ascertainment, the sourced population, the age of the patient (frequency is higher in younger age groups), and the definition of the disease.[14,15] Noninsulin-requiring diabetes with diabetes-associated autoantibodies is not confined to the age group of 30–70 years, and when found in children is called latent autoimmune diabetes of the young (LADY). The use of ICA in defining LADA or LADY patients further extends the percentage of patients with these clinical conditions as many patients with ICA do not have GAD autoantibodies and that percentage increases with the age at clinical onset of diabetes. The genetics of noninsulin-requiring autoimmune diabetes has yet to be well-characterized. In classical T1DM, HLA DR3, DQB1*0201 and DR4, DQB1*0302 are associated with increased disease susceptibility while HLA DR2, DQB1*0602, DRB1*0403 seem to confer protection.[8–10] In a substantial study, LADA was also associated with increased frequencies of HLA DR3 (28%), DR4 (27%), and DR3/4 (22%) and as with classical T1DM these risk allele frequencies declined with age at diagnosis.[16] As with adult-onset T1DM, however, HLA DR2 appears to play little role in disease protection. A feature of LADA is that following diagnosis some patients may progress over months or years toward insulin dependence.[14] As we shall discuss, this is not an invariant feature of LADA but it does reflect the propensity for autoimmune diabetes to show variable rates of disease progression even to insulin dependence.

We can summarize the analysis to date of patients with autoimmune diabetes defined solely by the presence of diabetes-associated autoantibodies as: those who are insulin-dependent at diagnosis or within a short period thereafter (called T1DM); those who are not insulin-dependent initially and for a period of at least 6 months (called LADA or LADY according to age at diagnosis); those who are not insulin-dependent initially but progress over a variable period to insulin dependence (called LADA, LADY, or slowly progressive insulin-dependent diabetes mellitus [SPIDDM]). Slowly progressing SPIDDM was originally described in Japanese adults.[17] In contrast to LADA, patients with SPIDDM are not confined by an age at diagnosis of 30–70 years, they may present at any age, and all of them progress to insulin dependence while only a proportion of LADA cases do so. Genetic features of SPIDDM and LADA are similar though HLA-DQA1*0301-DQB1*0401 is found in Japanese SPIDDM but not in Japanese patients with T1DM and the genetic features are similar to LADA.[17] Further, in contrast to TIDM patients, patients in Japan with SPIDDM have GADA with a unique N-terminal linear epitope located on the anchoring domain of the GAD65 molecules.[18] Recent study showed that SPIDDM patients tended to have unique (N-terminal) epitope of GAD65 antibody, thus such an association between GAD65 antibody targeted to this region and slowly progressive beta cell failure in SPIDDM.[17]

METABOLIC PROGRESSION OF AUTOIMMUNE DIABETES

Children and adults can have diabetes-associated autoantibodies; they occur in less than 5% of the normal population and in a higher percentage of twins (about 30%) and siblings (about 10%) of patients with T1DM. It is possible that some of these individuals will never develop diabetes but we will need long-term follow-up to confirm that this is the case. Some individuals with autoantibodies pass through a "prediabetic" stage of impaired glucose tolerance or even noninsulin-requiring diabetes before becoming frankly insulin dependent and this stage is more prevalent in adults than in children. Diabetes prevention trial of type 1 diabetes mellitus (DPT-T1DM) detected 585 relatives of T1DM patients who had ICA plus either IAA or low first-phase insulin response to intravenous glucose.[19] Of them, 427 had normal glucose tolerance, 87 had impaired glucose tolerance, and 61 were diabetic, yet asymptomatic, on glucose tolerance testing. Those subjects with asymptomatic autoimmune diabetes resemble LADA but their age was less than 30 years in this study precluding the diagnosis. It follows that some patients with autoimmune diabetes, pass through a phase of altered glucose levels including noninsulin-requiring diabetes before becoming insulin dependent.

GENETIC IMPACT ON DISEASE PROGRESSION

Metabolic changes during the prodrome of autoimmune diabetes are probably determined by nongenetic factors but their rate of progression is in part genetically determined. Changes in identical twins detected in the prediabetic period were not found in low-disease risk identical twins of patients with T1DM, so it is likely that these changes are nongenetically determined.[20] On the other hand, genetic factors determine when T1DM presents, probably by controlling disease progression. Identical twins develop the disease at a similar age, which is for them also at a similar time, with heritability for age at diagnosis of 74%.[21] The age at diagnosis, but not the time of diagnosis, in affected siblings is also strongly correlated. This observation argues against a common environmental exposure precipitating diabetes, which would be associated with clustering of time of diagnosis in siblings, and favors a distinct environmental event. Given clustering in time between siblings for immune activation, as judged by autoantibody seroconversion, as well as clustering by age at time of diagnosis, the rate of progression of the destructive process during the intervening prediabetic period is probably, to a degree, genetically determined in both children and adults.

The rate of progression to clinical diabetes is more rapid in patients presenting under 5 years of age than in those presenting much later.[7] Islet insulin secretory cells tend to be absent within 12 months of diagnosis in patients aged less than 7 years, but detected for longer periods in older patients.[22] Variability in progression to clinical diabetes has been noted, being more rapid in obese than lean children and in children than adults.[7,23] From these observations it follows that there is a spectrum in the rate of metabolic decompensation during the prediabetic period in autoimmune T1DM—this spectrum is evident at all age. No similar data are available in LADA or SPIDDM. In summary, there is a continuous spectrum of loss of insulin secretory capacity both pre- and postdiagnosis, the severity of which is age related, being more severe and generally, but not universally, more rapid in children than adults with T1DM, and more severe in the latter and in SPIDDM than in LADA subjects.

INSULIN RESISTANCE AND THE METABOLIC SYNDROME

Patients with T1DM can be insensitive to insulin and patients with LADA may well have more severe insulin insensitivity than that found in childhood-onset T1DM, though there have only been two small studies to date of LADA and none in SPIDDM and both these studies used the homeostasis model assessment (HOMA) and not the euglycemic clamp.[24,25] One feature of insulin resistance is the metabolic syndrome, a confederacy of cardiovascular risk factors including hypertension, dyslipidemia, hyperglycemia, and obesity, found in approximately 22% of the North American population. Perhaps surprisingly

TABLE 1. Criteria for autoimmune diabetes

	T1DM	SPIDDM	LADA
Age at onset	any age	any age	25–70 years (variable)
Initial insulin dependent	Yes	No	No
Ultimately insulin dependent	Yes	Yes	Maybe
Diabetes-autoantibodies	Yes	Yes	Yes

adult patients with T1DM diagnosed in childhood have a high frequency of the metabolic syndrome (about 40%),[26] and it has been detected in 77% and 42% of LADA cases; ascertainment biases dictating the differences in the frequency.[27,28] By implication insensitivity to insulin, whether estimated by conventional techniques or implied by the frequency of the metabolic syndrome, is a feature of autoimmune diabetes irrespective of the clinical form of that it might take.

It is likely, therefore, that within autoimmune diabetes there is an age-related spectrum of decreasing insulin secretory capacity, worst in children, and increasing severity of insulin insensitivity and metabolic syndrome, worst in adults. LADA occupies one end of this spectrum without any clear division between it and other forms of autoimmune T1DM. SPIDDM, on the other hand, occupies a position between the two, in that it always, by definition, progresses to insulin dependence but it does so more slowly than classical T1DM (TABLE 1). It should be evident that the loose term "autoimmune diabetes" encompasses many different clinical forms of a condition that may have several pathogenetic origins. Exercises in diagnostic and acronym gymnastics incorporating LADA and SPIDDM highlight the nature of this spectrum.

REFERENCES

1. KULMALA, P., K. SAVOLA, J.S. PETERSEN, *et al.* 1998. Prediction of insulin-dependent diabetes mellitus in siblings of children with diabetes; a population based study. J. Clin. Invest. **101:** 327–336.
2. ROSE, N.R. & C. BONA 1993. Defining criteria for autoimmune diseases (Witebsky's postulates revisited). Immunol. Today **14:** 426–430.
3. LAMPETER, E.F., M. HOMBERG, K. QUABECK, *et al.* 1993. Transfer of insulin-dependent diabetes between HLA-identical siblings by bone marrow transplantation. Lancet **34:** 1243–1244.
4. SIBLEY, R.K., D.E. SUTHERLAND, F. GOETZ, *et al.* 1985. Recurrent diabetes mellitus in the pancreas iso- and allograft. A light and electron microscopic and immunohistochemical analysis of four cases. Lab. Invest. **53:** 132–144.
5. FEUTREN, G., L. PAPOZ, R. ASSAN, *et al.* 1986. For the Cyclosporine/Diabetes French Study Group. Cyclosporine increases the rate and length of remissions in insulin dependent diabetes of recent onset: results of a multicentre double-blind trial. Lancet **II:** 119–124.

6. McEvor, R.C., B. Fedun, L.Z. Cooper, *et al.* 1988. Children at high risk of diabetes mellitus: New York studies of families with diabetes and of children with congenital rubella syndrome.Adv. Exp. Med. Biol. **246:** 221–227.
7. Leslie, R.D. & M. Delli Castelli. 2004. Age-dependent influences on the origins of autoimmune diabetes: evidence and implications. Diabetes **53:** 3033–3040.
8. Field, L.L. 2002. Genetic linkage and association studies of type 1 diabetes: challenges and rewards. Diabetologia **45:** 21–35.
9. Sabbah, E., K. Savola, T. Ebeling, *et al.* 2000. Genetic, autoimmune, and clinical characteristics of childhood- and adult-onset type 1 diabetes. Diabetes Care **23:** 1326–1332.
10. Vanderwalle, C.L., T. Cecraene, F.C. Schuit, *et al.* 1993. Insulin antibodies and high titre islet cell antibodies are preferentially associated with the HLA DQA1*03100-DQB1*0302 haplotype at clinical onset of type 1 (insulin-dependent) diabetes mellitus before age 10 years but not at onset between age 10 and 40 years. Diabetologia **36:** 1155–1162.
11. Imagawa, A., T. Hanafusa, J. Miyagawa, *et al.* 2000. A novel subtype of type 1 diabetes mellitus characterized by a rapid onset and an absence of diabetes-related antibodies. Osaka IDDM Study Group. N. Engl. J. Med. **342:** 301–307.
12. Proks, P., J.F. Antcliff, J. Lippiat, *et al.* 2004. Molecular basis of Kir6.2 mutations associated with neonatal diabetes or neonatal diabetes plus neurological features. Proc. Natl. Acad. Sci. USA **101:** 17539–17544.
13. Pozzilli, P. & U. Di Mario. 2001. Autoimmune diabetes not requiring insulin at diagnosis (Latent Autoimmune Diabetes of the Adult). Diabetes Care **24:** 1460–1467.
14. UKPDS 25. 1997. Autoantibodies to islet-cell cytoplasm and glutamic acid decarboxylase for prediction of insulin requirement in type 2 diabetes. UK Prospective Diabetes Study Group. Lancet **350:** 1288–1293.
15. Palmer, J.P., C.S. Hampe. *et al.* 2005. Is late autoimmune diabetes in adult distinct from type 1 diabetes or just type 1 diabetes at an older age? Diabetes **54**(Suppl. 2): S62–S67.
16. Horton, V., I. Stratton, G.F. Bottazzo, *et al.* 1999. UK Prospective Diabetes Study (UKPDS) Group. Genetic heterogeneity of autoimmune diabetes: age at presentation in adults is influenced by HLA DRB1 and DQB1 genotypes (UKPDS 43). Diabetologia **42:** 608–616.
17. Kobayashi, T., S. Tanaka, M. Okubo, *et al.* 2003. Unique epitopes of glutamic acid decarboxylase autoantibodies in slowly progressive type 1 diabetes. J. Clin. Endocrinol. Metab. **88:** 4768–4775.
18. Ohtsu, S., N. Takubo, M. Kazahari, *et al.* 2005. Slowly progressing form of type 1 diabetes mellitus in children: genetic analysis compared with other forms of diabetes mellitus in Japanese children. Pediatr. Diabetes **6:** 221–229.
19. Greenbaum, C.J., D. Cuthbertson & J.P. Krischer 2001. Disease prevention Trial of Type I Diabetes Study Group. Type I diabetes manifested solely by 2-h oral glucose tolerance test criteria. Diabetes **50:** 470–476.
20. Hawa, M.I., R. Bonfanti, C. Valeri, *et al.* 2005. No evidence for genetically determined alteration in insulin secretion or sensitivity predisposing to type 1 diabetes: a study of identical twins. Diabetes Care **28:** 1415–1418.
21. Gous, F.K. 1997. Diabetes registries and early biological markers of insulin-dependent diabetes mellitus. Belgian Diabetes Registry. Diabetes Metab. Rev. **13:** 247–274.

22. PIPELEERS, D. & Z. LING 1992. Pancreatic β cells in insulin-dependent diabetes. Diabetes Metab. Rev. **8:** 209–227.
23. KIBIRIGE, M., B. METCALF, R. RENUKA, *et al.* 2003. Testing the accelerator hypothesis; the relationship between body mass and age at diagnosis of type 1 diabetes. Diabetes Care **26:** 2865–2870.
24. BEHME, M.T., J. DUPRE, S.B. HARRIS, *et al.* 2003. Insulin resistance in latent autoimmune diabetes of adulthood. Ann. N. Y. Acad. Sci. **1005:** 374–377.
25. CARLSSON, A., G. SUNDKVIST, L. GROOP, *et al.* 2000. Insulin and glucagon secretion in patients with slowly progressing autoimmune diabetes (LADA). J. Clin. Endocrinol. Metab. **85:** 76–80.
26. THORN, L.M., C. FORSBLOM, J. FAGERUDD *et al.* 2005. FinnDiane Study Group. Metabolic syndrome in type 1 diabetes: association with diabetic nephropathy and glycemic control (the FinnDiane study). Diabetes Care **28:** 2019–2024.
27. HOSSZUFALUSI, N., A. VATAY, K. RAJCZY, *et al.* 2003. Similar genetic features and different islet cell autoantibody pattern of latent autoimmune diabetes in adults (LADA) compared with adult-onset type 1 diabetes with rapid progression. Diabetes Care **26:** 452–457.
28. ZINMAN, B., S.E. KAHN, S.M. HAFFNER, *et al.* 2004. ADOPT Study Group. Phenotypic characteristics of GAD antibody-positive recently diagnosed patients with type 2 diabetes in North America and Europe. Diabetes **53:** 3193–2004.

Immunomodulation for the Prevention of SPIDDM and LADA

P. POZZILLI[a,b] AND C. GUGLIELMI[a,b]

[a]*Department of Endocrinology and Diabetes, University Campus Bio-Medico 00155, Rome, Italy*

[b]*Institute of Cell and Molecular Science, Department of Diabetes and Metabolism, St Bartholomew's Hospital, London, UK*

ABSTRACT: Type 1 diabetes may occur at any age, in young individuals before or after adolescence, during middle age life, or even in the elderly. When diagnosed in adults it is characterized by the presence of islet cell-related autoantibodies (ICA), in particular GAD and IA2 (less common) and very rarely insulin autoantibodies (IAA). Baseline C-peptide at diagnosis of type 1 diabetes can identify different patient populations according to when the disease is diagnosed depending on age. A key question is whether the process of beta cell destruction follows the same pattern in patients diagnosed in young age, soon after adolescence, or in adult age. The terms *SPIDDM*—slowly progressive insulin-dependent diabetes mellitus and *LADA*—latent autoimmune diabetes in adults have been considered synonymous on most grounds based on the fact that with this form of diabetes we intend a form of diabetes that has an autoimmune basis that eventually will require insulin for its treatment sometime after diagnosis. Therapeutic approaches are similar for prevention and treatment of SPIDDM or LADA, including both specific and nonspecific immunomodulation. For specific immunomodulation the attention is focused on DiaPep277, GAD, and insulin, and for nonspecific immunomodulation on 1,25 dihydroxy-vitamin D3 (calcitriol) and thiazolidinediones. Current trials in SPIDDM/LADA with both specific and nonspecific immunomodulation seem promising. Response to therapy varies according to age and residual beta cell function at diagnosis of SPIDMM/LADA. Results in beta cell protection with different agents can also help to identify differences, if any, between SPIDMM and LADA.

KEYWORDS: LADA; SPIDDM; GAD antibodies; immunotherapy; diabetes

Address for correspondence: Paolo Pozzilli, M.D., Department of Endocrinology and Diabetes, University Campus Bio-Medico, Via E. Longoni, 83, 00155 Rome, Italy. Voice: +3906-22541-556; fax: +3906-22541-336.

e-mail: p.pozzilli@unicampus.it

Ann. N.Y. Acad. Sci. 1079: 90–98 (2006). © 2006 New York Academy of Sciences.
doi: 10.1196/annals.1375.012

INTRODUCTION

Among patients diagnosed with type 2 diabetes some of them develop insulin-requiring diabetes during follow-up and some of these patients can be identified earlier in the natural history of the disease by the presence of circulating islet autoantibodies.[1] This form of diabetes also referred to as latent autoimmune diabetes in adults (LADA),[2–5] according to the latest classification, is now considered a form of type 1 diabetes.[6]

Autoimmune diabetes is characterized by the presence of one or more islet-specific autoantibodies, including islet cell autoantibodies (ICA) and autoantibodies directed against the three major islet autoantigens, that is, glutamic acid decarboxylase (GAD), protein tyrosine phosphatase IA-2 (IA-2A), and its isoform IA-2β (IA-2βA), and insulin autoantibodies (IAA).[7–10] The detection of either ICA or GAD at the time of diagnosis of adult-onset diabetes identifies a subgroup of patients with clinical characteristics more similar to those of classical type 1 diabetes and is predictive of a more rapid progression to insulin requirement.[11]

Type 1 diabetes may occur at any age, in young individuals before and soon after adolescence, during middle age life, or even in the elderly. When diagnosed in adults it is characterized by the presence of GAD and IA2 (less common), very rarely insulin antibodies (IA) and by the occurrence of a less predominant HLA genetic susceptibility.

The terms *LADA* and *SPIDDM*[12] are considered synonymous on most grounds (especially for treatment) based on the fact that with this form of diabetes we intend a type of disease that has an autoimmune basis, which eventually will lead to insulin for its treatment.

Several studies have been performed to evaluate the prevalence of LADA in patients with adult-onset diabetes based on screening for ICA and/or GAD.[13]Some of these studies also evaluated the correlation between the presence of GAD and the clinical features of affected patients showing that the majority of patients have a clinical phenotype typical of type 1 diabetes.

A critical issue of type 1 diabetes/SPIDDM/LADA, when diagnosed, is to look for the residual beta cell function. As shown in FIGURE 1, baseline C-peptide at diagnosis of type 1 diabetes identifies different categories of patients according to the age at diagnosis.[14] For instance in children and young adolescents the baseline C-peptide is significantly lower than in patients diagnosed in adult age.

A key question is whether the process of beta cell destruction follows the same pattern in patients diagnosed in young age, after adolescence, or in adult age. The speed of beta cell loss probably varies according to genetic, environmental, and immunological features of affected individuals. Nevertheless, therapeutic approaches are similar for prevention and treatment of SPIDDM or LADA including both specific and nonspecific immunomodulation.

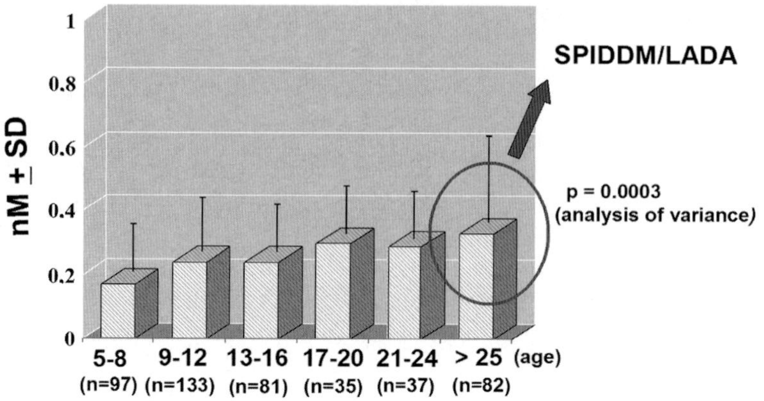

FIGURE 1. Basal C-peptide and age at diagnosis of type 1 diabetes (modified from Pozzilli P. *et al.*[14]).

Regarding specific immunomodulation current trials consider the use of DiaPep277, GAD, and insulin, for nonspecific immunomodulation 1,25 dihydroxy-vitamin D3 (calcitriol) and thiazolidinediones have been tested in preliminary trials with interesting results.

We now describe the major trials carried out in SPIDDM/LADA or those that are undergoing and whose results will be soon available (TABLE 1).

Peptide of Heat Shock Protein 60 (DiaPep277)

The basic mechanism of action of this compound is to induce tolerance to a peptide of 24 amino acids of heat shock protein 60 involved in the process of beta cell destruction.

DiaPep277 has been tested at diagnosis in the prevention of beta cell loss in subjects with recent-onset type 1 diabetes of both adolescence and young adult age. This peptide's effect probably involves either an inhibition of proinflammatory cytokines (IFN-γ) or an upregulation of anti-inflammatory cytokines in particular IL-10.[15]

Recent unpublished data on stratified analysis of adult newly diagnosed type 1 diabetic patients, 30–45 years of age treated with 1 mg of DiaPep277, suggest that this drug is able to preserve residual C-peptide secretion under base line or after mixed meal conditions.

A phase II trial with DiaPep277 has been completed in a group of LADA patients and results will be available very soon. This was a randomized, double-blind, placebo-controlled, multicenter, parallel group study to investigate safety and tolerability as well as the immunological and clinical effects of multiple subcutaneous doses of DiaPep277 in LADA patients. Importantly, safety and tolerability have been met so far. Patients diagnosed with LADA within 2 to

TABLE 1. Major trials in LADA patients

STUDY	PATIENTS	APPROACH	END POINTS
DiaPep277	60 patients	3 arm and 20 patients per arm. Randomization of GAD-antibodies positive patients per arm 15 with treatment + 5 placebo.	Evaluate safety, tolerability, and efficacy of DiaPep277, preservation of beta cell function, effects on glucose control and insulin requirement, and influence on immune response.
GAD	47 patients	4 dose groups: 1. 4 μg 2. 20 μg 3. 100 μg 4. 500 μg	Evaluate if alum-formulated human recombinant GAD is safe and does not compromise beta cell function.
Insulin	54 patients	2 treatment groups:1. subcutaneous insulin injection 2. sulfonylurea	Evaluate serum C-peptide response (CPR) and blood glucose level during 75 g oral glucose tolerancetest (OGTT).
1,25 dydroxy-vitamin D3 (Calcitriol)	62 patients	4 treatment groups: 1. calcitriol + oral hypoglycemic agents 2. calcitriol + insulin 3. insulin 4. oral hypoglycemic agents	Evaluate the effect of calcitriol intervention on pancreatic beta cell function.
Rosiglitazone	23 patients	2 treatment groups: 1. Insulin 2. Insulin + Rosiglitazone	Evaluate the impact on islet beta cell function using PCP(C-peptide after 2 h 75-g glucose load) and ΔCP (ΔCP =PCP-FCP [fasting C-peptide]).

60 months after diagnosis and of age between 30 and 50 years were included. It was a trial with three arms, 20 patients per arm, 15 patients treated with Diapep277 and 5 with placebo. Unpublished data showed that at entry into the trial a significant response to DiaPep277 was observed (24 out of 41: 59%). These data indicate that in patients with SPIDDM/LADA there is indeed recognition of DiaPep277 antigen and therefore induction of tolerance to this peptide may occur. A large action LADA intervention study, a phase IIb/III, multinational, randomized, double-blind, placebo-controlled, parallel-group study will be initiated soon in Europe to investigate the clinical efficacy and safety of DiaPep277 in patients with LADA. This large trial will be carried out in 10 European countries (Austria, Denmark, Italy, UK, Finland, Greece, Northern Ireland, Spain, Germany, and France) and will involve approximately 400 LADA patients.

GAD

An interesting antigen-specific immunomodulatory approach to SPIDDM/LADA is represented by the subcutaneous administration of GAD. This is probably the major antigen in type 1 diabetes of adults, and antibodies to GAD alone or in combination with other islet autoantibodies are currently used as marker for this disease. Preclinical studies in the spontaneously non-obese type 1 diabetes (NOD) mouse model demonstrated that the destruction of beta cells is associated with T cells recognizing GAD65. It has also been shown that the administration of small quantities of GAD65 effectively prevents autoimmune beta cell destruction and reduces or delays the development of spontaneous diabetes.[16–19]

Based on these preclinical data, a controlled clinical trial was initiated to assess the potential of GAD65 to halt beta cell destruction and prevent or delay insulin dependence. Following extensive preclinical safety evaluation and a phase I clinical trial with the Diamyd Bulk Drug (rhGAD65 without adjuvant; Diamyd Therapeutics, Stockholm, Sweden, unpublished), a phase II study with rhGAD65 formulated with alum was conducted in LADA patients.

The study objectives were to investigate the clinical safety of subcutaneously administered recombinant GAD65 and to assess its impact on the immune system and diabetes status. The results of this study have been recently published.[20]

The study was conducted in a total of 47 LADA patients who received either placebo or 4, 20, 100, or 500 μg GAD65 subcutaneously at weeks 1 and 4. Safety evaluations, including beta cell function tests, diabetes status assessment, hematology, biochemistry, and cellular and humoral immunological markers were repeatedly assessed over 24 weeks. The results of this study showed that a dose of 20 μg of GAD65 in LADA patients determines a significant rise in C-peptide 6–12 months following its administration. Such metabolic result is accompanied by an immunological effect as demonstrated by the increase of $CD4^+CD25^+/CD4^+CD25^-$ lymphocyte that indicates generation of immunoregulatory T cells. Based on these preliminary results, long-term studies using the effective dose should be carried out to assess the real effect of recombinant GAD on preservation of beta cell function.

Insulin for Tolerance

Insulin is a major antigen in the very young patients with type 1 diabetes.[10] Its role in SPIDDM and LADA is probably less relevant as IAA are seldom detected in this patient age group. However, studies in Japan suggest that insulin administration before the necessity of insulin therapy can protect beta cell mass in patients with SPIDDM/LADA.[21] The Tokyo study was later implemented to demonstrate whether insulin is more affective in protecting beta cell mass when compared to sulphonylureas. The purpose of the study was first to evaluate the frequency of GAD autoantibodies in patients not requiring insulin at diagnosis and their natural course and, second, to see whether insulin given not only as an agent to control blood glucose but also as tolerogen can halt the progressive beta cell failure in these patients.

The study was a randomized, multicenter prospective trial. Patients were randomly assigned to one of the two groups.[22] One group received subcutaneous insulin injections as therapy for hyperglycemia and the other group was treated with sulphonylurea. The insulin-treated group compared to the sulphonylurea group showed a reduction in the progression to insulin therapy as 2 out of 30 patients did so in the insulin group compared to 7 out of 30 in sulphonylurea-treated group. The results indicate that small doses of insulin effectively prevent progressive beta cell failure in SPIDDM/LADA, specifically in those patients with preserved beta cell function and high GAD titers at entry into the trial. The data are of great interest and suggest that by downregulating beta cell antigen release associated with endogenous insulin secretion, tolerance induction is possible and protection of beta cell function over a long period of time may be obtained.

Calcitriol

Calcitriol is the active form of vitamin D. It has been shown to a have a protective effect in preserving beta cell mass in the NOD mouse.[23] It has also an immunomodulatory function in particular on dendritic cells and it induces a significant reduction of MHC class 1 expression on pancreatic beta cells,[24] which suggests an interesting potential effect of this compound in controlling the beta cell autoimmune process.

Epidemiological data from EuroDiab study indicate that vitamin D supplementation at birth may protect later in life from developing type 1 diabetes.[25] Recent findings from the IMDIAB XI trial indicate that the administration of calcitriol at diagnosis in children with type 1 diabetes can be beneficial in protecting residual beta cell function 1 year later.[26]

Regarding SPIDDM/LADA a recent study carried out in 62 patients have evaluated four treatment groups: (*a*) calcitriol + oral hypoglycemic agents; (*b*) calcitriol + insulin; (*c*) insulin alone; and (*d*) oral hypoglycemic agents only.[27] The aim of the study was to evaluate the effect of calcitriol on beta cell function as assessed by measuring C- peptide secretion.

This pilot trial showed that after 6 months of therapy in patients receiving calcitriol residual C-peptide secretion tends to increase. It indicates that calcitriol can preserve beta cell function in SPIDDM/LADA patients as compared to oral hypoglycemic agents or insulin. More data are required to confirm whether this approach is feasible in SPIDDM/LADA.

Thiazolidinediones

Data in the experimental model of the NOD mouse have demonstrated a protective effect of thiazolidinediones on beta cell mass.[28] The insulin sensitizers rosiglitazone and pioglitazone have the potential to increase the islet cell insulin content probably by downregulating the local inflammatory process and thereby the autoimmune response.

As recently demonstrated, rosiglitazone therapy combined with insulin in LADA patients was able to protect residual beta cell function after 16 months of therapy.[29] This was a pilot randomized, unblinded, controlled trial where 23 LADA patients were randomly assigned to two different treatment regimes, one group receiving insulin alone (insulin group, $n = 12$) and the other receiving rosiglitazone plus insulin (insulin + RSG group, $n = 11$).

Patients in the insulin + RSG group were on rosiglitazone 4 mg/day. All patients were instructed on a diet containing 30 kcal per kg ideal body weight per day with 50–60% of carbohydrates. Target for glucose control was: fasting levels <6.1 mmol/L and 2-h postprandial > 8.0mmol/L. The dose of insulin was adjusted on the basis of blood glucose levels, while the dose of rosiglitazone was unchanged. Results from this pilot study indicated that rosiglitazone plus insulin had beneficial effects on beta cell function in LADA. The administration of thiazolidinediones, although recently introduced in the management of type 2 diabetes, may be therefore of value in LADA patients. Insulin treatment alone did not prevent the tendency toward beta cell dysfunction, in contrast with what was reported by the Tokyo study. The possible reason might be the different patient selection. For example, patients enrolled in the rosiglitazone study had high GAD-Ab titers and low C-peptide levels, which probably resulted in a rapid beta cell destruction during the follow- up.

CONCLUSIONS

SPIDMM and LADA represent an ideal test bed for trials aimed to protect beta cells so that gained information can offer new opportunities for trials to be implemented in younger patients.

Preservation of beta cells in SPIDDM/LADA remains a major effort in preventing long-term complications and current trials with both specific and nonspecific immunomodulation seem promising in this respect.

Response to different therapies varies according to age at diagnosis of SPIDMM/LADA and the results may help to define whether protection of beta cells can help to identify differences between SPIDMM and LADA.

ACKNOWLEDGMENTS

We wish to acknowledge the support of MIUR 40% project grants, EU Biomed programme, CISD and DEM Foundation, all contributing to our department for studies in LADA.

REFERENCES

1. Fourlanos, S., F. Dotta, C.J. Greenbaum, *et al.* 2005. Latent autoimmune diabetes in adults (LADA) should be less latent. Diabetologia **48:** 2206–2212.

2. TUOMI, T., L.C. GROOP, P.Z. ZIMMET, *et al.* 1993. Antibodies to glutamic acid decarboxylase reveal latent autoimmune diabetes mellitus in adults with a non insulin-dependent onset of disease. Diabetes **42:** 359–362.
3. ZIMMET, P., T. TUOMI, I.R. MACKAY, *et al.* 1994. Latent autoimmune diabetes mellitus in adult (LADA): the role of antibodies to glutamic acid decarboxylase in diagnosis and prediction of insulin dependency. Diabet. Med. **11:** 299–303.
4. LESLIE, R.D. & P. POZZILLI. 1994. Type I diabetes masquerading as type II diabetes. Possible implications for prevention and treatment. Diabetes Care **17:** 1214–1219.
5. POZZILLI, P. & U. DI MARIO. 2001. Autoimmune diabetes not requiring insulin at diagnosis (Latent Autoimmune Diabetes of the Adult): definition, characterization and potential prevention. Diabetes Care **24:** 1460–1467.
6. AMERICAN DIABETES ASSOCIATION. DIAGNOSIS AND CLASSIFICATION OF DIABETES MELLITUS. 2004. Diabetes Care. **27:** S5–S10.
7. BONIFACIO, E., S. GENOVESE, S. BRAGHI, *et al.* 1995. Islet autoantibody markers in insulin dependent diabetes: identification of screening strategies yielding high sensitivity. Diabetologia **38:** 816–822.
8. BONIFACIO, E., V. LAMPASONA, S. GENOVESE, *et al.* 1995. Identification of protein tyrosine phosphatase-like IA-2 (Islet Cell Antigen 512) as the insulin-dependent diabetes-related 37/40K autoantigen and a target of islet-cell antibodies. J. Immunol. **155:** 5419–5426.
9. BONIFACIO, E., V. LAMPASPONA & P.J. BINGLEY. 1998. IA-2 (islet cell antigen 512) is the primary target of humoral autoimmunity against type 1 diabetes mellitus-associated tyrosine phosphate autoantigens. J. Immunol. **161:** 2648–2654.
10. VERGE, C.F., D. STENGER, E. BONIFACIO, *et al.* 1998. Combined use of autoantibodies (IA-2autoantibody, GAD autoantibody, insulin autoantibody, cytoplasmic islet cell antibodies) in type 1 diabetes mellitus: combinatorial islet autoantibody workshop. Diabetes **47:** 1857–1866.
11. TURNER, R., I. STRATTON, V. HORTON, *et al.* for UK Prospective Diabetes Study (UKPDS) Group. 1997. UKPDS 25: autoantibodies to islet-cell cytoplasm and glutamic acid decarboxylase for prediction of insulin requirement in type 2 diabetes. Lancet **350:** 1288–1293.
12. KOBAYASHI, T., K. TAMEMOTO, K. NAKANISHI, *et al.* 1993. Immunogenetic and clinical characterization of slowly progressive IDDM. Diabetes Care **16:** 780–788.
13. POZZILLI, P. & U. DI MARIO. 2001. Autoimmune diabetes not requiring insulin at diagnosis (latent autoimmune diabetes of the adult): definition, characterization, and potential prevention. Diabetes Care **24:** 1460–1467.
14. POZZILLI, P., N. VISALLI, R. BUZZETTI, *et al.* 1998. Metabolic and immune parameters at clinical onset of insulin-dependent diabetes: a population-based study. IMDIAB Study Group. Immun. Diabetes Metab. **47:** 1205–1210.
15. RAZ, I., D. ELIAS, A. AVRON, *et al.* 2001. Beta-cell function in new-onset type 1 diabetes and immunomodulation with a heat-shock protein peptide (DiaPep277): a randomised, double-blind, phase II trial. Lancet **358:** 1749–1753.
16. KAUFMAN, D.L., M. CLARE-SALZLER, J. TIAN, *et al.* 1993. Spontaneous loss of T-cell tolerance to glutamic acid decarboxylase in murine insulin-dependent diabetes. Nature **366:** 69–72.
17. TIAN, J., M.A. ATKINSON, M. CLARE-SALZLER, *et al.* 1996. Nasal administration of glutamate decarboxylase (GAD65) peptides induces Th2 responses and prevents murine insulin-dependent diabetes. J. Exp. Med. **183:** 1–7.

18. Tian, J., M. Clare-Salzler, A. Herschenfeld, *et al.* 1996. Modulating autoimmune responses to GAD inhibits disease progression and prolongs islet graft survival in diabetes-prone mice. Nat. Med. **2:** 1348–1353.
19. Tisch, R., R.S. Liblau, X.D. Yang, *et al.* 1998. Induction of GAD65-specific regulatory T-cells inhibits on going autoimmune diabetes in non obese diabetic mice. Diabetes **47:** 894–899.
20. Agardh, C.D., C.M. Cilio, A. Lethagen, *et al.* 2005. Clinical evidence for the safety of GAD65 immunomodulation in adult-onset autoimmune diabetes. J. Diabetes Comp. **19:** 238–246.
21. Nakanishi, K., T. Kobayashi, H. Inoko, *et al.* 1995. Residual beta-cell function and HLA-A24 in IDDM. Markers of glycemic control and subsequent development of diabetic retinopathy. Diabetes **44:** 1334–1339.
22. Maruyama, T., A. Shimada, A. Kanatsuka, *et al.* 2003. Multicenter prevention trial of slowly progressive type 1 diabetes with small dose of insulin (the Tokyo study): preliminary report. Ann. N. Y. Acad. Sci. **1005:** 362–369.
23. Giulietti, A., C. Gysemans, K. Stoffels, *et al.* 2004. Vitamin D deficiency in early life accelerates type 1 diabetes in non-obese diabetic mice. Diabetologia **47:** 451–462.
24. DeLuca, H.F. & M.T. Cantorna. 2001. Vitamin D: its role and uses in immunology. FASEB J. **14:** 2579–2585.
25. Hypponen, E., E. Läärä, A. Reunanen, *et al.* 2001. Intake of vitamin D and risk of type 1 diabetes: a birth cohort study. Lancet **358:** 1500–1503.
26. Pitocco, D., A. Crinò, E. Di Stasio, *et al.* 2005. on behalf of the IMDIAB Group. A randomized pilot trial of calcitriol versus nicotinamide in patients with recent onset type 1 diabetes (IMDIAB XI). Diabetic Med. In press.
27. Zhou, Z., N. Liao, X. Li & M. Lei. 2005. Vitamin D supplementation in adults with latent autoimmune diabetes (LADA) [abstract]. Diabetologia **48:** A87.
28. Beales, P.E. & P. Pozzilli. 2002. Thiazolidinediones for the prevention of diabetes in the non-obese diabetic (NOD) mouse: implications for human type 1 diabetes. Diabetes Metab. Res. Rev. **18:** 114–117.
29. Zhou, Z., X. Li, G. Huang, *et al.* 2005. Rosiglitazone combined with insulin preserves islet beta cell function in adult-onset latent autoimmune diabetes (LADA). Diabetes Metab. Res. Rev. **21:** 203–208.

Heightened Interferon-α/β Response Causes Myeloid Cell Dysfunction and Promotes T1D Pathogenesis in NOD Mice

RUI HUA PENG, EDWARD PAEK, CHANQING Q. XIA, NATHAN TENNYSON, AND MICHAEL J. CLARE-SALZLER

Department of Pathology, Immunology, Laboratory Medicine, University of Florida, Gainesville, Florida 32610, USA

ABSTRACT: Increasing attention is drawn to the contributions of abnormalities in both innate and acquired immune responses to the pathogenesis of autoimmune diseases, such as type 1 diabetes (T1D). Dendritic cells (DC) are critical immune cells linking innate and acquired immune responses and previous studies in NOD mice suggest abnormalities in these cells. To address DC dysregulation we examined kinetic global gene expression in NOD and B6 GM-CSF/IL-4-induced bone marrow-derived DC following lipopolysaccharide (LPS)-stimulation. We identified expression differences in over 300 genes including a cluster of 16 interferon (IFN-α/β) target genes overexpressed in NOD DC. Mechanistically, heightened IFN-α/β responses were not due to increased production of this cytokine, IFN-γ priming or increased Syk kinase activity. We found, however, heightened responses to IFN-α/β in NOD versus B6 as demonstrated by increased type 1 IFN target gene expression, for example, IRF-7, in NOD DC and macrophages. Analysis of multiple congenic strains demonstrated that the *Idd5* susceptibility region largely governed heightened IFN-α responses. Of interest, heightened IFN-α/β response in NOD mice was not confined to hematopoietic cells but was also seen in the pancreas and β cells. Compounding the IFN-α response defect, NOD mice harbor significantly more PDC in spleen in comparison to B6 and produce four- to sixfold more IFN-α when stimulated with CpG. Finally, treatment of NOD mice with IFN-α inducing agents, for example, high-dose poly I:C accelerates diabetes in both female and male mice. The abnormalities in the IFN-α/β axis appear to play a significant role in T1D pathogenesis.

KEYWORDS: type 1 interferon-α/β; dendritic cell; type 1 diabetes

Address for correspondence: Dr. Michael J. Clare-Salzler, Department of Pathology, Immunology, Laboratory Medicine, University of Florida, P.O. Box 100275, Gainesville, FL 32610. Voice: 352-392-9885; fax: 352-392-5393.
e-mail: salzler@pathology.ufl.edu

**Ann. N.Y. Acad. Sci. 1079: 99–102 (2006). © 2006 New York Academy of Sciences.
doi: 10.1196/annals.1375.013**

INTRODUCTION

Individuals at increased-risk for type 1 diabetes (T1D) likely inherit multiple disease susceptibility genes imparting systemic immunoregulatory abnormalities in the innate and acquired immune systems. Dendritic cells (DC) are important bridges between innate and acquired immunity. Interferon (IFN-α/β) target genes play a critical role in the transition from innate to acquired immunity by driving development of immunogenic DC with high-level costimulatory molecule expression and enhanced antigen presentation.[1,2] These events also make DC potent antigen-presenting cells (APC) for stimulating Th1 lymphocytes. Because IFN-α/β potently affect the immune response, strict regulation of these cytokines is likely essential to avoid autoimmunity. Indeed, it has been reported that high-level expression of IFN-α/β or high level and dysregulated signaling both accelerate or induce autoimmune diseases including T1D.[3,4] In this article, we demonstrate a dysregulation of type 1 IFN response and its contributions to the expression of type 1 diabetes in NOD mice.

EXPERIMENTAL METHODS

1. Global gene expression analysis by affymetrix cDNA array.
2. Real-time PCR for quantification of IRF-7 and other type 1 IFN gene targets following stimulation with lipopolysaccharide (LPS) or IFN-α/β.
3. Western blotting for phosphor-STAT1/2 activated by IFN-β.
4. Pancreatic histology and immunochemistry examining plasmacytoid dendritic cells (PDC) infiltration of islets and pathology induced by poly I:C treatment.
5. Flow cytometry for examining the DC maturation and frequency of PDC in splenocytes of NOD and B6 mice.
6. Intraperitoneal (i.p.) injection of poly I:C to induce T1D. Mice were treated for 7 days with daily injection of poly I:C or phosphate buffered saline (PBS). Diabetes was monitored daily by urine glucose testing and was confirmed by blood glucose >300 mg/dL.

RESULTS AND DISCUSSION

Global gene expression in myeloid DC induced by LPS stimulation: identification of heightened type 1 IFN-related genes in NOD mice: We analyzed global gene expression using affymetrix-based gene array systems in bone marrow-derived myeloid DC at 0, 6, 12, 24 h after LPS stimulation. Over 300 genes were identified to differ between NOD and B6 mice. A distinct cluster of 16 type 1 IFN-targeted genes were significantly upregulated in NOD DC ($P < 0.005$) including IRF-7, recently reported as an essential factor in regulation of type 1 IFN responses.[5] We confirmed heightened IRF-7 expression in NOD DC by quantitative RT-PCR in bone marrow-derived DC (15-fold increase in NOD versus. twofold in B6) as well as in purified splenic CD11c$^+$ DC (20-fold increase in NOD versus 2.5-fold in B6) following IFN-β stimulation. We also demonstrated heightened IFN-α/β target gene responses in macrophages of NOD mice. In separate studies, we find IFN-α/β readily induces Cox-2 expression in bone marrow-derived macrophages of NOD mice in contrast to B6.

To further evaluate IFN-α/β responses in DC we examined phospho-STAT1/2 in DC and found higher levels of these transcription factors in NOD than in B6. These findings demonstrate heightened type 1 IFN responses in myeloid APC in NOD mice. Studies of IFN signaling in several congenic B6 strains mice demonstrated that chromosome 1 encompassing the *Idd5* susceptibility region largely contributed to the abnormalities in type 1 IFN responses.

Splenic CD11c$^+$ DC Show Heightened Responses to IFN-α/β in NOD Mice

Because type 1 IFN plays a central role in promoting DC maturation we postulated that DC in lymphoid tissues may enhance maturation due to heightened IFN-α/β signaling. We injected NOD mice with poly I:C and examined CD86 expression on splenic CD11c$^+$ DC. We found NOD DC express markedly higher levels of CD86 expression in response to poly I:C than B6. These data suggest NOD DC demonstrate a heightened maturation response to agents that induce IFN-α/β.

Increased IFN-α/β-Producing PDC in NOD Mice

It was reported recently that type 1 IFN plays a central role in PDC activation and migration and that mouse strains differ in PDC numbers.[6] We found that PDC number is significantly increased in NOD spleen in comparison to B6. We also found CpG stimulation of NOD spleen leads to four- to sixfold higher levels of IFN-α production than in B6 and that PDC are the source for IFN-α production.

Poly I:C Induces Rapid Onset of Diabetes

To determine whether type 1 IFN play an important role in T1D pathogenesis, we treated female NOD mice with daily poly I:C injections for 7 days. This treatment rapidly precipitated the onset of diabetes in 50% of treated female and male NOD mice within 7 days of treatment.

CONCLUSIONS

NOD mice demonstrate a heightened responsiveness to type 1 IFN that contributes to enhanced DC maturation and expression of proinflammatory genes in macrophages. Furthermore, agents that induce type 1 IFN rapidly precipitate diabetes in the NOD mouse and induce type 1 responsive antigens in β cells.

REFERENCES

1. MONTOYA, M., G. SCHIAVONI, F. MATTEI, *et al.* 2002. Type I interferon produced by dendritic cells promote their phenotypic and functional activation. Blood **99:** 3263–3271.
2. LUFT, T., K.C. PANG, E. THOMAS, *et al.* 1998. Type I IFNs enhance the terminal differentiation of dendritic cells. J. Immunol. **161:** 1947–1953.
3. VASSILEVA, G., S.C. CHEN, M. ZENG, *et al.* 2003. Expression of a novel murine type I IFN in the pancreatic islets induces diabetes in mice. J. Immunol. **170:** 5748–5755.
4. HUANG, X., J. YUANG, A. GODDARD, *et al.* 1995. Stewart interferon expression in the pancreases of patients with type I diabetes. Diabetes **44:** 658–664.
5. HONDA, K., H. YANAI, H. NEGISHI, *et al.* 2005. IRF-7 is the master regulator of type-I interferon-dependent immune responses. Nature **434:** 772–777.
6. ASSELIN-PATUREL, C., G. BRIZARD, K. CHEMIN, *et al.* 2005. Type I interferon dependence of plasmacytoid dendritic cell activation and migration. Exp. Med. **201:** 1157–1167.

Immunolocalization of Monocyte Chemoattractant Protein-1 in Islets of NOD Mice during Cyclophosphamide Administration

SHIVA REDDY,[a] YAN BAI,[a] ELIZABETH ROBINSON,[b] AND JACQUELINE ROSS[c]

[a]*School of Biological Sciences,* [b]*School of Population Health, and* [c]*Department of Anatomy with Radiology, University of Auckland, 92019 Auckland, New Zealand*

ABSTRACT: The molecular processes that initiate insulitis in type 1 diabetes remain unclear. Chemokines, such as monocyte chemoattractant protein-1 (MCP-1), mediate chemotaxis and leukocyte migration to inflammatory sites. Although MCP-1 mRNA has been shown in islets isolated from NOD mice at 2 weeks of age and at later stages, the cellular sources of this chemokine, at the protein level, and its role in insulitis are unclear. The aims of the present study were to employ immunohistochemical techniques to examine the expression of MCP-1 and quantify its cellular sources in islets of NOD mice both after cyclophosphamide (Cy) administration and in spontaneous diabetes. Tissues were examined at days 1 (=day 73, first day of Cy), 4, 7, 11, and 14 and in age-matched control NOD mice. Pancreatic sections from NOD mice without Cy administration were also studied between days 21–65 and at onset of diabetes and from adult CD-1 mice. In the Cy group, a small number of peri-islet macrophages were immunopositive for MCP-1 at day 1 whereas at day 4, the number declined but increased subsequently at day 7. In the same group, it increased markedly at days 11 and 14 compared with age-matched control NOD mice. In young NOD mice, MCP-1 was present in selective macrophages in islets with early insulitis (day 45) but was absent at diabetes onset. MCP-1 was undetectable in beta cells and in most T cells. Islets from adult CD-1 mice did not show immunostaining for MCP-1. We conclude that MCP-1 is expressed in a proportion of islet and exocrine macrophages. This expression increases during the later stages of Cy-induced diabetes. Thus, MCP-1 positive macrophages that migrate to the islet periphery during the early stages of Cy-induced

Address for correspondence: Shiva Reddy, Ph.D., School of Biological Sciences, University of Auckland, Private Bag 92019, Auckland, New Zealand. Voice: +64-9-3737599; ext.: 82917; fax: +64-9-3737668.

e-mail: s.reddy@auckland.ac.nz

Ann. N.Y. Acad. Sci. 1079: 103–108 (2006).
doi: 10.1196/annals.1375.014

diabetes and preceding spontaneous diabetes may augment insulitis by further attracting macrophages and T cells.

KEYWORDS: **NOD mice; MCP-1; immunohistochemistry; islets**

INTRODUCTION

The processes that control the early influx of immune cells into pancreatic islets in type 1 diabetes are poorly understood. Various adhesion molecules expressed by endothelial cells and by blood trafficking lymphocytes may act in concert with a special class of molecules, known as chemokines, and their cognate receptors in facilitating islet-directed leukocyte migration.[1] Thus, in the early prediabetic stage, a complex interplay between such molecules, in concert with certain signals from the beta cell, may provide essential cues for directing blood-borne mononuclear cell migration toward the islets.[2]

Chemokines elicit important pleotropic effects, including their role in leukocyte chemotaxis, inflammation, and angiogenesis.[3] Monocyte chemoattractant protein-1 (MCP-1), also known as CCL2, is produced by a variety of cells, including lymphocytes, monocytes, endothelial cells, mesangial cells, and fibroblasts, in response to proinflammatory stimuli.[4]

Although MCP-1 mRNA has been shown to be present in isolated islets of the NOD mouse, direct evidence for its expression at the protein level and its cellular sources are lacking.[5] In this study, the expression of MCP-1 protein was investigated immunohistochemically in pancreatic sections of the NOD mouse at various time points following acceleration of diabetes with cyclophosphamide (Cy). Dual- and triple-label immunohistochemistry were employed to establish and quantify the cellular sources of the protein at various time points following Cy administration and in spontaneous diabetes.

METHODS

Pancreatic cryosections from the NOD mouse were immunohistochemically stained with antibodies to MCP-1 at various time points following Cy administration (300 mg/kg body weight) to days 73 female NOD mice. Following Cy administration, pancreatic tissues were collected at days 1 (first day of study and without Cy injection), 4, 7, 11, and 14 and at similar time points from diluent-injected NOD mice. Pancreatic tissues were also studied at various stages of spontaneous diabetes in the NOD mouse (days 21–65) and at onset of spontaneous diabetes. Dual- and triple-label immunohistochemistry were used to establish the cellular source of MCP-1 with antibodies to insulin, CD3 cells, and macrophages. The number of MCP-1 positive macrophages within the islets was expressed as a mean percentage per islet ± SEM for each time point.

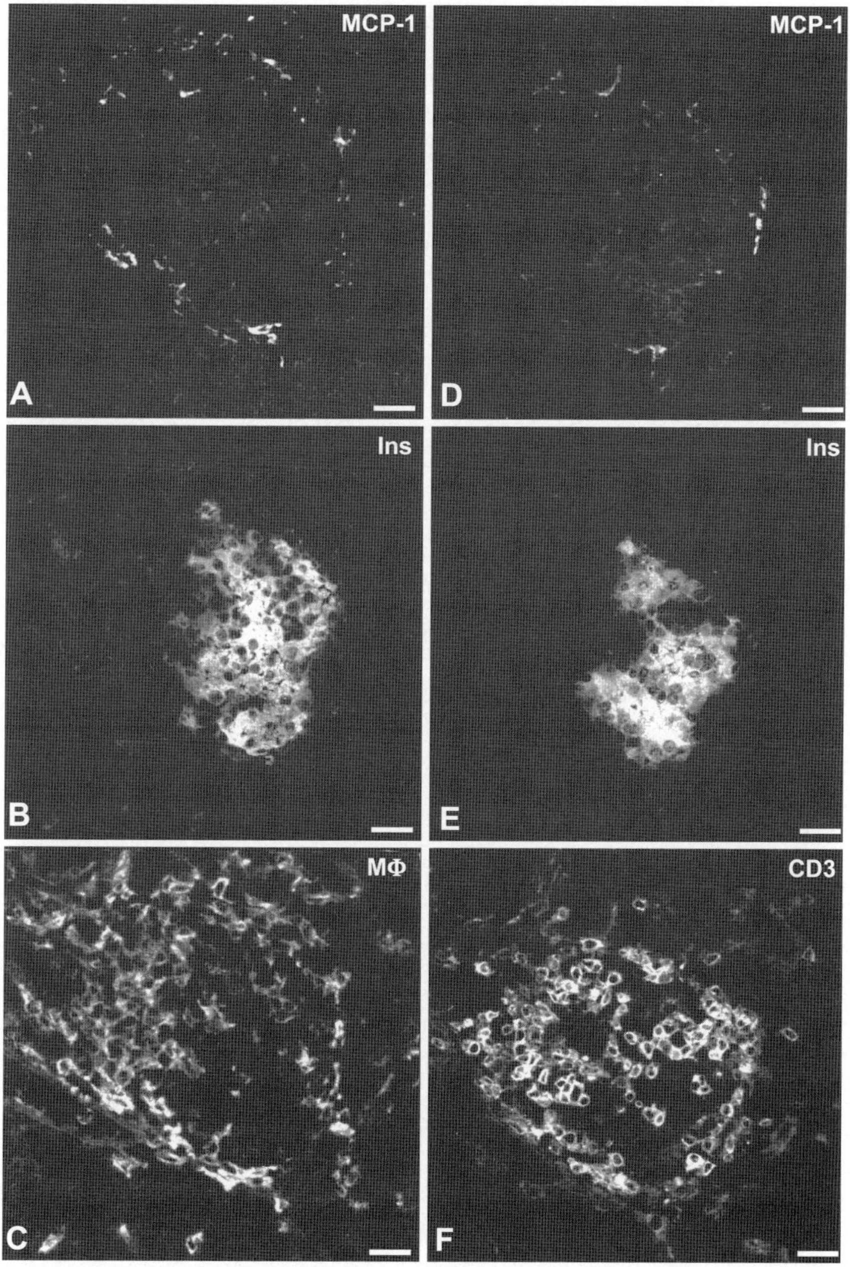

FIGURE 1. Confocal images of islets from day 7 Cy-treated NOD mice triple-labeled for MCP-1 (**A**) + insulin (**B**) + macrophages (**C**) and for MCP-1 (**D**) + insulin (**E**) + CD3 T cells (**F**). Note MCP-1 expression is seen in selective peri-islet macrophages. Scale bars: 20 microns.

RESULTS

In the Cy-treated and untreated mice, a small number of peri-islet macrophages were immunopositive for MCP-1 at days 1 and 4, but the number increased at day 7. It increased markedly at days 11 and 14 (Cy group) compared with control NOD mice. In young NOD mice, MCP-1 was present in selective macrophages in islets with early insulitis (day 45) but was absent at diabetes onset. MCP-1 was undetectable in beta cells and in most T cells in the Cy and spontaneous models. Islets from adult CD-1 mice did not show immunostaining for MCP-1.

Representative islets from the Cy group (7 days after Cy treatment) following triple-labeling (MCP-1 + macrophages + insulin or MCP-1 + T cells + insulin) are shown in FIGURE 1 A–F.

The presence of macrophages expressing MCP-1 had a different pattern over time in the Cy and control groups ($P = 0.002$, logistic regression model; FIG. 2). In the Cy group, there was a change over time ($P = 0.007$) and, in particular, there was an increase at day 11. In the control group, there was little evidence of change over time ($P = 0.07$). There was no significant difference in the mean percentage of MCP-1 positive macrophages between Cy-treated mice which developed diabetes and those which did not ($P = 0.6$). However, there was a difference between the time points, with the chemokine more likely to be present at day 11 than at day 14 ($P = 0.046$).

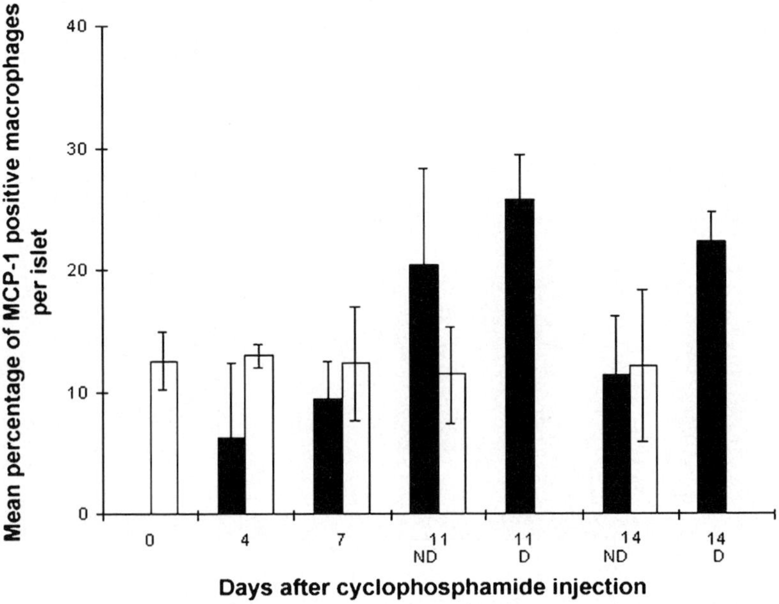

FIGURE 2. Mean percentage ± SEM MCP-1 positive macrophages per islet at various stages of Cy-treated and age-matched diluent-treated NOD mice. Open bars: diluent-treated group; solid bars: Cy-treated group. D = diabetic, Cy treated; ND = nondiabetic;, Cy treated.

DISCUSSION

The present studies in the Cy model show that MCP-1 is expressed almost exclusively in a proportion of intra-islet and peri-islet macrophages. The number of MCP-1 positive macrophages showed a marked increase towards the latter stages of Cy-induced diabetes. The distribution of MCP-1 positive cells in a proportion of perivascular and exocrine-located macrophages in association with an intra-islet location suggests that the extra-islet-located chemokine may provide signals for directing leukocyte trafficking from vascular sites toward the islets.

Previous reports indicate that mRNA for MCP-1 is detectable in isolated islets from NOD mice, as early as 2 weeks of age.[5] In addition, MCP-1 mRNA showed an increase in rat and human beta cells following exposure to interleukin-1β (IL-1β).[5] Reasons for the apparent differences between our findings and this previous study are unclear and may suggest the relative insensitivity of the immunohistochemical technique or that mRNA and protein expression data may not always be concordant. By immunohistochemistry and *in situ* hybridization, MCP-1 was reported to be expressed constitutively in pancreatic beta cells and isolated islets from the human and the levels increased following exposure to proinflammatory cytokines and lipopolysaccharide.[6] Thus, there may be species differences in the cellular sources of chemokines within the islets. Our present findings concur with a recent report that employed a mouse model of insulitis and demonstrated that MCP-1 immunolabeling corresponded to macrophages within the peri-islet region.[2] The expression of MCP-1 in macrophages has also been demonstrated in other disease systems, such as in artherosclerosis.[7] We speculate that a proportion of early islet-infiltrating macrophages may express MCP-1 in response to specific signals, probably from beta cells that have sustained limited injury. Macrophages positive for MCP-1 within the islet may then attract additional immune cells and enhance the inflammatory "build-up" that leads to further destruction of beta cells.

ACKNOWLEDGMENTS

Financial assistance from the Auckland Medical Research Foundation, the Child Health Research Foundation, and the Paykel Trust is gratefully acknowledged. We thank Lorraine Rolston and Beryl Davy for histological assistance.

REFERENCES

1. BENDALL, L. 2005. Chemokines and their receptors in disease. Histol. Histopathol. **20:** 907–926.
2. FRIGERIO, S. *et al.* 2002. β-Cells are responsible for CXCR3-mediated T-cell infiltration in insulitis. Nat. Med. **12:** 1414–1420.

3. BORING, L. *et al.* 1999. MCP-1 in human disease: insights gained from animal models. *In* Chemokines in Disease, Biology and Clinical Research. C.A. Hebert. Ed.: 53-65. Human Press. Totowa, New Jersey.
4. OPPENHEIM, J.J. *et al.* 1991. Properties of the novel proinflammatory supergene 'intercrine' cytokine family. Ann. Rev. Immunol. **9:** 617–648.
5. CHEN, M-C. *et al.* 2001. Monocyte chemoattractant protein-1 is expressed in pancreatic islets from prediabetic and in interleukin-1β-exposed human and rat pancreatic islet cells. Diabetologia **44:** 325–338.
6. PIEMONTI, L. *et al.* 2002. Human pancreatic islets produce and secrete MCP-1/CCL2: relevance in human islet transplantation. Diabetes **51:** 55–65.
7. YLA-HERTTUALA, S. *et al.* 1991. Expression of monocyte chemoattractant protein-1 in macrophage-rich areas of human and rabbit atherosclerotic lesions. Proc. Nat. Acad. Sci. USA **188:** 5252–5256.

Young NOD Mice Show Increased Diabetes Sensitivity to Low Doses of Streptozotocin

SHIVA REDDY,[a] MIKE CHANG,[a] AND ELIZABETH ROBINSON[b]

[a]*School of Biological Sciences, and* [b]*School of Population Health, University of Auckland, 92019 Auckland, New Zealand*

ABSTRACT: In type 1 diabetes, environmentally induced early-limited beta cell damage may pre-empt the subsequent immune-mediated beta cell destruction. Low doses of streptozotocin (Stz), given early to diabetes-prone mice, may cause limited beta cell destruction during the early phase and precipitate diabetes. Here, we aimed to see if young NOD mice are more diabetes-sensitive to various multiple low doses of Stz than nondiabetes-prone mice. We also determined the molecular pathology of islets following administration of the diabetogen. Female NOD and CD-1 mice received 5 daily doses of Stz at day 21 (20, 30, and 40 mg/kg body weight; 18 mice per group) or diluent, and diabetes was monitored. Pancreas were studied histochemically and immunohistochemically at various time points after Stz administration. Following administration of Stz, NOD mice showed a much earlier onset and increased diabetes rate, at all three doses, than CD-1 mice. By day 80, the final diabetes rates following the 40, 30, and 20 mg dose in NOD mice were 95%, 85%, and 33%, respectively, compared with 33%, 28%, and 5.5%, respectively, in CD-1 mice. However, following the 20 mg dose, only 2 of the 12 remaining NOD mice developed the disease between 90 and 250 days compared with 19 of 24 NOD mice that did not receive Stz at day 21. Stz-administered NOD and CD-1 mice showed an initial loss of beta cells, with redistribution of islet endocrine cells, early macrophage infiltration, and increasing insulitis.

KEYWORDS: NOD mice; streptozotocin; beta cell sensitivity; type 1 diabetes

INTRODUCTION

Type 1 diabetes is a chronic disease characterized by progressive destruction of beta cells by immune mechanisms.[1] Epidemiological evidence suggests

Address for correspondence: Shiva Reddy, Ph.D., School of Biological Sciences, University of Auckland, Private Bag 92019, Auckland, New Zealand. Voice: +64-9-3737599; ext.: 82917; fax: +64-9-3737668.
e-mail: s.reddy@auckland.ac.nz

**Ann. N.Y. Acad. Sci. 1079: 109–113 (2006). © 2006 New York Academy of Sciences.
doi: 10.1196/annals.1375.015**

that the disease may be initiated by environmental factors, such as certain viruses or toxins in genetically-prone individuals.[2–4] The identity of specific environmental agents and the processes by which they interact with diabetes-susceptibility genes to induce type 1 diabetes are under intense study. Previous studies have shown that beta cells are more deficient in mounting an adequate defense following injury than other cell types, such as hepatocytes.[5] Our studies with isolated islets from NOD mice suggest that the diabetes-prone beta cells may be more sensitive to injury than nondiabetes-prone beta cells.[6] It is possible that the increased sensitivity and limited injury of diabetes-prone beta cell, provoked by certain environmental toxins in early life, may precede the more protracted immune phase of beta cell destruction, culminating in diabetes. The aims of the present article were, therefore, to test whether newly weaned NOD mice were more diabetes-sensitive to various low doses of streptozotocin (Stz), a beta cell toxin, *in vivo*, than nondiabetes-prone mice.

MATERIALS AND METHODS

Female NOD and control CD-1 mice received five daily doses of Stz at day 21 (20, 30, and 40 mg/kg body weight; 18 mice per group) or diluent. Following the fifth injection, all mice were monitored for the development of diabetes. Diabetes was defined as the presence of a hyperglycemic value of greater than 12 mM in tail blood samples over 3 consecutive days. Pancreas was studied histochemically and immunohistochemically at various time points after Stz administration.

RESULTS

The incidence of diabetes in NOD and CD-1 mice, following administration of three low doses of Stz on 5 consecutive days is shown in FIGURE 1 A and B. By day 80, the final diabetes rates following the 40, 30, and 20 mg dose in NOD mice were 95%, 85%, and 33%, respectively. In comparison, the 40, 30, and 20 mg dose in CD-1 mice resulted in a diabetes rate of 33%, 28%, and 5.5%, respectively, during the same period of observation. In addition, following Stz administration, there was a greater delay in the onset of diabetes in CD-1 mice than in NOD mice. Following the 20 mg dose, only 2 of the 12 remaining NOD mice subsequently developed diabetes between 90 and 250 days (FIG. 1 C). In comparison, 19 of 24 NOD mice, which did not receive Stz at weaning, developed spontaneous disease (FIG. 1 C).

Stz-treated NOD and CD-1 mice showed an initial loss of beta cells, with redistribution of islet endocrine cells, differential immunolabeling for insulin in the beta cell cytoplasm, early macrophage infiltration, and increasing insulitis (FIG. 2).

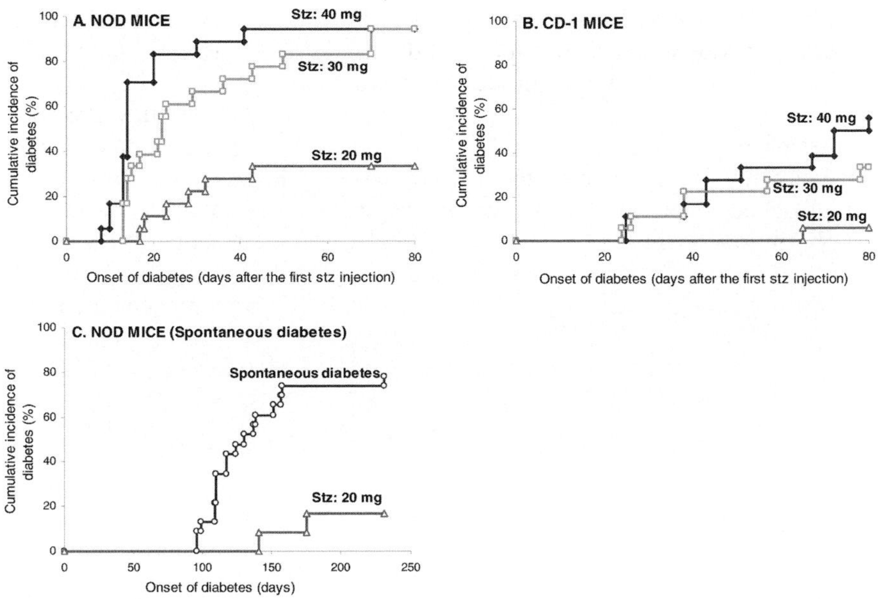

FIGURE 1. Cumulative incidence of diabetes following administration of three different low doses of Stz to day 21 female NOD mice (**A**) and CD-1 mice (**B**) (18 mice per dose of Stz). Panel **C** shows cumulative incidence of diabetes in the remaining 12 NOD mice previously injected with 20 mg/kg body weight of Stz on 5 consecutive days from weaning and in 24 female NOD mice that did not receive the drug at day 21. Note only 2/12 Stz-injected mice developed diabetes between days 90–250 whereas 19/24 NOD mice that did not receive Stz developed the disease spontaneously during the same period.

DISCUSSION

This study shows that beta cells from young NOD mice are more sensitive to low doses of Stz than nondiabetes-prone CD-1 mice. Beta cells have been shown to be poorly equipped with defense processes against free radical-induced injury.[5] Indeed, studies have shown that stable overexpression of the free radical scavenging enzymes, such as glutathione peroxidase, catalase, and superoxide dismutase, in RINm5F cells resulted in protection against the cooperative toxicity of nitric oxide and oxygen-free radicals.[7] Beta cell expression of thioredoxin prevents diabetes in NOD mice and also in mice given multiple low doses of Stz.[8] The greater early sensitivity of beta cells from young NOD mice to low doses of the diabetogen may be due to their diminished capacity to mount adequate protection. Our present *in vivo* studies support our previous findings with isolated islets from young NOD mice, which showed a similar enhanced sensitivity of beta cells to low and graded doses of Stz.[6]

In the present study, early exposure of young NOD mice to the lowest dose of Stz tested had a profound and paradoxical effect in preventing the subsequent

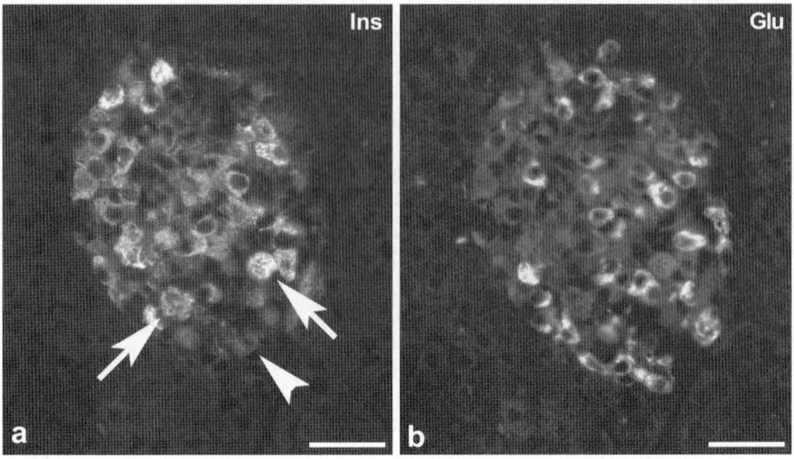

FIGURE 2. An islet from a 47-day-old diabetic NOD mouse following injection with 30 mg/kg body weight of Stz at weaning, immunohistochemically stained for insulin (**A**) and glucagon (**B**). Note the presence of several beta cells in the islet showing differential immunolabeling for insulin; arrows point to bright insulin cells whereas an arrowhead points to weaker immunolabeling for insulin. In panel **B** a marked redistribution of glucagon cells toward the central region of the islet is seen. Scale bars = 20 microns; Ins = insulin; Glu = glucagon.

spontaneous onset of diabetes. The mechanisms underlying these unexpected findings are unclear. We speculate that a critical low threshold of Stz¨ may invoke repair processes in the beta cell that may inhibit future development of diabetes. Alternatively, low-dose Stz may cause limited beta cell apoptosis and release previously sequestered neoantigens that may reshape the immune repertoire.[9] Our present findings may have important implications for the initiation and prevention of human type 1 diabetes.

ACKNOWLEDGMENTS

Financial assistance from the Auckland Medical Research Foundation, the Child Health Research Foundation, and the Paykel Trust is gratefully acknowledged. We thank Jacqueline Ross for assistance with image preparation and Lorraine Rolston and Beryl Davy for histological support.

REFERENCES

1. Eisenbarth, G.S. *et al.* 1987. The "natural" history of type 1 diabetes. Diabetes Metab. Rev. **3:** 873–891.

2. LESLIE, R.D.G. & R.B. ELLIOTT. 1994. Early environmental events as a cause of IDDM: evidence and implications. Diabetes **43:** 843–850.
3. AKERBLOM, H.K. *et al.* 2002. Environmental factors in the etiology of type 1 diabetes. Am. J. Med. Genet. **115:** 18–29.
4. TAURIAI, S. *et al.* 2003. Can enteroviruses cause type 1 diabetes? Ann. N. Y. Acad. Sci. **1005:** 13–22.
5. MALAISSE, W.J. *et al.* 1982. Determinants of the selective toxicity of alloxan to the pancreatic B cell. Proc. Natl. Acad. Sci. USA **79:** 927–930.
6. REDDY, S. & S. SANDLER. 1996. Age-dependent sensitivity to streptozotocin of pancreatic islets isolated from female NOD mice. Autoimmunity **22:** 121–126.
7. TIEDGE, M. *et al.* 1999. Protection against the co-operative toxicity of nitric oxide and oxygen free radicals by overexpression of antioxidant enzymes in bioengineered insulin-producing RINm5F cells. Diabetologia **42:** 849–855.
8. HOTTA, M. *et al.* 1998. Pancreatic beta cell-specific expression of thioredoxin, an antioxidative and antiapoptotic protein, prevents autoimmune and streptozotocin-induced diabetes. J. Exp. Med. **188:** 1445–1451.
9. HUGUES, S. *et al.* 2002. Tolerance to islet antigens and prevention from diabetes induced by limited apoptosis of pancreatic β cells. Immunity **16:** 169–181.

Contribution of Class III MHC to Susceptibility to Type 1 Diabetes in the NOD Mouse

KAORI YAMAJI,[a] HIROSHI IKEGAMI,[a,b] TOMOMI FUJISAWA,[a] SHINSUKE NOSO,[a] KOJI NOJIMA,[a] NARU BABAYA,[a,b] MICHIKO ITOI-BABAYA,[a] MISATO KOBAYASHI,[a] YOSHIHISA HIROMINE,[a] SUSUMU MAKINO,[a,b] AND TOSHIO OGIHARA[a]

[a]*Department of Geriatric Medicine, Osaka University Graduate School of Medicine, Osaka 565-0871, Japan*

[b]*Department of Endocrinology, Metabolism and Diabetes, Kinki University School of Medicine, Osaka-sayama, Osaka 589-8511, Japan*

ABSTRACT: A recombinant major histocompatibility complex (MHC) with the same class III region as the NOD mouse, but different class II region from the NOD mouse was identified in the NON mouse, and NOD mice congenic for this recombinant MHC, NOD.NON-*H2*, was established. None of the congenic mice homozygous for the NON MHC developed type 1 diabetes, indicating that the NOD MHC is necessary for the development of type 1 diabetes. A small portion of MHC heterozygotes developed late-onset type 1 diabetes, suggesting the contribution of class III MHC to type 1 diabetes susceptibility.

KEYWORDS: type 1 diabetes; major histocompatibility complex (MHC); gene; autoimmunity; NOD mouse

INTRODUCTION

To further localize and characterize a second component of the major histocompatibility complex (MHC)-linked susceptibility to type 1 diabetes in the NOD mouse, we adopted "ancestral haplotype congenic mapping," which we previously reported and successfully applied for genetic dissection of *Idd1* on chromosome 17[1,2] and *Idd10* on chromosome 3.[3] To this end, we screened NOD-related strains for a strain possessing the same non-class II region as the NOD mouse, but a different class II region in both the *A* and *E* genes from

Address for correspondence: Hiroshi Ikegami, Department of Endocrinology, Metabolism and Diabetes, Kinki University School of Medicine, 377-2 Ohno-higashi, Osaka-Sayama, Osaka. 589-8511, Japan
e-mail: ikegami@med.kindai.ac.jp

**Ann. N.Y. Acad. Sci. 1079: 114–117 (2006). © 2006 New York Academy of Sciences.
doi: 10.1196/annals.1375.016**

the NOD mouse. The non-obese nondiabetic (NON) mouse was suggested to possess such a recombinant MHC with the same alleles in the class III region as the NOD mouse, but different alleles in the class II region from the NOD mouse.[4] We introgressed this recombinant MHC onto NOD background genes to establish a congenic NOD line carrying the MHC (*H2*) region from the NON mouse, the NOD.NON-*H2* congenic mice, and studied the development of type 1 diabetes in comparison with NOD mice.

METHODS

The NOD.NON-*H2* congenic mice were established by mating NON mice with NOD mice and repeated backcrossing to NOD mice with selection for the NON MHC. Heterozygous NOD.NON-*H2* mice were intercrossed to produce the NON MHC homozygotes, MHC heterozygotes, and the NOD MHC homozygotes, and the development of type 1 diabetes was monitored relative to the MHC genotypes.

RESULTS

In the process of repeated backcrossing to establish NOD.NON-*H2* congenic mice, we noticed that a few female heterozygous mice developed late-onset type 1 diabetes. The present study, although still preliminary, confirmed this in that the MHC heterozygotes of the congenic mice developed type 1 diabetes, although the frequency was very low. Phenotypes of the NOD MHC homozygotes were indistinguishable from NOD parental strain, indicating that genetic background of the congenic mice were successfully replaced by the NOD genome. None of the NON MHC homozygotes developed type 1 diabetes, confirming that the NOD MHC is necessary for the development of type 1 diabetes.

DISCUSSION

NOD mice congenic for the MHC from control strains were reported to be protective against type 1 diabetes.[5] The NON MHC homozygotes of the NOD.NON-*H2* in the present study were also completely protected from type 1 diabetes, indicating that the NOD MHC is necessary for the development of type 1 diabetes and the NON MHC is protective against type 1 diabetes. In contrast to the complete protection from type 1 diabetes in the NON MHC homozygotes, MHC heterozygotes of the NOD.NON-*H2* mice developed type 1 diabetes, although the frequency was very low and the onset was delayed, suggesting that the NON MHC is weakly susceptible to type 1 diabetes (Yamaji *et al.* manuscript in preparation).

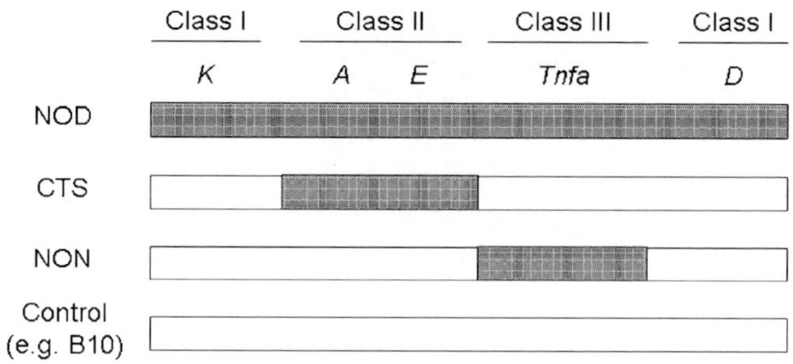

FIGURE 1. MHC region of NOD, CTS, NON, and control strains. Regions identical by descent (IBD) with NOD in CTS and NON strains are shaded.

We previously reported that the Cataract Shionogi (CTS) MHC, which is identical to the NOD MHC in the class II A and E genes, but different from the NOD MHC outside of this region[1,6] (FIG. 1), confers susceptibility to type 1 diabetes, even in homozygous state.[2] This strongly suggested that class II *A* and *E* genes are responsible for *Idd1*, the MHC-linked susceptibility to type 1 diabetes in the NOD mouse. The frequency of type 1 diabetes, however, were significantly lower in the CTS MHC homozygotes than in the NOD MHC homozygotes, indicating that the CTS MHC is weaker in conferring susceptibility to type 1 diabetes than the NOD MHC. Weaker susceptibility conferred by the CTS MHC as compared with the NOD MHC despite sharing the same class II MHC at both *A* and *E* genes indicated that *Idd1* in the class II MHC is not sufficient for type 1 diabetes susceptibility in the NOD mouse and that the MHC-linked susceptibility to type 1 diabetes consisted of multiple components with *Idd1* in the class II A and E regions and a second component, termed *Idd16*, located adjacent to, but distinct from, *Idd1*.[2] The NOD MHC possesses susceptibility alleles at both *Idd1* and *Idd16*, while the CTS MHC possesses susceptibility allele only at *Idd1*, but resistant allele at *Idd16*, resulting in weaker susceptibility to type 1 diabetes (TABLE 1). The data in the present study together with the previous studies on the CTS MHC[1,2]

TABLE 1. Hierarchy of susceptibility to type 1 diabetes conferred by the MHC

Strain	MHC	IBD* with NOD	Type 1 diabetes susceptibility	*Idd1*	*Idd16*
NOD	NOD (g7)	all	strong	susceptible	susceptible
NOD.CTS-*H2*	CTS	Class II	intermediate	susceptible	protective
NOD.NON-*H2*	NON	Class III	weak	protective	susceptible
NOD.B10-*H2*	B10 (b)	none	protective	protective	protective

*IBD = identical by descent.

IBD was judged by sharing the same alleles and/or genomic sequences with the NOD mouse in strains derived from the same closed colony as the NOD mouse.

suggest that the NON MHC, which confers susceptibility to type 1 diabetes only when combined with one dose of the NOD MHC, may possess susceptibility allele at *Idd16*, resulting in the weak susceptibility despite the presence of resistant allele at *Idd1* (TABLE 1) (Yamaji *et al.* manuscript in preparation). The NON MHC shares the same alleles in class III region with the NOD MHC[4] (FIG. 1), suggesting that class III region of the MHC may contribute to type 1 diabetes susceptibility and *Idd16* may be located in the class III region. Further studies with a large number of subcongenic strains with different segments of the MHC from NON and CTS mice are necessary to confirm this.

ACKNOWLEDGMENTS

We thank Y. Tsukamoto and M. Miyuki for their skillful technical assistance. This work was supported by a Grant-in-Aid for Scientific Research from the Ministry of Education, Science, Sports, Culture, and Technology, Japan.

REFERENCES

1. IKEGAMI, H., G.S. EISENBARTH & M. HATTORI. 1990. Major histocompatibility complex-linked diabetogenic gene of the nonobese diabetic mouse. Analysis of genomic DNA amplified by the polymerase chain reaction. J. Clin. Invest. **85:** 18–24.
2. IKEGAMI, H., S. MAKINO, E. YAMATO, *et al.* 1995. Identification of a new susceptibility locus for insulin-dependent diabetes mellitus by ancestral haplotype congenic mapping. J. Clin. Invest. **96:** 1936–1942.
3. INOUE, K., H. IKEGAMI, T. FUJISAWA, *et al.* 2005. Evidence for *CD101* but not *Fcgr1* as candidate for type 1 diabetes locus, *Idd10*. Biochem. Biophys. Res. Commun. **331:** 536–542.
4. IKEGAMI, H., T. FUJISAWA, S. MAKINO, *et al.* 2003. Congenic mapping and candidate sequencing of susceptibility genes for type 1 diabetes in the NOD mouse. Ann. N. Y. Acad. Sci. **1005:** 196–204.
5. IKEGAMI, H., S. MAKINO & T. OGIHARA. 1996. Molecular genetics of insulin-dependent diabetes mellitus: analysis of congenic strains. *In* Frontiers in Diabetes Research: Lessons from Animal Diabetes VI. Shafrir E. Ed.: 33–46. Birkhauser. Boston.
6. IKEGAMI, H., S. MAKINO, M. HARADA, *et al.* 1988. The cataract Shionogi mouse, a sister strain of the non-obese diabetic mouse: similar class II but different class I gene products. Diabetologia **31:** 254–258.

MHC-Linked Susceptibility to Type 1 Diabetes in the NOD Mouse

Further Localization of *Idd16* by Subcongenic Analysis

TOMOMI FUJISAWA,[a] HIROSHI IKEGAMI,[a,b] SHINSUKE NOSO,[a] KAORI YAMAJI,[a] KOJI NOJIMA,[a] NARU BABAYA,[a] MICHIKO ITOI-BABAYA,[a] YOSHIHISA HIROMINE,[a] MISATO KOBAYASHI,[a] SUSUMU MAKINO,[a] AND TOSHIO OGIHARA[a]

[a]*Department of Geriatric Medicine, Osaka University Graduate School of Medicine, Suita, Osaka 565-0871, Japan*

[b]*Department of Endocrinology, Diabetes and Metabolism, Kinki University School of Medicine, Sayama, Osaka 589-8511, Japan*

ABSTRACT: Although major histocompatibility complex (MHC)-linked susceptibility is the strongest component, recent studies demonstrated that MHC-linked susceptibility to type 1 diabetes consists of multiple components both in humans and non-obese diabetic (NOD) mouse. In the NOD mouse, *Idd16* has been mapped to the region adjacent to, but distinct from *Idd1* in the MHC class II region. Establishment of subcongenic NOD.CTS-*H2* lines that possess the same MHC class II as the NOD mouse but non-NOD-derived chromosomal region in its adjacent regions, would facilitate further narrowing down of the localization of *Idd16*.

KEYWORDS: type 1 diabetes mellitus; genetics; major histocompatibility complex (MHC); susceptibility gene; NOD mouse

INTRODUCTION

Type 1 diabetes mellitus is a polygenetic disorder with the strong susceptibility linked to human leukocyte antigen (HLA) region.[1] A number of studies so far consistently demonstrated that the HLA class II genes, DR and DQ genes in particular, are strongly associated with the disease, and HLA class II genes

Address for correspondence: Dr. Hiroshi Ikegami, Department of Endocrinology, Diabetes and Metabolism, Kinki University School of Medicine, 377-2 Ohno-higashi, Sayama, Osaka 589-8511, Japan. Voice: +81-72-366-0221; ext.: 3123; fax: +81-72-366-2095.
e-mail: ikegami@med.kindai.ac.jp

**Ann. N.Y. Acad. Sci. 1079: 118–121 (2006). © 2006 New York Academy of Sciences.
doi: 10.1196/annals.1375.017**

are widely recognized as *IDDM1*. Recent accumulating lines of evidence, however, demonstrated that HLA-linked strong susceptibility consists of multiple components; several data suggested the contribution of HLA class I region[2] or class III region in addition to class II genes in conferring susceptibility to and/or clinical heterogeneity in type 1 diabetes. Strong linkage disequilibrium across the HLA region, however, makes it difficult to genetically dissect a nonclass II gene(s) contributing to the HLA-linked strong susceptibility in humans.

Non-obese diabetic (NOD) mouse is an inbred strain of mice established from the outbred colony Jcl:ICR.[3] The NOD mice exhibit invasion of immune T cells to pancreatic islets, termed *insulitis*, and autoimmunity against islet beta cells, whose characteristics closely resemble to those in humans, making NOD mice serve as an animal model for type 1 diabetes. Genetic analyses of NOD mice have also pointed to a similarity in genetic susceptibility between human and the NOD mouse. In particular, the major histocompatibility complex (MHC), corresponding to HLA in humans, has been shown as the strongest component of the susceptibility to diabetes in the NOD mouse.[4] In the NOD mouse, lack of class II I-E molecule due to a deletion within its promotor region and unique amino acid sequence of I-A, another class II molecule, are shown be involved in susceptibility to type 1 diabetes, and designated as *Idd1*. Given that these class II genes are orthologue of human HLA class II genes (*IDDM1*) and the strong similarity between human *IDDM1* and mouse *Idd1*, genetic dissection of *Idd1* will contribute to better understanding of the genetic predisposition to type 1 diabetes in humans.

Accumulating data demonstrated that the MHC-linked strong susceptibility of the NOD mouse is not solely explained by the MHC class II genes, as in the case of humans. MHC region contains many genes, including MHC genes as well as other genes functionally relevant to immune and inflammation systems. Previously, we established a congenic line of mice by introgressing a CTS-derived MHC region[5] onto NOD genetic background.[6] The NOD congenic line, NOD.CTS-*H2*, possessed the class II region identical to that of the NOD,[5] but their chromosomal region adjacent to class II region was different from that of the NOD mouse. The development of diabetes in the NOD.CTS-*H2* mice was reduced, indicating the contribution of a second gene, in the region adjacent to but distinct from *Idd1* in the class II region, designated *Idd16*, to the disease susceptibility.[6] Susceptibility gene(s) outside the MHC class II in NOD mice has been further supported by other experimental results.

In this article, we established a subcongenic line of mice to fine map the *Idd16*. Given a similar genetic structure of MHC between humans and mice as well as multiple components in susceptibility genes for type 1 diabetes both in humans and mice, the information obtained from the congenic analysis would facilitate the genetic dissection of the HLA-linked susceptibility in humans.

METHODS

Heterozygous NOD.CTS-*H2* mice were repeatedly backcrossed to NOD mice with the selection for the CTS MHC, and a subcongenic line, NOD.CTS-*H2*R1, was established from the original congenic NOD.CTS-*H2* line that possesses the same MHC class II as the NOD mouse.[6] These mice were subjected to weekly monitoring for the development of diabetes up to 1 year.

RESULTS

One congenic NOD line, NOD.CTS-*H2*R1, was established whose congenic interval shared centromeric end with the original NOD.CTS-*H2* but with a shorter chromosomal segment (6.4 cM). Preliminary data suggested that the frequency of diabetes in the NOD.CTS-*H2*R1 was not significantly different from that of their *NOD*-type littermates ($P > 0.3$).

DISCUSSION

To fine map *Idd16*, we have established a new subcongenic line of mice whose centromeric end was identical to the original congenic NOD.CTS-*H2*.[6] As the development of diabetes in the original congenic NOD.CTS-*H2* line (whose congenic interval of 8.5 cM)[6] was significantly reduced in our present colony as compared with *NOD*-type littermates (unpublished), no reduction in diabetes development in the new subcongenics suggests that *Idd16* is mapped to the 4.1 cM region encompassing the class II region, including class I *K* gene.[7] From statistical point of view, however, a large number of mice are needed to *exclude* the existence of a susceptibility gene in some chromosomal region, especially one with a modest effect. The present results should therefore be interpreted as little effect, if any, of the present subcongenic interval (6.4 cM) on susceptibility to type 1 diabetes.

ACKNOWLEDGMENTS

We thank Y. Tsukamoto and M. Moritani for their skillful technical assistance. This work was supported by a Grant-in-Aid for Scientific Research from the Ministry of Education, Science, Sports, Culture, and Technology, Japan.

REFERENCES

1. Ikegami, H. & T. Ogihara. 1996. Genetics of insulin-dependent diabetes mellitus. Endocr. J. **43:** 605–613.

2. FUJISAWA, T., H. IKEGAMI, *et al.* 1995. Class I HLA is associated with age-at-onset of IDDM, while class II HLA confers susceptibility to IDDM. Diabetologia **38:** 1493–1495.
3. MAKINO, S. *et al.* 1980. Breeding of a non-obese, diabetic strain of mice. Exp. Anim. **29:** 1–13.
4. HATTORI, M. *et al.* 1986. The NOD mouse: recessive diabetogenic gene in the major histocompatibility complex. Science **231:** 733–735.
5. IKEGAMI, H., G.S. EISENBARTH & M. HATTORI. 1990. Major histocompatibility complex-linked diabetogenic gene of the nonobese diabetic mouse. Analysis of genomic DNA amplified by the polymerase chain reaction. J. Clin. Invest. **85:** 18–24.
6. IKEGAMI, H. *et al.* 1995. Identification of a new susceptibility locus for insulin-dependent diabetes mellitus by ancestral haplotype congenic mapping. J. Clin. Invest. **96:** 1936–1942.
7. INOUE, K., H. IKEGAMI, T. FUJISAWA, *et al.* 2004. Allelic variation in class I K gene as candidate for a second of MHC-linked susceptibility to type 1 diabetes in non-obese diabetic mice. Diabetologia **47:** 739–747.

Long-Term Prevention of Diabetes and Marked Suppression of Insulin Autoantibodies and Insulitis in Mice Lacking Native Insulin B9–23 Sequence

M. NAKAYAMA, N. BABAYA, D. MIAO, R. GIANANI, E. LIU, J.F. ELLIOTT, AND G.S. EISENBARTH

Barbara Davis Center for Childhood Diabetes, University of Colorado Health Sciences Center, Aurora, Colorado 80045, USA
Alberta Diabetes Institute and MMI, University of Alberta, Edmonton, Alberta T6G 2H7, Canada

ABSTRACT: We analyzed double native insulin gene knockout NOD mice with a mutated (B16:alanine) proinsulin transgene at multiple ages for the development of insulin autoantibodies, insulitis, and diabetes. In contrast to mice with at least one copy of a native insulin gene that expressed insulin antibodies, only 2 out of 21 (10%) double native insulin gene knockout mice with a mutated insulin transgene developed insulin autoantibodies. Of 21 double insulin knockout mice sacrificed between 10 to 48 weeks of age, only 5 showed minimal insulitis versus 100% of wild-type NOD and more than 90% of insulin 1 knockout mice. Consistent with robust suppression of insulin autoantibodies and insulitis, no double insulin knockout mice developed diabetes. In that the B9–23 peptide with B16A is an altered peptide ligand inducing Th2 responses, we analyzed transfer of splenocytes into NOD.SCID mice. There was no evidence for regulatory T cells able to inhibit transfer of diabetes by diabetogenic NOD splenocytes. Insulin peptide B9–23 is likely a crucial target for initiation of islet autoimmunity and further mutation of the sequence will be tested to attempt to eliminate all anti-islet autoimmunity.

KEYWORDS: NOD mouse; insulin knockout; insulin B9–23 peptide; insulin autoantibodies

INTRODUCTION

Insulin is one of the major autoantigens of type 1A diabetes for both human and animal models, such as the NOD mouse.[1–3] There are several insulin epitopes reported to be targets of anti-islet autoreactive CD4 T cells (e.g., insulin

Address for correspondence: George S. Eisenbarth, Barbara Davis Center for Childhood Diabetes, University of Colorado Health Sciences Center, Mail Stop B-140, P.O. Box 6511, Aurora, CO 80045. Voice: 303-724-6842; fax: 303-724-6839.
e-mail: George.Eisenbarth@uchsc.edu

Ann. N.Y. Acad. Sci. 1079: 122–129 (2006). © 2006 New York Academy of Sciences.
doi: 10.1196/annals.1375.018

A chain amino acids 1–15 peptide, insulin B chain 9–23 peptide [insulin B9–23], and insulin B chain 24 to connecting peptide 36).[4–6] In NOD mice, the insulin peptide B9–23 has been a focus of study with T cells from islets recognizing insulin B9–23 (both insulin B9–16 and insulin B13–23 sequences for CD4 T cells) and insulin B15–23 peptide (CD8 T cells).[5,7,8]

Mice have two insulin genes: preproinsulin 1 and preproinsulin 2. Insulin 1 differs by two amino acids from insulin 2 and the position 9 of the B chain is a serine for insulin 2 and proline in insulin 1. The knockout of each insulin gene results in opposite effects on development of diabetes. Namely, NOD mice lacking the preproinsulin 1 gene exhibit "normal" development of insulin autoantibodies (IAA) with delayed but progressive insulitis, but approximately 90% of mice are protected from diabetes.[9] On the other hand, knockout of the preproinsulin 2 gene results in acceleration of the development of diabetes and increased levels of insulin autoantibodies.[9,10] Recently, we reported that NOD mice lacking native insulin 1 and insulin 2 genes but bearing a mutated insulin transgene (B16:alanine) are strongly protected from anti-islet autoimmunity.[11] This double insulin knockout NOD mouse has only a mutated insulin that possesses alanine rather than tyrosine at position 16 of the insulin B chain. B16:alanine insulin retains insulin metabolic activity, but the peptide B9–23 with B16A does not stimulate proliferation of a series of NOD T cell clones, and is an altered peptide ligand of the B9–23 peptide.[12] In this article, we have prospectively analyzed over time a cohort of these knockout mice till 48 weeks of age.

METHODS

Mice

NOD mice with mutated preproinsulin (B16:A insulin) transgene and with or without insulin 1 and/or insulin 2 genes were established as previously described.[12,13] Briefly, insulin 1 and insulin 2 knockout NOD mice were established by breeding the original insulin knockouts kindly provided by J. Jami onto NOD/Bdc mice using speed congenic techniques.[9] B16:A insulin-transgenic NOD mice were produced by microinjection of mutated preproinsulin 2 (alanine rather than tyrosine at position 16 of B chain) cDNA constructs ligated to the pRIP7 (rat insulin 7) promotor directly into NOD fertilized oocytes and four different founder strains were established.[13] Insulin 1 knockout NOD mice, insulin 2 knockout NOD mice, and mutated preproinsulin (B16:A insulin)-transgenic mice are combined to obtain NOD mice with various insulin genotypes. Genotyping for the native insulin 1 and insulin 2 gene and mutated insulin transgene was performed using polymerase chain reaction (PCR) amplification as previously described.[13] Double insulin knockout NOD mice with mutated insulin transgene from two of the mutated B16:A insulin-transgenic founder strains (strain B and F) produced sufficient insulin to prevent metabolic diabetes and female mice with the transgene from these two strains were used for the study. Severe combined immunodeficient NOD mice (NOD.SCID) for the transfer experiment were purchased from The Jackson Laboratory. All mice were housed in a pathogen-free animal colony at Center for Comparative Medicine in University of Colorado Health Sciences Center with an approved protocol from the University of Colorado Health Sciences Center Animal Care and Use Committee.

Insulin Autoantibody (IAA) Assay

Mice were bled every 2 to 3 weeks between 8 to 26 weeks of age. IAA were measured with a 96-well filtration plate micro-IAA assay as previously described[14] and expressed as an index. A value of 0.01 or greater is considered positive.

Histology

The pancreata obtained from the mice were fixed in 10% formalin and paraffin embedded. Paraffin-embedded tissue sections were stained with hematoxylin and eosin. For the scoring of insulitis, each islet was scored as no infiltration, peri-islet infiltration, and intraislet infiltration by a reader blinded to the category of mice.

Diabetes

Glucose was measured weekly with the FreeStyle blood glucose monitoring system (TheraSense, Alameda, CA), and the mice are considered diabetic after two consecutive blood glucose values >250 mg/dL.

Diabetes Transfer to NOD.SCID Mice

Splenocytes (3×10^7) from diabetic NOD mice were injected intravenously to 8-week-old NOD.SCID mice along with splenocytes (3×10^7) from double insulin knockout NOD mice or regular NOD mice.

Statistics

The development of insulin autoantibodies and the presence of insulitis were analyzed with the Fisher's exact test. Survival curves were analyzed with the log rank test. Statistical tests used PRISM software (Graphpad, San Diego, CA).

RESULTS

Establishing Mice with Various Insulin Genotypes

We combined insulin 1 knockout, insulin 2 knockout, and mutated B16:A mutated insulin-transgenic mice, and obtained NOD mice lacking both insulin 1 and insulin 2 genes but with mutated insulin transgene (*ins1-, ins2-, mutated ins+*) along with NOD mice bearing both insulin 1 and insulin 2 genes with mutated insulin transgene (*ins1+, ins2+, mutated ins+*), insulin 1 but not insulin 2 gene with transgene (*ins1+, ins2-, mutated ins+*), and insulin 2 but not insulin 1 gene with transgene (*ins1-, ins2+, mutated ins+*).

Development of Insulin Autoantibodies

We tested 21 double insulin knockout NOD mice with mutated B16:A insulin transgene and their littermates with at least one copy of native insulin gene and the mutated B16:A insulin for the development of insulin autoantibodies. As shown in FIGURE 1, 87% of mice with insulin 1 and insulin 2 genes, 82% of mice with only the insulin 1 gene, and 49% of mice with only the insulin 2 gene developed insulin autoantibodies. In contrast, only 2 out of 21 double insulin knockout mice with mutated B16:A insulin transgene developed insulin autoantibodies and the peak value of insulin autoantibodies of both mice was low (note log scale of FIG. 1). The lack of native insulin significantly prevented the development of insulin autoantibodies for as long as the mice were followed ($P < 0.0001$, $P < 0.0001$, and $P < 0.01$ versus mice bearing both native insulin 1 and insulin 2 genes, only the insulin 1 gene, and only the insulin 2 gene, respectively).

Histological Analysis of Double Insulin Knockout Mice

We analyzed pancreas histology obtained from female mice between 10 and 48 weeks of age. A mouse was categorized as peri-insulitis if one or more islets had peri-islet lymphocytic infiltration but not intraislet infiltration, and insulitis if a mouse has at least one islet with intra-infiltration. As shown in FIGURE 2, all tested wild-type NOD mice bearing both native insulin 1 and insulin 2 genes had either peri-insulitis or insulitis and even 92% of insulin 1 knockout NOD mice (most of which are protected from the development of diabetes) developed peri-insulitis/insulitis. On the other hand, double insulin knockout NOD mice were strongly protected from the development of insulitis (5/26 with any peri-insulitis/insulitis, $P < 0.0001$ versus wild-type NOD or insulin 1 knockout NOD mice). In addition, even in the double insulin knockout mice with any insulitis, greater than 70% of islets had no infiltration, whereas

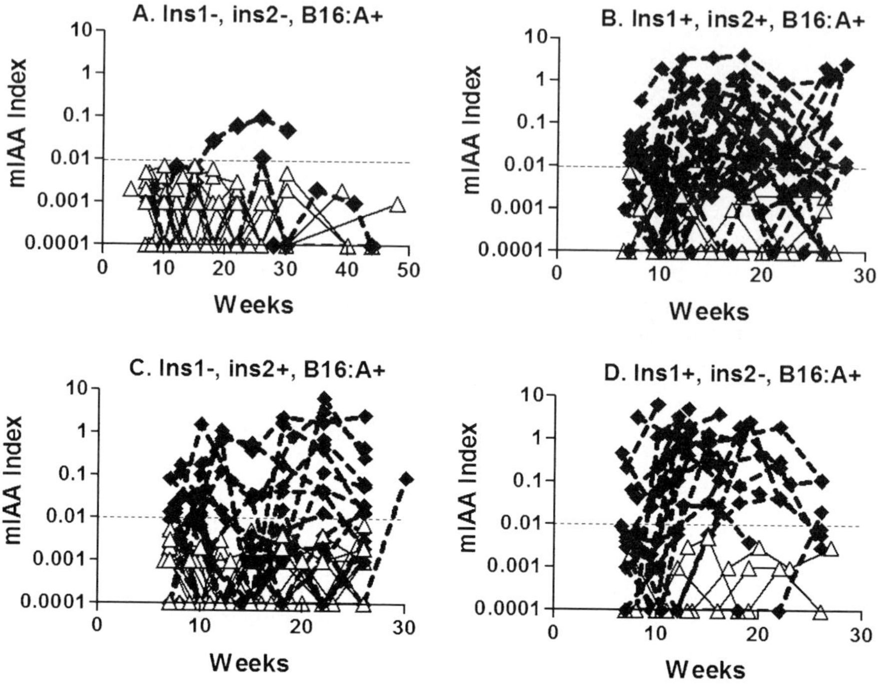

FIGURE 1. Each line represents sequential values over time for one mouse. Red dashed line represents mIAA (microinsulin autoantibodies) index of a mouse whose insulin autoantibodies were positive at least once (>0.010). Black solid line represents mIAA of a mouse whose insulin autoantibodies were always negative. Only 2 out of 21 mice lacking native insulin 1 and insulin 2 genes developed low level of insulin autoantibodies (*panel A*).

less than 20% of islets are free of infiltration in wild-type NOD mice and insulin 1 knockout mice. Consistent with robust suppression of insulitis, no double insulin knockout mouse has progressed to diabetes (FIG. 2 B).

No Evidence for Regulatory Splenocytes Inhibiting Transfer of Diabetes by NOD Splenocytes

The B16:A insulin 2 peptide can be recognized by NOD T cells as an "altered peptide ligand." To see whether double insulin knockout mice with mutated B16:A preproinsulin transgene have enhanced regulatory function, we tested whether splenocytes of double insulin knockout mice can prevent diabetes induced in NOD.SCID mice. Splenocytes of new onset diabetic NOD mice were transferred into NOD.SCID mice with and without splenocytes from the B16:A transgene double insulin knockout mice. No delay of diabetes transfer was observed (FIG. 2 C).

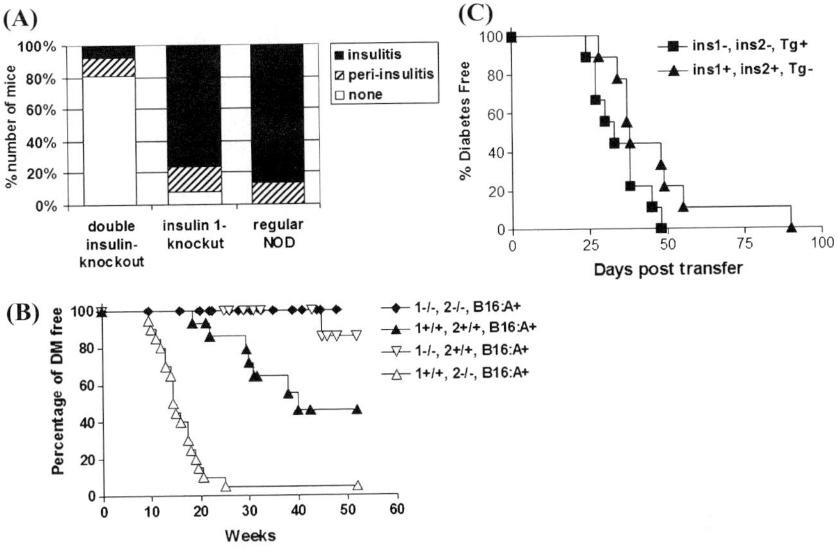

FIGURE 2. (**A**) The percentage of mice carrying insulitis. White, striped, and black column represents the percentage of mice with no insulitis, peri-insulitis, and insulitis, respectively. The percentage of double insulin knockout mice without any insulitis was significantly higher than that of insulin 1 knockout mice and regular NOD mice ($P < 0.0001$). (**B**) The development of diabetes of NOD mice with various insulin genotypes. NOD mice bearing both insulin 1 and insulin 2 plus the mutated B16:A insulin transgene gene (closed triangles, $n = 16$), only insulin 2 gene plus B16:A insulin (open inverted triangles, $n = 16$), only insulin 1 gene plus B16:A insulin (open triangles, $n = 20$), and mice lacking insulin 1 and insulin 2 gene plus B16:A insulin (closed diamonds, $n = 31$) were followed the development of diabetes. (**C**) No prevention of transferred diabetes in NOD.SCID mice by double insulin knockout splenocytes. NOD.SCID mice that received splenocytes from diabetic NOD mice along with splenocytes from double insulin knockout mice (square, $n = 9$) or regular NOD mice (triangle, $n = 9$) developed diabetes.

DISCUSSION

NOD mice lacking native insulin 1 and insulin 2 genes but with a mutated B16:A insulin transgene are strongly protected from the development of insulin autoantibodies, insulitis, and diabetes. NOD mice bearing at least one copy of native insulin 1 or 2 gene, with or without the mutated B16:A insulin transgene, develop diabetes and marked anti-islet autoimmunity. Insulin 2 is expressed within the thymus and islets, while insulin 1 is expressed only within the islets. Lack of thymic insulin 2 expression is probably related to acceleration of disease when native insulin 2 is absent and native insulin 1 is present. Transgene mutated B16:A insulin expression in thymus does not influence the development of diabetes of insulin 2 knockout NOD mice,[15] indicating that the altered B9–23 sequence in the thymus cannot replace the native insulin sequence.

With long-term follow-up, diabetes did not develop in mice lacking native insulin B:9–23 sequences. The presence of minimal insulitis in 5 out of 21 mice and insulin autoantibodies in 2 out of 21 mice lacking native insulin genes with only the B16:A insulin transgene is of interest. The insulin B9–23 mutation, B16:A, was chosen to retain insulin metabolic activity and to abrogate stimulation of proliferation of NOD anti-B:9–23 CD4 T cell clones.[12] The mutation changed but did not abrogate T cell responses to the B9–23 peptide in terms of cytokine secretion. This mutated insulin 2 B9–23 peptide, B16:A is an altered peptide ligand relative to the native sequence favoring Th2 responses.[12] Nevertheless, splenocytes from double insulin knockout NOD mice with B16:A insulin did not inhibit disease transfer consistent with the absence of enhanced T regulation inhibiting islet autoimmunity. We have recently developed NOD T cell receptor (BDC 12–4.1)-transgenic mice where the T cell receptor recognizes insulin peptide B9–23. We are testing the ability of such transgenic T cells to target double knockout islets with B16:A insulin. We hypothesize that the minimal insulitis of the double native insulin knockout with B16:alanine transgene results from decreased recognition of the mutated insulin. This hypothesis will be directly tested by generation of mice with additional B9–23 amino acid mutations, which cannot be even weakly recognized by B9–23 reactive NOD T cells.

ACKNOWLEDGMENT

This work was supported by grants from the NIH (DK55969, DK32083, DK62718, DK32493), Diabetes Endocrine Research Center (P30 DK57516), the American Diabetes Association, the Juvenile Diabetes Foundation, and the Children's Diabetes Foundation. M.N. was supported by a fellowship from the Juvenile Diabetes Foundation and has been awarded an advanced fellowship from the Juvenile Diabetes Foundation.

REFERENCES

1. Wegmann, D.R., M. Norbury-Glaser & D. Daniel. 1994. Insulin-specific T cells are a predominant component of islet infiltrates in pre-diabetic NOD mice. Eur. J. Immunol. **24:** 1853–1857.
2. Pugliese, A., M. Zeller, A. Fernandez Jr., *et al.* 1997. The insulin gene is transcribed in the human thymus and transcription levels correlated with allelic variation at the INS VNTR-IDDM2 susceptibility locus for type 1 diabetes. Nat. Genet. **15:** 293–297.
3. Jaeckel, E., M.A. Lipes & H. von Boehmer 2005. Recessive tolerance to preproinsulin 2 reduces but does not abolish type 1 diabetes. Nat. Immunol. **5:** 1028–1035.
4. Kent, S.C., Y. Chen, L. Bregoli, *et al.* 2005. Expanded T cells from pancreatic lymph nodes of type 1 diabetic subjects recognize an insulin epitope. Nature **435:** 224–228.

5. DANIEL, D., R.G. GILL, N. SCHLOOT & D. WEGMANN. 1995. Epitope specificity, cytokine production profile and diabetogenic activity of insulin-specific T cell clones isolated from NOD mice. Eur.J. Immunol. **25:** 1056–1062.
6. CHEN, W., I. BERGEROT, J.F. ELLIOTT, *et al.* 2001. Evidence that a peptide spanning the B-C junction of proinsulin is an early autoantigen epitope in the pathogenesis of type 1 diabetes. J. Immunol. **167:** 4926–4935.
7. ABIRU, N., D. WEGMANN, E. KAWASAKI, *et al.* 2000. Dual overlapping peptides recognized by insulin peptide B:9–23 T cell receptor AV13S3 T cell clones of the NOD mouse. J. Autoimmun. **14:** 231–237.
8. WONG, F.S., J. KARTTUNEN, C. DUMONT, *et al.* 1999. Identification of an MHC class I-restricted autoantigen in type 1 diabetes by screening an organ-specific cDNA library. Nat. Med. **5:** 1026–1031.
9. MORIYAMA, H., N. ABIRU, J. PARONEN, *et al.* 2003. Evidence for a primary islet autoantigen (preproinsulin 1) for insulitis and diabetes in the nonobese diabetic mouse. Proc. Natl. Acad. Sci. USA **100:** 10376–10381.
10. THÉBAULT-BAUMONT, K., D. DUBOIS-LAFORGUE, P. KRIEF, *et al.* 2003. Acceleration of type 1 diabetes mellitus in proinsulin 2–deficient NOD mice. J. Clin. Invest. **111:** 851–857.
11. NAKAYAMA, M., N. ABIRU, H. MORIYAMA, *et al.* 2005. Prime role for an insulin epitope in the development of type 1 diabetes in NOD mice. Nature **435:** 220–223.
12. ALLEVA, D.G., A. GAUR, L. JIN, *et al.* 2002. Immunological characterization and therapeutic activity of an altered-peptide ligand, NBI-6024, based on the immunodominant type 1 diabetes autoantigen insulin B-chain (9–23) peptide. Diabetes **51:** 2126–2134.
13. NAKAYAMA, M., H. MORIYAMA, N. ABIRU, *et al.* 2004. Establishment of native insulin-negative NOD mice and the methodology to distinguish specific insulin knockout genotypes and a B:16 alanine preproinsulin transgene. Ann. N. Y. Acad. Sci. 1037: 193–198.
14. YU, L., D.T. ROBLES, N. ABIRU, *et al.* 2000. Early expression of antiinsulin autoantibodies of humans and the NOD mouse: evidence for early determination of subsequent diabetes. Proc. Natl. Acad. Sci. USA **97:** 1701–1706.
15. NAKAYAMA, M., N. BABAYA, D. MIAO, *et al.* 2005. Thymic expression of mutated B16:A preproinsulin messenger RNA does not reverse acceleration of NOD diabetes associated with insulin 2 (thymic expressed insulin) knockout. J. Autoimmun. **25:** 193–198.

Eicosanoid Imbalance in the NOD Mouse Is Related to a Dysregulation in Soluble Epoxide Hydrolase and 15-PGDH Expression

MICHELLE RODRIGUEZ AND MICHAEL CLARE-SALZLER

Department of Pathology, Immunology, and Laboratory Medicine, College of Medicine, University of Florida, Gainesville Florida 32610, USA

ABSTRACT: Eicosanoids promote or resolve inflammation depending on the class produced. Macrophage from nonobese diabetic (NOD) mouse produce increased proinflammatory lipid mediators and low levels of antiinflammatory lipoxin A4 (LXA4). The enhanced proinflammatory eicosanoids is secondary to increased cyclooxygenase-2 (Cox-2) expression and low levels of prostaglandin/leukotriene catabolic enzyme, 15-hydroxyprostaglandin dehydrogenase (15-PGDH). Deficient LXA4 production is not due to deficient lipoxygenase (LO) activity, but is related to increased soluble epoxide hydrolase (sEH), involved in metabolism of anti-inflammatory epoxyeicosatrienoic acids (EET). These aberrations in eicosanoid biology suggest that inflammation in the NOD mouse is likely to be prolonged and robust and may contribute to type 1 diabetes (T1D) pathogenesis.

KEYWORDS: epoxide hydrolase; 15-PGDH; lipoxin A4; inflammation; type 1 diabetes; eicosanoids

INTRODUCTION

The regulation of inflammatory and anti-inflammatory eicosanoids is complex and involves several enzyme systems and lipid intermediates. Cyclooxygenase-2 (Cox-2) is induced during inflammation and leads to high-level production of inflammatory prostaglandins and thromboxane.[1] Leukotriene biosynthesis is initiated by the enzyme 5-lipoxygenase (LO), which converts arachidonic acid (AA) to highly proinflammatory mediator, leukotriene B4 (LTB4), while 15-LO is responsible for production of 15-hydroxyeicosatetraenoic acid (15-HETE).[2] Lipoxin A4 (LXA4), is

Address for correspondence: Michelle Rodriguez, Department of Pathology, Immunology, and Laboratory Medicine, College of Medicine, University of Florida, 1600 SW Archer Road No. D11-41, Gainesville, FL 32610. Voice: 352-392-4887; fax: 352-392-5393.
e-mail: rodrigm@pathology.ufl.edu

Ann. N.Y. Acad. Sci. 1079: 130–134 (2006). © 2006 New York Academy of Sciences.
doi: 10.1196/annals.1375.019

generated from AA via sequential actions of 5-, and 15-LO and is a potent anti-inflammatory eicosanoid that acts to promote resolution of inflammation.[2] Other enzyme systems are involved in eicosanoid breakdown, such as 15-hydroxyprostaglandin dehydrogenase (15-PGDH) enzyme which catabolizes prostaglandin E-2 (PGE-2), LTB4, and also converts LXA4 to inactive oxo- and dihydro products.[3] A critical lipid mediator pathway still relatively unexplored is the cytochrome P450 epoxygenases. These enzymes are responsible for the production of epoxyeicosatrienoic acids (EET), which are derived from AA and possess anti-inflammatory activity.[4] Previous work demonstrated that 14,15 EET inhibits PGE-2 production via suppression of Cox-2 activity.[5] Interestingly, the soluble epoxide hydrolase (sEH) transforms EETs into their corresponding diols (DHET),[5] which have limited anti-inflammatory activity. Moreover, sEH inhibitors promote the formation of both EETs and LXA4, thus supporting inflammatory resolution.[6]

Previous studies in type 1 diabetes (T1D) demonstrated increased Cox-2 expression in subjects with or at risk for T1D and in macrophages from nonobese diabetic (NOD) mouse, leading to enhanced inflammatory responses.[7] Additionally, products of the LO metabolism, such as LTB4, are also increased in the NOD mouse.[8] We have also recently found a relative deficiency in the production of anti-inflammatory LXA4 in this same model. The expression of 15-PGDH and sEH, however, has not been examined. In this article we demonstrate that macrophages from NOD mouse express heightened levels of sEH in combination with decreased expression of 15-PGDH which together, may limit anti-inflammatory LXA4 production and enhance inflammatory lipid mediators, respectively, and thus promote inflammation and perhaps T1D pathogenesis.

METHODS

Cell Culture and Eicosanoid Analysis

Bone marrow cells from NOD/LtJ and C57BL/6 were isolated from femur and tibia by standard procedures. Cells were cultured in enriched RPMI 1640 at a concentration of 1.75×10^6/mL in the presence of M-CSF for 4 days. Supernatants were assayed for PGE-2, and LTB4 using commercially available kits from Amersham Biosciences (Pittsburgh, PA). ELISA kits for LXA4 were obtained from Cayman Chemical (Ann Arbor, MI).

RNA Quantification by PCR

Macrophages received lipopolysaccharide (LPS) (1 μg/mL) challenge for 12 h. The RNeasy® Mini Kit (QIAgen, Valencia, CA) was used for the ex-

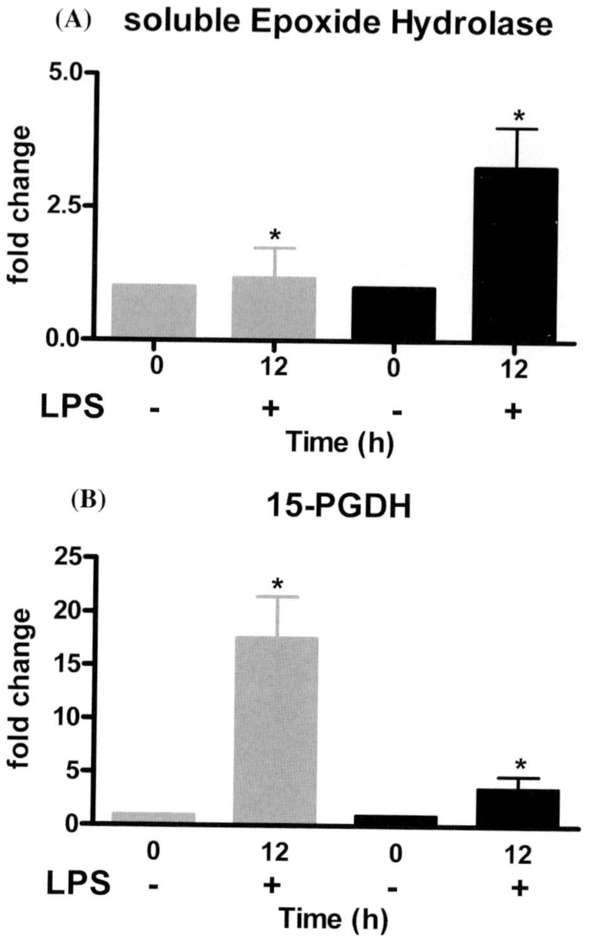

FIGURE 1. (**A**) and (**B**) Quantitation of soluble sEH, and 15-PGDH by reverse transciption polymerase chain reaction (RT-PCR) from bone marrow-derived macrophages from C57BL/6 (gray bars) and NOD/LtJ (black bars). Data is a mean ± SEM of at least three independent experiments. The data were analyzed by two-tailed Student's *t*-test. $P < 0.05$ was considered statistically significant. $^*P < 0.05$.

traction of total RNA from cell pellets. A total of 0.4 μg total RNA concentration was measured with the Jenway 6305 spectrophotometer (Model 6305 UV/Visible range spectrophotometer [190–1000 nm]; Barloworld Scientific Ltd. T/AS, Jenway, England). cDNA was obtained using the TaqMan® Reverse Transcription Kit (Applied Biosystems, Foster City, CA). For the TaqMan® assay the TaqMan® Universal PCR Master Mix Kit (Applied Biosystems) was used. The probe was labelled with the 5′ reporter dye 6-carboxyfluorescein (FAM). β-Actin was used as internal control. The reactions were run on the

ABI PRISM^{TM} 7700 Sequence Detection System (Applied Biosystems). The amplification program was: 50°C for 2min, 95°C for 10 min, followed by 45 cycles of 95°C for 15 s, 60°C for 1 min.

RESULTS AND CONCLUSIONS

Our previous studies and those of others demonstrated increased PGE-2 and LTB4 production with a relative deficiency in LXA4. We found markedly reduced levels of 15-PGDH (FIG. 1 A) in macrophages from NOD mice in comparison to C57BL/6. This is significant because 15-PGDH is the key enzyme responsible for metabolic inactivation of PGE-2, LTB4, and LXA4. Despite low levels of 15-PGDH, the production of LXA4 is still limited in the NOD mouse suggesting that LXA4 deficiencies are not secondary to increased 15-PGDH. However, quantitation of sEH showed increased mRNA expression in macrophages from NOD mouse, which would result in enhanced metabolism of anti-inflammatory EET, for example, 14,15 EET, to less active products (FIG. 1 B), thus failing to suppress COX-2 activity, and allowing for increased PGE-2 production as reported. Interestingly, limited LXA4 production was overcome by *in vitro* administration of a specific sEH inhibitor. Although not determined, this inhibitor would also increase anti-inflammatory EETs. Taken together, these results suggest the combinatorial effect of sustained expression of sEH, with decreased expression of 15-PGDH contributes to limited LXA4 synthesis and elevated levels of PGE2, and LTB4, respectively. These defects would therefore sustain the enhanced or prolonged inflammatory responses and potentially contribute to islet inflammation. Further studies are needed to determine whether treatment with selective sEH inhibitors and or replacement of LXA4 with stable analogues alters T1D.

REFERENCES

1. FITZPATRICK, F.A. 2004. Cyclooxygenase enzymes: regulation and function. Curr. Pharm. Des. **10:** 577–588.
2. NASSAR, G.M. & K.F. BADR. 1995. Role of leukotrienes and lipoxygenases in glomerular injury. Miner. Electrolyte Metab. **21:** 262–270.
3. CLISH, C.B., B.D. LEVY, *et al.* 2000. Oxidoreductases in lipoxin A4 metabolic inactivation: a novel role for 15-onoprostaglandin 13-reductase/leukotriene B4 12-hydroxydehydrogenase in inflammation. J. Biol. Chem. **275:** 25372–25380.
4. NODE, K., Y. HUO, *et al.* 1999. Anti-inflammatory properties of cytochrome P450 epoxygenase-derived eicosanoids. Science **285:** 1276–1279.
5. SPECTOR, A.A., X. FANG, *et al.* 2004. Epoxyeicosatrienoic acids (EETs): metabolism and biochemical function. Prog. Lipid Res. **43:** 55–90.
6. SCHMELZER, K.R., L. KUBALA, *et al.* 2005. Soluble epoxide hydrolase is a therapeutic target for acute inflammation. Proc. Natl. Acad. Sci. USA.

102: 9772–9777. Available at http://www.ncbi.nlm.nih.gov/entrez/query.fcgi?db=pubmed&cmd=Search&term=%22Nicolaou±KC%22%5BAuthor%5D.

7. LITHERLAND, S., T. XIE, *et al.* 2000. Aberrant prostaglandin synthase 2 expression defines an antigen-presenting cell defect for insulin-dependent diabetes mellitus. J. Clin. Invest. **104:** 515-523.
8. LETY, M.A., J. COULAUD, *et al.* 1992. Enhanced metabolism of arachidonic acid by macrophages from nonobese diabetic (NOD) mice. Clin. Immunol. Immunopathol. **64:** 188–196.

Pancreatic Autoimmunity Induction with Insulin B:9–23 Peptide and Viral Mimics in the NZB Mouse

DEVASENAN DEVENDRA,[a,b] DONGMEI MIAO,[a] MAKI NAKAYAMA,[a] GEORGE S. EISENBARTH,[a] AND EDWIN LIU[a]

[a]*Barbara Davis Center for Childhood Diabetes, University of Colorado Health Sciences Center, Aurora, Colorado 80010, USA*

[b]*Imperial College School of Medicine, London NW10 7NS, UK*

ABSTRACT: To create a new experimental model of diabetes, we used the New Zealand Black (NZB) mouse as a potential model. NZB mice were immunized with B:9–23 insulin peptide in IFA and the viral mimic, poly(A:U). No diabetes was observed but blood glucose was significantly higher in the B:9–23 peptide group compared to controls. Insulin autoantibodies (IAA) were only induced in groups given the B:9–23 peptide. B:9–23 alone induced peri-insulitis. We demonstrate insulin autoimmunity in the NZB mouse using the insulin peptide B:9–23 and viral mimics. The reason for the protection from diabetes despite the presence of autoimmunity is currently not established.

KEYWORDS: viral mimic; autoimmunity; diabetes; NZB; insulin B:9–23

INTRODUCTION

Type 1 diabetes results from T cell-mediated destruction of β cells of the pancreas with evidence of islet-specific autoimmunity.[1] Autoimmune mouse strains provide well-characterized models for the study of human autoimmune diseases. The New Zealand Black (NZB) mouse has an interferon-inducible gene (*Ifi202*) that acts as an immune response gene that influences antigen-driven B cell responses to self and possibly exogenous antigens.[2] Based on prior success with insulitis induction with insulin peptide B:9–23 and poly(I:C) in the Balb/c mouse,[3] we hypothesized that the NZB mouse would be more susceptible to develop autoimmune diabetes.

Address for correspondence: Dr. Edwin Liu, Barbara Davis Center for Childhood Diabetes, P.O. Box 6511, Mail Stop B140, Aurora, CO 80010. Voice: +1-303-724-6851; fax: +1-303-724-6839.
e-mail: Edwin.liu@UCHSC.edu

Ann. N.Y. Acad. Sci. 1079: 135–137 (2006).
doi: 10.1196/annals.1375.020

MATERIALS AND METHODS

NZB/BinJ female mice (Jackson Laboratories, Bar Harbor, Maine) were housed in a pathogen-free animal colony at the Barbara Davis Center for Childhood Diabetes with approved protocols from the University of Colorado Health Sciences Center Animal Care and Use Committee. B:9–23 insulin or TT peptide (100 μg/mouse) (SynPep Corporation, Dublin, CA) in incomplete Freund's adjuvant (IFA) was given subcutaneously (sq) once at 4 and 16 weeks of age. Additionally poly(A:U) (Sigma, St. Louis, MO) was administered intraperitoneally (i.p.), on days 1–5 and 8–14 (starting at 4 weeks of age) at a concentration of 7.5 μg/g body weight. Pancreata was microscopically examined at 16, 18, 30, and 32 weeks of age. Insulin autoantibody (IAA) expression was measured with the micro IAA assay[4] and a value of 0.01 or greater is considered positive.

RESULTS

TABLE 1 summarizes the major outcome of the study in the NZB mice. There were no detected cases of diabetes in all the groups of mice that were followed up to the age of 32 weeks. However, the group of mice given insulin peptide B:9–23 peptide alone had higher mean peak blood glucose levels when compared to TT peptide immunized mice (164 mg/dL versus 98 mg/dL, $P < 0.01$). Insulin peptide B:9–23 + poly(A:U) induced an even higher mean peak blood glucose level 171 mg/dL. Mice given B:9–23 + poly(A:U), induced high and persistent IAA. At 18 weeks of age, marked (peri)insulitis is observed in all the groups given B:9–23 insulin peptide only. However, insulitis almost disappeared when the islets were inspected at 32 weeks of age.

CONCLUSION

In conclusion, we demonstrate that the insulin B:9–23 peptide alone is able to induce a transient hyperglycemia, IAA, and insulitis in NZB mice. We are

TABLE 1. Summary of the findings using B:9–23 insulin peptide and viral mimic in the NZB mice. Mean peak glucose (mg/dL), mean glucose (mg/dL) levels at 20 weeks and mean peak IAA levels (index >0.01 considered positive)

	B:9–23 only	TT only	B:9–23 + p(A:U)	TT + p(A:U)
Number	10	10	10	10
Mean peak glucose	164 (21)	98 (17)	171 (28)	113 (22)
Median glucose at 20 weeks	144 (26)	96 (12)	162 (24)	104 (16)
Mean peak IAA levels	0.14 (0.04)	<0.01	1.38 (0.12)	<0.01

Values in brackets represent Standard Error of the mean.
TT = tetanus toxoid peptide, p(A:U) = poly A:U.

uncertain of the mechanisms accounting for the protection from diabetes in the NZB mice despite the presence of insulitis and IAA. We speculate that the NZB mice may have the potential to abrogate progressive islet autoimmunity despite initial activation.

ACKNOWLEDGMENTS

Research supported by grants from the NIH (DK 3202, DK 055969, DK 062718, AI 055466), Autoimmunity Prevention Center U19 (AI 050864), Diabetes Endocrine Research Center (P30 DK57516), the American Diabetes Association, the Juvenile Diabetes Foundation, and the Children's Diabetes Foundation. DD is supported by an Eli Lilly fellowship award and EL is supported by a NIH grant (DK 06405).

REFERENCES

1. ATKINSON, M.A. & N.K. MACLAREN. 1994. The pathogenesis of insulin-dependent diabetes mellitus. N. Engl. J. Med. **331:** 1428–1436.
2. ROZZO, S.J., J.D. ALLARD, D. CHOUBEY, *et al.* 2001. Evidence for an interferon-inducible gene, Ifi202, in the susceptibility to systemic lupus. Immunity **15:** 435–443.
3. MORIYAMA, H., L. WEN, N. ABIRU, *et al.* 2002. Induction and acceleration of insulitis/diabetes in mice with a viral mimic (polyinosinic-polycytidylic acid) and an insulin self-peptide. Proc. Natl. Acad. Sci. USA **99:** 5539–5544.
4. YU, L., D.T. ROBLES, N. ABIRU, *et al.* 2000. Early expression of anti-insulin autoantibodies of man and the NOD mouse: evidence for early determination of subsequent diabetes. Proc. Natl. Acad. Sci. USA **97:** 1701–1706.

Viruses Cause Type 1 Diabetes in Animals

JI-WON YOON AND HEE-SOOK JUN

Rosalind Franklin Comprehensive Diabetes Center, Chicago Medical School, North Chicago, Illinois 60064, USA

ABSTRACT: More than 10 viruses have been reported to be associated with the development of type 1 diabetes-like symptoms in animals, with the best evidence coming from studies on the D variant of encephalomyocarditis (EMC-D) virus in mice and Kilham rat virus (KRV) in rats. A high titer of EMC-D viral infection results in the development of diabetes within 3 days, primarily due to the rapid destruction of β cells by viral replication within the cells. A low titer of EMC-D viral infection results in the recruitment of macrophages to the islets. Soluble mediators produced by activated macrophages play a critical role in the destruction of residual β cells. A single amino acid at position 776 of the EMC viral genome controls the diabetogenicity of the virus. In contrast, KRV causes autoimmune type 1 diabetes in diabetes-resistant BioBreeding (DR-BB) rats without direct infection of β cells. Macrophages play an important role in the development of diabetes in KRV-infected DR-BB rats. As well, KRV infection preferentially activates effector T cells, such as Th1-like $CD45RC^+CD4^+$ T cells and $CD8^+$ T cells, and downregulates regulatory T cells, such as Th2-like $CD45RC^-CD4^+$ T cells. This results in the breakdown of the immune balance, contributing to the development of diabetes in KRV-infected DR-BB rats.

KEYWORDS: type 1 diabetes; Kilham rat virus; encephalomyocarditis virus; macrophages; T cells; cytokines; pancreatic β cells

INTRODUCTION

Over the last several decades, at least 10 viruses have been reported to be associated with the development of type 1 diabetes-like syndromes in animals. These viruses are coxsackie B viruses in mice and/or nonhuman primates, encephalomyocarditis (EMC) virus in mice, mengo virus in mice, foot-and-mouth disease virus in pigs and/or cattle, retrovirus in mice, rubella virus in hamsters and rabbits, bovine viral diarrhea-mucosal disease virus in cattle, reovirus in mice, Kilham rat virus (KRV) in rats, and cytomegalovirus in the

Address for correspondence: Hee-Sook Jun, Rosalind Franklin Comprehensive Diabetes Center, Chicago Medical School, North Chicago, IL 60064. Voice: 847-578-8341; fax: 847-578-3432.
e-mail: hee-sook.jeon@rosalindfranklin.edu

**Ann. N.Y. Acad. Sci. 1079: 138–146 (2006). © 2006 New York Academy of Sciences.
doi: 10.1196/annals.1375.021**

TABLE 1. Viruses associated with the development of type 1 diabetes in animals

Virus type	Virus	Host	Involvement of genetic factors
RNA viruses	Coxsackie B virus	Mice, nonhuman primates	Yes
	Encephalomyocarditis virus	Mice	Yes
	Mengo virus	Mice	Yes
	Foot-and-mouth disease virus	Pigs, cattle	Not determined
	Retrovirus	Mice	Yes
	Rubella virus	Hamsters, rabbits	Not determined
	Bovine viral diarrhea-mucosal disease virus	Cattle	Not determined
	Reovirus	Mice	Yes
DNA viruses	Kilham rat virus	Rats	Yes
	Cytomegalovirus	Degu	Not determined

Degu (TABLE 1).[1] Among those viruses, the most clear and unequivocal evidence that a virus induces type 1 diabetes in animals comes from studies on EMC virus in mice[2] and KRV in rats.[3] EMC virus is considered to be a primary agent that is selectively injurious to pancreatic β cells, whereas KRV is considered to be a triggering agent of β cell-specific autoimmunity without infection of β cells. In this brief article, we will focus on these two models of virus-induced diabetes.

EMC Virus-Induced Diabetes in Mice

EMC virus is a picornavirus with naked, single-stranded RNA and a genome size of about 7.8 kB. The capsid comprises four polypeptides; VP1, VP2, VP3, and VP4. EMC virus selectively infects pancreatic β cells and has been the most thoroughly studied diabetogenic virus in animals. When genetically susceptible animals were infected with the M variant of EMC virus, diabetes was inconsistently induced.[4,5] Plaque purification of the M variant found two stable variants, EMC-D and EMC-B, that could not be antigenically distinguished by plaque neutralization assay, competitive radioimmunoassay, or molecular hybridization studies with radiolabeled DNA complementary to EMC-D and EMC-B RNAs. Nevertheless, the EMC-D virus produced type 1 diabetes in over 90% of infected animals, whereas mice inoculated with EMC-B virus did not acquire diabetes.[6,7]

Nucleotide sequence analysis showed that EMC-D virus (7829 bases) differs from EMC-B virus (7825 bases) by only 14 nucleotides: two deletions totaling 5 nucleotides, 1 base insertion, and 8 point mutations.[8] The first deletion of 3 nucleotides and the second deletion of 2 nucleotides are located in the 5′-poly(C) tract and the 3′-end polyadenylation site, respectively. One base insertion in EMC-B occurs in the 5′-noncoding region. The 8 point mutations are located in the polyprotein coding region. Two of these are silent, whereas the remaining 6 mutations, 1 located on the L gene and 5 on the VP1 gene, result in amino acid changes. Further studies of 21 different nondiabetogenic and 15 different diabetogenic viruses derived from stocks of the EMC-B and EMC-D variants revealed that only the 776th amino acid, alanine (Ala-776), of the EMC virus polyprotein, located on the major capsid protein VP1, is common to all diabetogenic variants. In contrast, threonine in this position (Thr-776) is common to all nondiabetogenic variants.[9]

Point mutation at nucleotide position 3155 to substitute Ala-776 (GCC) with various other amino acids, including threonine (ACC), serine (TCC), proline (CCC), aspartic acid (GAC), or valine (GTC), resulted in the loss of diabetogenicity.[10] Three-dimensional molecular modeling of the VP1 protein showed greater van der Waals interactions and closer packing of residues surrounding position 776 of the EMC virus polyprotein in viruses that contained Thr-776 than viruses that contained Ala-776. This results in more accessible surface areas surrounding Ala-776, which increases the number of binding sites for viral attachment to β cell receptors and promotes viral infection, the destruction of β cells, and subsequently the development of type 1 diabetes.[11]

The genetic background of the host also influences the diabetogenicity of EMC-D virus, as only certain inbred strains of mice develop diabetes when infected. Susceptibility to EMC-D virus appears to be determined by a single autosomal recessive gene,[12] which may operate by modulating the levels of the expression of viral receptors on β cells.

Infection of genetically susceptible mouse strains with a high dose (5×10^5 plaque-forming units/mouse) of EMC-D virus results in the development of diabetes within 3–4 days. Several lines of evidence show that the development of diabetes in high-dose EMC-D virus-infected mice is mainly due to the acute destruction of β cells by viral replication within the cells,[5] rather than to involvement of the immune system. Treatment of EMC-D virus-infected mice with anti-L3T4 (anti-CD4) antibody and/or anti-Lyt2 (anti-CD8) antibody did not alter the incidence of diabetes.[13] In addition, athymic nude mice, which lack functional lymphocytes, had an incidence of diabetes similar to their heterozygous littermates when infected with EMC-D virus, indicating that T cells do not play a significant role in the destruction of β cells by a high dose of EMC-D virus.

Natural viral infections in animals and man generally involve exposure to relatively low numbers of virus, rather than the high viral titers used in the experiments described above. Thus, studies were conducted in mice infected with a low dose (50–100 plaque-forming units/mouse) of EMC-D virus.[14] In contrast to the situation in high-dose-infected mice, it was found that the immune system, especially macrophages, plays a central role in the destruction of pancreatic β cells in mice infected with a low dose of EMC-D virus. Activation of macrophages prior to viral infection resulted in a significant increase in the incidence of diabetes, whereas inactivation of macrophages prior to viral infection completely prevented EMC-D virus-induced diabetes.[14] Further studies showed that exposure to a low dose of EMC-D virus resulted in initial, selective infection of pancreatic β cells and recruitment of macrophages into the islets, followed by infiltration of other immunocytes including T cells, natural killer cells, and B cells.[15] In this situation, replication of the virus within the β cells plays a minor role in β cell destruction, whereas the cascade of events initiated by macrophages causes most of the β cell damage.[16]

To elucidate the mechanisms by which macrophages trigger β cell destruction in mice infected with a low dose of EMC-D virus, several studies examined the role of macrophage-derived soluble mediators, such as interleukin-1β (IL-1β), tumor necrosis factor-α (TNF-α), and nitric oxide (NO). The expression of IL-1β, TNF-α, and inducible nitric oxide synthase (iNOS) was detected in the pancreatic islets of mice infected with a low dose of EMC-D virus, and inhibition of these molecules resulted in a significant decrease in the incidence of diabetes.[17] However, the molecular mechanism involved in the destruction of β cells by these soluble mediators is not known. IL-1β induces apoptosis through the induction of iNOS expression and NO production in rat islet cells.[18] Therefore, IL-1β and TNF-α, produced by activated macrophages in the pancreatic islets after the infection of mice with a low dose of EMC-D virus, may induce iNOS expression and NO production and contribute to β cell death through apoptosis. Infection of macrophages isolated from DBA/2 mice with EMC-D virus induced a significant expression of iNOS and a high level of NO production.[19] Further experiments showed that a tyrosine kinase signaling pathway is clearly involved in the EMC-D virus-induced activation of macrophages, since inactivation of tyrosine kinase activity by treatment of EMC-D virus-infected mice with a tyrosine kinase inhibitor, tyrphostin AG126, prevented macrophage activation, resulting in the protection from β cell destruction.[19] Studies that examined the role of various tyrosine kinase families in EMC-D virus-induced macrophage activation revealed that the Src family of kinases, $p59/p56^{hck}$, plays a major role in the activation of macrophages, which subsequently produce IL-1β, TNF-α, and NO, leading to the destruction of pancreatic β cells.[20]

On the basis of these observations, it appears that infection of genetically susceptible strains of mice with EMC-D virus initially results in the replication of the virus in pancreatic β cells and recruitment of macrophages that are activated by the EMC-D virus into the pancreatic islets. These activated macrophages produce soluble mediators, such as IL-1β, TNF-α, and NO in the islets, which induce apoptosis in the β cells. The tyrosine kinase signaling pathway, particularly the Src family of kinases, $p59/p56^{hck}$, play a major role in the activation of macrophages, resulting in the production of IL-1β, TNF-α, and NO, leading to the destruction of β cells and subsequent development of diabetes in mice.

KRV-Induced Diabetes in Rats

KRV is a small DNA parvovirus that causes diabetes by inducing autoimmune responses against the β cell, rather than by direct β cell cytolysis, in diabetes-resistant BioBreeding (DR-BB) rats. These rats are derived from diabetes-prone progenitors, but do not normally develop the disease. When infected with KRV at 3 weeks of age, about 30% of DR-BB rats develop autoimmune diabetes within 2–4 weeks and a further 30% show insulitis without diabetes.[3] However, the incidence of diabetes can be increased to 80–100% if DR-BB rats are injected with poly (I:C) along with KRV.[3] It was later found that activation of the innate immune system through toll-like receptor (TLR) plays a crucial role in KRV-induced diabetes.[21]

KRV infects lymphoid organs, such as the spleen, thymus, and lymph nodes, but not β cells. The mechanisms by which KRV causes the destruction of β cells in DR-BB rats without infection are unclear. Macrophages appear to play an important role in KRV-induced diabetes in DR-BB rats. The production of macrophage-derived proinflammatory cytokines, such as TNF-α, IL-1β, and IL-12 was closely correlated with an elevated Th1 immune response in KRV-infected DR-BB rats.[22] Further studies found that NO produced from activated macrophages played a critical role in the regulation of immune responses, such as the upregulation of the Th1 immune response and activation of β cell-specific cytotoxic T lymphocytes, resulting in the development of autoimmune diabetes in KRV-infected DR-BB rats.[23]

The presence of a common epitope between a KRV-specific peptide and a β cell autoantigen, so-called "molecular mimicry," has been suggested as a mechanism for the initiation of β cell-specific autoimmune diabetes.[3,22] If this is the case, then KRV antigen-specific T cells generated by KRV peptides might cross-react with β cells and attack them, resulting in the development of insulitis and, subsequently, diabetes. However, experimental data showed that infection of DR-BB rats with recombinant vaccinia viruses expressing the KRV capsid proteins or nonstructural proteins did not cause insulitis or diabetes, even though each viral peptide was clearly expressed in the infected DR-BB rats, viral peptide-specific T cells were generated, and antibodies against the KRV peptides were induced.[24] This result suggests that molecular mimicry between KRV peptides and β cell-specific autoantigens in DR-BB rats is unlikely to be a mechanism by which KRV induces β cell-specific autoimmune diabetes.

An alternative hypothesis is that KRV infection disturbs the finely tuned immune balance and activates autoreactive T cells that are cytotoxic to β cells, resulting in T cells-mediated autoimmune diabetes similar to that seen in diabetes-prone BioBreeding (DP-BB) rats. Several observations support this hypothesis. In DR-BB rats infected with KRV, the absolute number of both $CD4^+$ and $CD8^+$ T cells in splenocytes increased, however, the proportion of $CD4^+$ T cells in splenocytes decreased, whereas the proportion of $CD8^+$ T cells increased as a result of preferential proliferation of $CD8^+$ T cells. In addition, treatment of KRV-infected DR-BB rats with OX-8 (anti-CD8) monoclonal antibody decreased the incidence of diabetes.[22] These results indicate that $CD8^+$ T cells are clearly involved in the destruction of β cells.

In the rat, $CD4^+$ T cells can be divided into Th1-like $CD45RC^+CD4^+$ T cells, which express IL-2 and interferon-γ (IFN-γ) and play an important role in cell-mediated immune responses, and Th2-like $CD45RC^-CD4^+$ T cells, which express IL-4 and IL-10 and play an important part in humoral immune responses.[25] It has been suggested that dominance of Th1 cells over Th2 cells is associated with the development of autoimmune type 1 diabetes, whereas the dominance of Th2 cells over Th1 cells is associated with the prevention of type 1 diabetes.[26] KRV infection in DR-BB rats significantly decreased the number of Th2-like $CD45RC^-CD4^+$ T cells and increased the number of Th1-like $CD45RC^+CD4^+$ T cells as compared with uninfected controls.[24] Furthermore, adoptive transfer of both Th1-like $CD45RC^+CD4^+$ T cells and $CD8^+$ T cells, isolated from DR-BB rats after KRV infection, into young DP-BB rats resulted in the development of diabetes in 88% of the recipients. The incidence of diabetes in DP-BB rats that received either $CD45RC^+CD4^+$ or $CD8^+$ T cells alone was significantly less than rats that received a combination of $CD45RC^+CD4^+$ and $CD8^+$ T cells. A combination of $CD45RC^+CD4^+$ T cells from infected rats and $CD8^+$ T cells from uninfected rats or a combination of $CD8^+$ T cells from infected rats and $CD45RC^+CD4^+$ T cells from uninfected rats did not change the incidence of diabetes.[24] These results indicate that Th1-like $CD4^+$ and $CD8^+$ T cells from KRV-infected rats work synergistically to destroy β cells. In contrast, none of the recipients of both $CD45RC^-CD4^+$ and $CD8^+$ T cells developed diabetes, indicating that $CD45RC^-CD4^+$ T cells may play a role as regulatory T cells. Additional studies also showed that the development of KRV-induced diabetes could be due to the failure to maintain the function of regulatory T cells ($CD4^+CD25^+$ T cells).[27] On the basis of these observations, it appears that infection of DR-BB rats with KRV results in the preferential activation of effector T cells, such as Th1-like $CD45RC^+CD4^+$ T cells and $CD8^+$ T cells, and the downregulation of Th2-like $CD45RC^-CD4^+$ and $CD4^+CD25^+$ T cells, and the activated effector T cells kill the β cells, similar to the case in DP-BB rats.

In this brief review of virus-induced diabetes, we have discussed how two distinct viruses, a small RNA virus (EMC-D virus) and a small DNA parvovirus (KRV), can kill pancreatic β cells in mice and rats, resulting in type 1 diabetes. Infection of genetically susceptible strains of mice (SJL/J, SWR, DBA/2) with a high dose of EMC-D virus results in the development of diabetes by the acute destruction of β cells through rapid replication of the virus within the β cells. However, infection of genetically susceptible mouse strains with a low dose of EMC-D virus results in the initial replication of the virus in β cells, followed by recruitment of macrophages to the infected pancreatic islets. These activated macrophages secrete soluble mediators, such as cytokines (IL-1, TNF-α, IFN-γ) and oxygen-free radicals (NO), which destroy

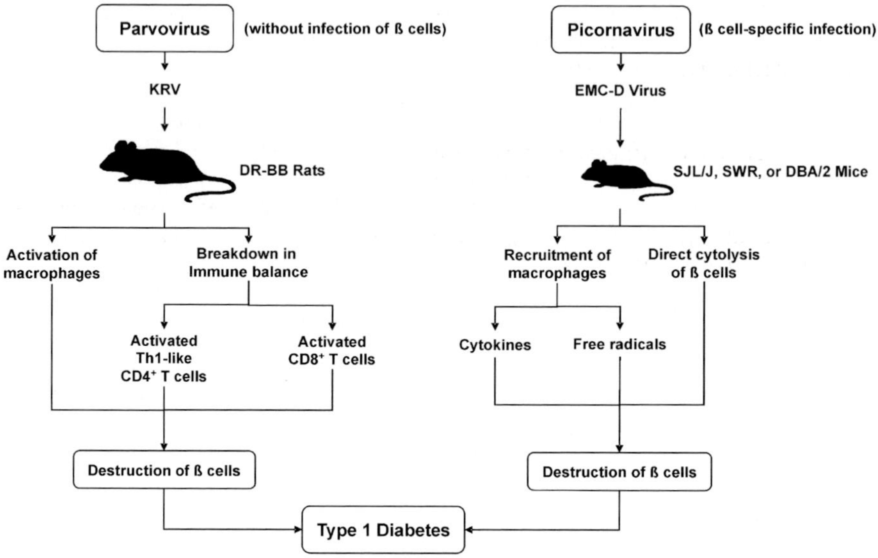

Figure 1. Two distinct pathogenic mechanisms of virus-induced type 1 diabetes in animals. KRV, a parvovirus, causes autoimmune diabetes without infection of β cells, whereas EMC virus, a picornavirus, directly infects and destroys β cells. Infection of DR-BB rats with KRV results in the activation of macrophages and breakdown of the finely tuned immune balance between Th1-like $CD45RC^{+}CD4^{+}$ and Th2-like $CD45RC^{-}CD4^{+}$ T cells, resulting in the activation of β cell-specific, Th1-like $CD4^{+}$ and $CD8^{+}$ T cells. These cells act synergistically to destroy β cells, which contributes to the development of diabetes. Infection of genetically susceptible strains of mice with a high dose of EMC-D virus destroys β cells by direct cytolysis, and activated macrophages play a minor role in β cell destruction. However, infection with a low dose of EMC-D virus results in the initial replication of the virus in β cells, followed by recruitment of macrophages to the infected islets. The activated macrophages produce cytokines and free radicals and contribute to the destruction of β cells, and subsequently the development of diabetes.

the residual β cells by apoptosis (FIG. 1). In contrast to EMC-D virus-induced diabetes, KRV can cause type 1 diabetes by inducing autoimmune responses against pancreatic β cells, rather than by direct infection of β cells. Infection of DR-BB rats with KRV results in the breakdown of immune tolerance by the downregulation of the Th2-type immune response, including a decrease in the regulatory T cell population, and/or the upregulation of the Th1-type immune response, including an increase in the autoreactive effector T cell population, leading to autoimmune type 1 diabetes (FIG. 1).

REFERENCES

1. JUN, H.S. & J.W. YOON. 2003. A new look at viruses in type 1 diabetes. Diabetes Metab. Res. Rev. **19:** 8–31.

2. Craighead, J.E. & M.F. McLane. 1968. Diabetes mellitus: induction in mice by encephalomyocarditis virus. Science **162:** 913–914.
3. Guberski, D.L. *et al.* 1991. Induction of type I diabetes by Kilham's rat virus in diabetes-resistant BB/Wor rats. Science **254:** 1010–1013.
4. Ross, M.E. *et al.* 1976. Virus-induced diabetes mellitus. IV. Genetic and environmental factors influencing the development of diabetes after infection with the M variant of encephalomyocarditis virus. Diabetes **25:** 190–197.
5. Yoon, J., T. Onodera & A.L. Notkins. 1977. Virus-induced diabetes mellitus: VIII. Passage of encephalomyocarditis virus and severity of diabetes in susceptible and resistant strains of mice. J. Gen. Virol. **37:** 225–232.
6. Yoon, J.W. *et al.* 1980. Virus-induced diabetes mellitus. XVIII. Inhibition by a nondiabetogenic variant of encephalomyocarditis virus. J. Exp. Med. **152:** 878–892.
7. Ray, U.R. *et al.* 1983. Virus-induced diabetes mellitus. XXV. Difference in the RNA fingerprints of diabetogenic and non-diabetogenic variants of encephalomyocarditis virus. J. Gen. Virol. **64**(Pt 4)**:** 947–950.
8. Bae, Y.S., H.M. Eun & J.W. Yoon. 1989. Genomic differences between the diabetogenic and nondiabetogenic variants of encephalomyocarditis virus. Virology **170:** 282–287.
9. Bae, Y.S. & J.W. Yoon. 1993. Determination of diabetogenicity attributable to a single amino acid, Ala776, on the polyprotein of encephalomyocarditis virus. Diabetes **42:** 435–443.
10. Jun, H.S. *et al.* 1997. Gain or loss of diabetogenicity resulting from a single point mutation in recombinant encephalomyocarditis virus. J. Virol. **71:** 9782–9785.
11. Jun, H.S. *et al.* 1998. Determination of encephalomyocarditis viral diabetogenicity by a putative binding site of the viral capsid protein. Diabetes **47:** 576–582.
12. Onodera, T. *et al.* 1978. Evidence for a single locus controlling susceptibility to virus-induced diabetes mellitus. Nature **274:** 693–696.
13. Yoon, J.W. *et al.* 1985. Virus-induced diabetes mellitus. No evidence for immune mechanisms in the destruction of beta-cells by the D-variant of encephalomyocarditis virus. Diabetes **34:** 922–925.
14. Baek, H.S. & J.W. Yoon. 1991. Direct involvement of macrophages in destruction of beta-cells leading to development of diabetes in virus-infected mice. Diabetes **40:** 1586–1597.
15. Baek, H.S. & J.W. Yoon. 1990. Role of macrophages in the pathogenesis of encephalomyocarditis virus-induced diabetes in mice. J. Virol. **64:** 5708–5715.
16. Jun, H.S. & J.W. Yoon. 2001. The role of viruses in type I diabetes: two distinct cellular and molecular pathogenic mechanisms of virus-induced diabetes in animals. Diabetologia **44:** 271–285.
17. Hirasawa, K. *et al.* 1997. Possible role of macrophage-derived soluble mediators in the pathogenesis of encephalomyocarditis virus-induced diabetes in mice. J. Virol. **71:** 4024–4031.
18. Kaneto, H. *et al.* 1995. Apoptotic cell death triggered by nitric oxide in pancreatic beta-cells. Diabetes **44:** 733–738.
19. Hirasawa, K. *et al.* 1999. Prevention of encephalomyocarditis virus-induced diabetes in mice by inhibition of the tyrosine kinase signalling pathway and subsequent suppression of nitric oxide production in macrophages. J. Virol. **73:** 8541–8548.
20. Choi, K.S. *et al.* 2001. Role of Hck in the pathogenesis of encephalomyocarditis virus-induced diabetes in mice. J. Virol. **75:** 1949–1957.

21. ZIPRIS, D. *et al.* 2005. TLR activation synergizes with Kilham rat virus infection to induce diabetes in BBDR rats. J. Immunol. **174:** 131–142.
22. CHUNG, Y.H. *et al.* 1997. Role of macrophages and macrophage-derived cytokines in the pathogenesis of Kilham rat virus-induced autoimmune diabetes in diabetes-resistant BioBreeding rats. J. Immunol. **159:** 466–471.
23. MENDEZ, I.I. *et al.* 2004. Immunoregulatory role of nitric oxide in Kilham rat virus-induced autoimmune diabetes in DR-BB rats. J. Immunol. **173:** 1327–1335.
24. CHUNG, Y.H. *et al.* 2000. Cellular and molecular mechanism for Kilham rat virus-induced autoimmune diabetes in DR-BB rats. J. Immunol. **165:** 2866–2876.
25. FOWELL, D. *et al.* 1991. Subsets of CD4+ T cells and their roles in the induction and prevention of autoimmunity. Immunol. Rev. **123:** 37–64.
26. LIBLAU, R.S., S.M. SINGER & H.O. MCDEVITT. 1995. Th1 and Th2 CD4+ T cells in the pathogenesis of organ-specific autoimmune diseases. Immunol. Today **16:** 34–38.
27. ZIPRIS, D. *et al.* 2003. Infections that induce autoimmune diabetes in BBDR rats modulate $CD4^+CD25^+$ T cell populations. J. Immunol. **170:** 3592–3602.

Characterization of *PAF-AH Ib1* in NOD Mice

PAF-AH May Not Be a Candidate Gene of the Diabetes Susceptibility *Idd4.1* Locus

QING-SHENG MI,[a,b] LI ZHOU,[a,c] MARSHA GRATTAN,[b] ZAI-ZHAO WANG,[a] M. SIVILOTTI,[b] JING-XIANG SHE,[a] AND TERRY L. DELOVITCH[b,d]

[a]*Center for Biotechnology and Genomic Medicine, Medical College of Georgia, Augusta, Georgia 30912, USA*

[b]*Laboratory of Autoimmune Diabetes, Robarts Research Institute, University of Western Ontario, London, Ontario, Canada N6A 5K8*

[c]*TaiShan Medical College, 271000 Taian, China*

[d]*Department of Microbiology and Immunology, University of Western Ontario, London, Ontario, Canada N6A 5C1*

ABSTRACT: We recently mapped *Idd4* to a 5.2 cM interval on chromosome 11 with two subloci, *Idd4.1* and *Idd4.2*, in nonobese diabetic (NOD) mice. Based on the localization of platelet-activating factor acetylhydrolase Ib1 (*PAF-AHIb1*) and the decreased activity of PAF-AH in type 1 diabetes (T1D) patients, we hypothesized that *PAF-AHIb1* in *Idd4.1* is a candidate gene. The *PAF-AHIb1* gene in NOD mice was cloned and sequenced, and its expression and function were studied. No polymorphisms were detected in *PAF-AHIb1* cDNA between NOD and B6 mice. The expression of *PAF-AH Ib1* at the mRNA and protein levels was found to be similar in different tissues between NOD and B6 mice. PAF-AH activity does not differ in the pancreatic islets or spleen between NOD and B6 mice. Our findings suggest that *PAF-AH Ib1* may not be a diabetes-susceptibility gene in the *Idd4.1* sublocus.

KEYWORDS: platelet-activating factor acetylhydrolase Ib1 gene; *Idd4*; nonobese diabetic mice; diabetes; genetic susceptibility

Address for correspondence: Dr. Terry L. Delovitch, Laboratory of Autoimmune Diabetes, Robarts Research Institute, 100 Perth Drive, London, Ontario, Canada, N6A 5K8. Voice: 519-663-3846; fax: 519-663-3847.

e-mail: del@robarts.ca

Ann. N.Y. Acad. Sci. 1079: 147–152 (2006).
doi: 10.1196/annals.1375.022

INTRODUCTION

Platelet-activating factor (PAF) is a potent proinflammatory phospholipid and is inactivated by the PAF acetylhydrolase (PAF-AH) enzyme present in many tissues, blood cells, and plasma. PAF-AH cleaves the acetyl moiety at the *sn*-2 position of the glycerol backbone and modifies PAF to lyso-PAF, and this self-protective mechanism limits the damaging effect of PAF.[1] Interestingly, serum levels of PAF are elevated in patients with type 1 diabetes (T1D) but not type 2 diabetes (T2D), and PAF-AH activity is significantly decreased in the plasma of T1D but not T2D patients.[2–4] PAF inhibitors can reduce the severity of insulitis and frequency of T1D in Bio Breeding (BB) rats.[5] Intraperitoneal injection of recombinant PAF-AH reduces the incidence of T1D in diabetes-prone BB rats.[6] These findings suggest that the elevated levels of PAF in T1D may be due to a decrease in PAF-AH activity. Mammalian PAF-AH is classified into two types, plasma (extracellular) and tissue (intracellular). The former is a 43-kDa monomeric enzyme that effectively abolishes the inflammatory effects of PAF on leukocytes and the vasculature. Tissue cytosol contains at least two types of intracellular PAF-AH, isoforms Ib and II. Isoform Ib is a heterotrimeric enzyme that consists of two 26-kDa catalytic subunits, $\alpha 1$ and $\alpha 2$, and a regulatory 45-kDa β subunit ([platelet-activating factor acetylhydrolase Ib1] *PAF-AHIb1*).[1] Biochemical analyses have revealed that the $\alpha 1/\alpha 2$ heterodimer and $\alpha 2/\alpha 2$ homodimer are the major catalytic units of embryonic and adult brain PAF-AHs, respectively. These activities have substrate specificities very similar to that of plasma PAF-AH. The nonobese diabetic (NOD) mouse spontaneously develops autoimmune T1D with an immunopathological profile similar to the human disease. Recently we limited diabetes susceptibility *Idd4* locus to a 5.2 cM interval with two subloci, *Idd4.1* and *Idd4.2*.[7] *Idd4.1* is localized in the *D11Nds1* interval containing the intracellular PAF-AH Ib regulator subunit *PAF-AH Ib1* gene. Based on the localization of *PAF-AH Ib1* in *Idd4.1* and the function of PAF-AH, we hypothesized that *PAF-AH Ib1* could be a candidate gene in *Idd4.1* that confers protection from insulitis and T1D.

MATERIALS AND METHODS

Mice

B6, NOD/Del and NOD.*Scid* mice were bred in our specific pathogen-free barrier facility. The use of animals was in accordance with NIH guidelines.

RNA Isolation and RT-PCR Amplification

Total RNA from thymus, spleen, pancreatic islets, and brain was extracted using an RNeasy Kit (Qiagen, Valencia, CA). Primers for PAF-AH were from separate exons and yielded specific reverse transcription polymerase chain reaction (RT-PCR) products.[8] To sequence the *PAF-AH Ib1* gene open reading frame, 5′- and 3′-untranslated region (UTR), multiple PCR primers were designed based on the *PAF-AH Ib1* cDNA sequence from B6 mice. PCR fragments were cloned and sequenced.

Protein Extraction and Western Blotting

Pancreas, thymus, spleen, and brain from age-matched mice were snap-frozen in liquid nitrogen. Tissues were thawed, homogenized, and sonicated in an antiprotease buffer (Roche, Laval, PQ, Canada). Proteins were separated by 12.5% SDS-PAGE and identified by Western blotting. Monoclonal anti-LIS1 (*PAF-AH Ib1*) antibody clone 210 (1:5000 dilution) was a kind gift from Dr. Orly Reiner (Weizmann Institute of Science, Rehovot, Israel).

Assay of PAF-AH Activity

PAF-AH activity was analyzed using a PAF-AH assay kit (Cayman Chemical, Ann Arbor, MI) according to the manufacturer's recommendations.

Statistical Analysis

Levels of gene expression were compared using the Student's *t*-test. A $P < 0.05$ value was chosen as the level of significance.

RESULTS AND DISCUSSION

We initially investigated whether transcripts of the *PAF-AH Ib* catalytic (α1, α2) and regulatory subunit *PAF-AH Ib1* genes are differentially expressed between NOD and B6 mice. RT-PCR analyses demonstrated that mRNAs encoding *PAF-AH Ib* α1, α2 and *PAF-AH Ib1* are expressed in the spleen, thymus, brain, and islets. Although the level of PAF-AH subunit expression varies in these tissues, the expression level of a given subunit does not differ significantly between NOD and B6 tissues (FIG. 1 A). Because T1D develops in an age-dependent manner in NOD mice, we further analyzed whether altered levels of *PAF-AH Ib* expression occur in islets of female NOD mice at different ages and whether such alterations correlate with the onset of insulitis or T1D. *PAF-AH Ib* α1, α2 and *PAF-AH* Ib1 genes were found to be expressed at similar levels in the islets of 3, 9, 13, and 25-week-old diabetes-free NOD mice as well as newly diabetic NOD mice (FIG. 1 B). We further determined whether interleukin (IL)-1β plus interferon (IFN)-γ elicits a different level of expression of PAF-AH in islets from NOD and B6 mice. No significant difference in expression of *PAF-AH Ib1* mRNA was detected at 12 or 24 h after cytokine treatment (FIG. 1 C). Given that the

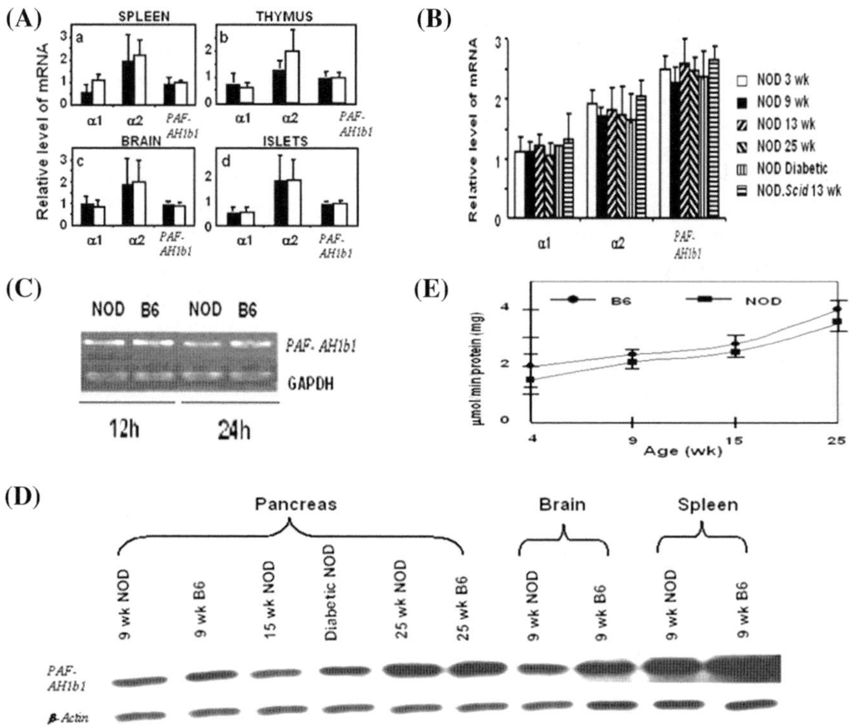

FIGURE 1. *PAF-AH Ib* subunit genes are expressed in different lymphoid and non-lymphoid tissues. (**A**) Total RNA isolated from the spleen, thymus, brain, and pancreas of 6- to 8-week-old female NOD and B6 mice ($n = 5$) was used to detect *PAF-AH1b* α1, α2 and *PAF-AH Ib1* expression by RT-PCR analysis. The relative levels of expression of *PAF-AH Ib* subunit genes are equivalent in different NOD (black bar) and B6 (white bar) tissues, and the quantity of individual transcripts was normalized to the glyceraldehyde-3-phosphate dehydrogenase (GAPDH) transcript internal control. The results are presented as relative levels of mRNA ($P > 0.05$). (**B**) Total islet RNA was isolated from 3-, 9-, 13-, and 25-week-old female NOD mice, 13-week-old female NOD.*Scid* mice, and 16- to 20-week-old diabetic female NOD mice ($n = 5$–10) for analyses of *PAF-AH Ib* expression. (**C**) Expression of *PAF-AH Ib1* in cytokine-treated islet cells. Islet cells from 4-week-old NOD and B6 mice ($n = 8$–10) were treated with IL-1β (50 units/mL) and IFN-γ (1000 units/mL) for 12 h or 24 h. (**D**) Relative levels of *PAF-AH Ib1* protein expression are similar in tissues of NOD and B6 mice of different ages. Pancreata were isolated from 9, 15, and 25-week-old nondiabetic female NOD and B6 mice and 15 to 20-week-old female diabetic NOD mice ($n = 3$–5). Brain and spleen tissues were isolated from 9-week-old NOD and B6 mice ($n = 3$–5). Western blot analysis of protein samples (40 μg/lane) was performed using anti-*LIS1/PAF-AHIb1* and anti-β-actin antibodies. (**E**) Intracellular PAF-AH activity in the pancreatic islets is similar between NOD and B6 mice. Pancreatic islets were isolated from female NOD and B6 mice ($n = 10$) at 4, 9, 15, and 25 weeks of age. PAF-AH activity was analyzed in islet protein extracts using a PAF-AH assay kit (Cayman Chemical) according to the manufacturer's recommendations. PAF-AH activity is expressed as mmol/min/protein.

posttranscriptional regulation may affect the level of protein expression, we next analyzed whether any mutations in potential regulatory sequences alter the level of *PAF-AH Ib1* protein expression in the pancreas and spleen. Similar levels of *PAF-AH Ib1* protein expression were detected in Western blots of pancreas and spleen cell lysates from NOD and B6 mice at different ages (FIG. 1 D). Thus, *PAF-AH Ib1* mRNA and protein expression does not differ between NOD and B6 mice, and variability in *PAF-AH Ib1* expression does not appear to correlate with the onset of either insulitis or T1D. To test the possibilities that polymorphisms of *PAF-AH Ib1* in NOD mice may alter the structure and function of *PAF-AH Ib1*, we cloned and sequenced NOD *PAF-AH Ib1* in order to determine whether a polymorphism(s) exits in the coding sequence, particularly the binding site, of the NOD and B6 *PAF-AH Ib1* genes. We did not detect any polymorphism in either the coding sequences of the NOD and B6 *PAF-AH Ib1* genes or in the 186 bp (base pairs) 5′-UTR and 1.5 kb 3′-UTR regions. To further test the possibility that a difference in *PAF-AH Ib1* crystal structure between these two strains could affect its function, we assayed the functional activity of intracellular PAF-AH. No significant differences in PAF-AH activity were detected in the islets (FIG. 1 E), whole pancreas, spleen, or thymus (our unpublished observations) of NOD and B6 mice at 4, 9, 15, or 25 weeks of age. These results are consistent with the lack of coding polymorphism between the NOD and B6 *PAF-AH Ib1* genes and the similar levels of *PAF-AH Ib1* protein expression in the pancreas of 4 to 25-week-old NOD and B6 mice.

In the present study, we demonstrate that the *PAF-AH Ib1* gene does not exhibit any polymorphisms between NOD and B6 mice. In addition, the relative levels of *PAF-AH Ib1* mRNA and protein expression in the pancreas and spleen as well as the intrapancreatic PAF-AH functional activity are comparable in diabetes-susceptible NOD and diabetes-resistant B6 mice. Thus, based on these data, the *PAF-AH Ib1* gene does not appear to be a candidate gene in the *Idd4.1* locus that contributes to reduced insulitis and protection from T1D. Additional fine mapping and characterization of genes in *Idd4.1* may identify an *Idd4*-linked T1D susceptibility gene(s) and further elucidate the mechanisms involved in the genetic control of diabetes resistance.

ACKNOWLEDGMENTS

We thank Dr. Orly Reiner for monoclonal anti-LIS1 (*PAF-AH Ib1*) antibody clone 210. This work was supported by grants from the American Diabetes Association and Juvenile Diabetes Research Foundation International (Q. S. M.), the National Natural Science Foundation of China (L. Z., 30370683), Canadian Institutes of Health Research, and the Ontario Research and Development Challenge Fund (T. L. D.).

REFERENCES

1. TJOELKER, L.W. & D.M. STAFFORINI. 2000. Platelet-activating factor acetylhydrolases in health and disease. Biochim. Biophys. Acta **1488:** 102–123.
2. NATHAN, N., Y. DENIZOT, M.C. HUC, *et al.* 1992. Elevated levels of paf-acether in blood of patients with type 1 diabetes mellitus. Diabetes Metab. **18:** 59–62.
3. CAVALLO-PERIN, P., E. LUPIA, G. GRUDEN, *et al.* 2000. Increased blood levels of platelet-activating factor in insulin-dependent diabetic patients with microalbuminuria. Nephrol. Dial. Transplant. **15:** 994–999.
4. MEMON, R.A., S.A. SAEED, A. JABBAR, *et al.* 1995. Altered platelet activating factor metabolism in insulin dependent diabetes mellitus. J. Pak. Med. Assoc. **45:** 122–125.
5. JOBE, L.W., R. UBUNGEN, C.J. GOODNER, *et al.* 1993. Protection from BB rat diabetes by the platelet-activating factor inhibitor BN50730. Autoimmunity **16:** 259–266.
6. LEE, E.S., J. JIANG, G.C. SUND, *et al.* 1999. Recombinant human platelet-activating factor acetylhydrolase reduces the frequency of diabetes in the diabetes-prone BB rat. Diabetes **48:** 43–49.
7. GRATTAN, M., Q.S. MI, C. MEAGHER & T.L. DELOVITCH TL. 2002. Congenic mapping of the diabetogenic locus *Idd4* to a 5.2-cM region of chromosome 11 in nonobese diabetic mice: identification of two potential candidate subloci. Diabetes **51:** 215–223.
8. HATTORI, M., H. ARAI & K. INOUE. 1993. Purification and characterization of bovine brain platelet-activating factor acetylhydrolase. J. Biol. Chem. **268:** 18748–18753.

Peptide-Pulsed Immature Dendritic Cells Reduce Response to β Cell Target Antigens and Protect NOD Recipients from Type I Diabetes

JEANNETTE LO, RUI HUA PENG, TOLGA BARKER, CHANG-QING XIA, AND MICHAEL J. CLARE-SALZLER

Department of Pathology, Immunology, and Laboratory Medicine, University of Florida, Gainesville, Florida 32610, USA

ABSTRACT: Our previous work demonstrated peptide-pulsed mature myeloid dendritic cells (DC) presenting β cell antigens induce tolerance. Here we determine whether immature DC (iDC) presenting dominant (insulin β9–23 chain, proinsulin C19–A3) or ignored (glutamic acid decarboxylase 65_{78-97}) antigen determinants promote tolerance. Nonobese diabetic (NOD) mice were given injections of either unpulsed or peptide-pulsed myeloid iDC beginning at 9 weeks of age for 3 consecutive weeks. Diabetes incidence in recipients of unpulsed iDC was comparable to unmanipulated animals (∼80%), whereas $GAD65_{78-97}$ pulsed iDC recipients were protected from the disease ($P = 0.05$). We also analyzed splenic T cell proliferation responses to the panel of studied peptides in diabetic and nondiabetic recipients. When stimulated with insulin or proinsulin peptide, nondiabetic mice receiving the peptide-pulsed iDC had a 21- to 31-fold or 3.9- to 9.0-fold reduction in T cell response, respectively, as compared to the response of diabetic unpulsed recipients. However, only a 2.6- to 3.1-fold reduction in response to β chain peptide, and a 1.5- to 3.4-fold reduction in proinsulin response were observed in diabetic mice receiving peptide-pulsed iDC. The reduction was not specific to the immunizing peptide, as reduced proliferation was observed to other diabetes-target peptides. We conclude that protective iDC-based therapies require target antigen presentation, and ignored determinants may be preferable perhaps due to an available naïve T cell repertoire. In addition, iDC presenting peptides induce a nonspecific reduction in T cell responses to β cell antigens, possibly through the induction of regulatory T cells.

KEYWORDS: immature dendritic cell; ignored determinant; diabetes; NOD; therapy

Address for correspondence: Michael J. Clare-Salzler, Department of Pathology, Immunology, and Laboratory Medicine, University of Florida, 1600 SW Archer Road, Gainesville, FL 32610. Voice: 352-392-9885; fax: 352-392-5393.
e-mail: salzler@ufl.edu

Ann. N.Y. Acad. Sci. 1079: 153–156 (2006).
doi: 10.1196/annals.1375.023

INTRODUCTION

Type I diabetes (TID) is an autoimmune disease characterized by a T cell-mediated destruction of insulin-producing β cells. The destructive response is believed to be mediated by a Th1-dominant immune attack targeted to several autoantigens including glutamate decarboxylase (GAD) and insulin in the presence of an ineffective regulatory response.[1] Our previous studies with nonobese diabetic (NOD) mice demonstrated that mature myeloid dendritic cells (DC) lacking interleukin (IL)-12 production and presenting β cell antigens induce tolerance through activation of regulatory cells.[2] However, the efficacy of mature DC for tolerance induction in clinical applications remains unclear. Additionally, recent evidence suggests that the use of an ignored-determinant antigen peptide may be more effective in the recruitment of naïve T cells for regulatory function.[3] Here we demonstrate that NOD recipients of immature DC (iDC) presenting an ignored determinant were significantly protected from the disease ($P = 0.05$). We also show a reduction in T cell response to target autoantigens in nondiabetic mice that received diabetes-target peptide-pulsed iDC.

METHODS

Animals

Female NOD/LtJ donor mice ranged from 5 to 8 weeks of age. Recipient nondiabetic female NOD/LtJ mice were 9 weeks of age. All mice were housed under specific pathogen-free conditions. Recipient mice received weekly footpad injections of either unpulsed or peptide-pulsed immature myeloid DC (10^5) for 3 consecutive weeks. Mice were monitored for diabetes weekly. Diabetes was diagnosed when glucose was >300 dg/mL on two occasions. Antigen responsiveness was tested in a subset of DC recipients by testing recall antigen response following ovalbumin/Alum immunizations.

iDC Preparation

Bone marrow (BM) was obtained from the tibia and femur of the donor mice. BM-derived DC were grown in RPMI/10% FCS (fetal calf serum), 500 U/mL granulocyte macrophage colony-stimulating factor, and 1000 u/mL IL-4, with media changed on day 2. On day 6, dendritic cells were harvested and DC purified with CD11c magnetic beads (MiltenyiBiotec, Auburn, CA). iDC were pulsed with 3 uM of peptide for 2 h at 37°C. Cells were then washed thrice and resuspended in PBS at 10^6 cells/mL. DC purity was >90% as determined by flow cytometry for cd11c + cells.

Proliferation Assay

Suspensions of spleen cells were cultured in serum-free HL-1 media in triplicate with peptide (25 uM). At 72 h of culture, 3H-thymidine was added and allowed to incorporate for 12–16 h. Cells were harvested, washed, and analyzed using a liquid scintillation counter.

RESULTS

No adverse immune reaction was observed following peptide-pulsed iDC injections. Mice were monitored weekly for diabetes through 27 weeks of age. Diabetes incidence in recipients of unpulsed DC was comparable to unmanipulated animals (~80%), whereas GAD-pulsed DC recipients were significantly protected from the disease (FIG. 1). Mice receiving insulin and proinsulin-pulsed DC showed some protection (not statistically significant). We also analyzed splenic T cell proliferation responses to the panel of study peptides in diabetic and nondiabetic recipients. When stimulated with insulin or proinsulin peptide, nondiabetic mice receiving the peptide-pulsed DC had a 14- to 24-fold or 2.6- to 7.3-fold reduction in T cell response, respectively, as compared to the response of diabetic-unpulsed recipients. However, only a 1.9–2.8 fold reduction in response to β chain peptide, and a 1.3- to 2.8-fold reduction in proinsulin response were observed in diabetic mice receiving peptide-pulsed DC. This reduction was not specific to the immunizing peptide, as reduction was observed to other study peptides tested. We found no cases of enhanced

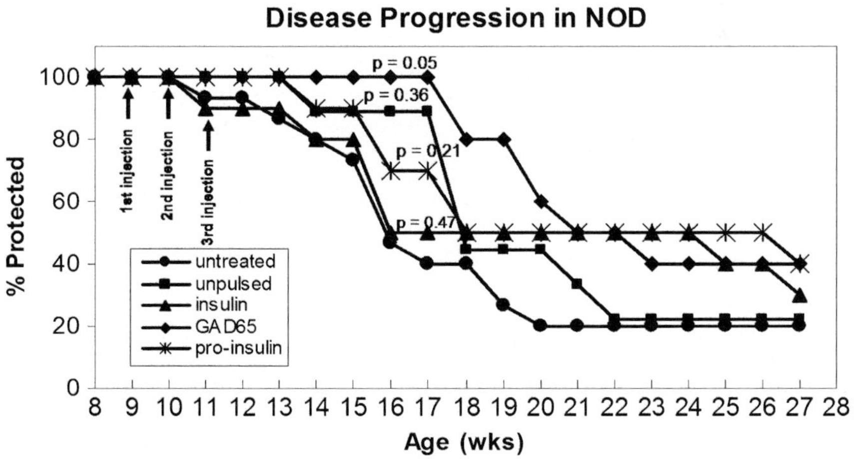

FIGURE 1. Disease progression in NOD. NOD/LtJ mice were given footpad injections of unpulsed or peptide-pulsed iDCs once a week for 3 weeks beginning at 9 weeks of age, then monitored for disease progression through 27 weeks of age.

response to the immunizing peptide including the ignored GAD determinant. We conclude that protective DC-based therapies require target antigen presentation, and ignored determinants may be preferable, perhaps due to an available repertoire. In addition, DC presenting peptides induce a nonspecific reduction in T cell responses to β cell antigens, possibly through the induction of regulatory T cells.

ACKNOWLEDGMENT

This study was supported by NIH/NIDDK/NIAID R21/R33 research grant to Michael J. Clare-Salzler.

REFERENCES

1. Morel, P.A., A.C. Vasquez & M. Feili-Hariri. 1999. Immunobiology of DC in NOD mice. J. Leukoc. Biol. **66:** 276–280.
2. Clare-Salzler, M.J. *et al*. 1992. Prevention of diabetes in nonobese diabetic mice by dendritic cell transfer. J. Clin. Invest. **90:** 741–748.
3. Olcott, A.P. *et al*. 2005. Antigen-based therapies using ignored determinants of beta cell antigens can more effectively inhibit late-stage autoimmune disease in diabetes-prone mice. J. Immunol. **175:** 1991–1999.

New Members of the Interleukin-12 Family of Cytokines: IL-23 and IL-27 Modulate Autoimmune Diabetes

E.P.K. MENSAH-BROWN,[a] A. SHAHIN,[b] M. AL-SHAMSI,[b] AND M.L. LUKIC[b]

[a]*Department of Anatomy, Faculty of Medicine and Health Sciences, UAE University, Al Ain, United Arab Emirates*

[b]*Departments of Microbiology and Immunology, Faculty of Medicine and Health Sciences, UAE University, Al Ain, United Arab Emirates*

ABSTRACT: **Multiple low doses of streptozotocin (5 × 40 mg/kg) given to susceptible male C57BL6 mice induced delayed and sustained hyperglycemia accompanied by body weight loss, mononuclear cell infiltration in the islet, and apoptosis of β cells. Shorter regimes (4 × 40 mg/kg) did not have such effect. Administration of IL-23 at a dose of 400 ng/mL for 10 consecutive days concomitantly with this subdiabetogenic regimen of STZ, however, induced significant hyperglycemia, weight loss, and mononuclear cellular infiltration. The same regimen of IL-27 induced milder effect on glycemia and no weight loss inspite of a massive peri-islet and intra-islet infiltration of mononuclear cells. The molecular mechanisms underlying the actions of these cytokines on diabetogenesis is under study.**

KEYWORDS: **Diabetes; interleukin-17; interleukin-23; interleukin-27; interferon-γ**

INTRODUCTION

Interleukin-23 (IL-23) and -27 are heterodimeric IL-12-related cytokines that play decisive roles in the development of autoimmune inflammation in the central nervous system (CNS).[1,2] While the former influences the expansion of $CD4^+$ T cell producing IL-17 and tumor necrosis factor alpha-α (TNF-α),[3] the latter synergizes with IL-12 to trigger the production of interferon-γ (IFN-γ) in naïve $CD4^+$ T cells, driving these cells toward a Th1 phenotype and suppresses basal expression of GATA-3, the critical Th2-specific transcription factor that

Address for correspondence: Prof. M.L. Lukic, Department of Microbiology and Immunology, Faculty of Medicine and Health Sciences, UAE University, P.O. Box 17666, Al Ain, United Arab Emirates.
e-mail: m.lukic@uaeu.ac.ae

Ann. N.Y. Acad. Sci. 1079: 157–160 (2006).
doi: 10.1196/annals.1375.024

inhibits Th1 development.[4] We have employed the model of disease induced by multiple doses of streptozotocin in susceptible male C_{57}Bl/6 mice, which offers a tool to study the effect of cytokines on synchronized groups of diabetic mice. We have previously demonstrated that in contrast to five injections, four (40 mg/kg body weight) doses of STZ do not induce diabetes as evaluated by glycemia and body weight.[5,6] The roles of IL-23 and IL-27 in autoimmune inflammation of islets and selective β cell destruction has been determined by administration of recombinant IL-23 and IL-27 concomitantly with regimen of STZ (4 × 40 mg/kg body weight). Using immunohistological techniques we have assessed the effect of the cytokine on the level of mononuclear cellular infiltration, percentage insulin immunopositive β cell, and apoptosis of β cells.

MATERIALS AND METHODS

Injections of recombinant IL-23 and IL-27 at a dose of 400 ng in 0.5 mL of 0.1% BSA/saline were administered intraperitoneally (i.p.) in C57Bl/6 male mice 8–10 weeks of age as previously reported by us.[6] Briefly, 10 daily injections started on the first day of MLD-STZ treatment (STZ + IL-23; STZ + IL-27) and the levels of glycemia and weights of mice were determined weekly over a period of 31 days. Pancreata of both groups as well as those that had been treated only with STZ were taken 31 days post induction and routinely embedded in paraffin wax. Noncontiguous wax sections of thickness 7 μm were then either examined after H&E staining or immunostained by the direct FITC-immunofluorescent technique using prediluted polyclonal guinea pig anti-insulin primary antibody (DAKO, Copenhagen) followed by incubation in propidium iodide (PI) nuclear staining to determine the percentage insulin-producing β cells per total PI nuclear content of islet. Wax sections were also stained by the indirect ABC method technique using rabbit anti-human cleaved caspase-3 antibody (Cell Signaling Technology, New England Biolabs, Ipswich, MA) to determine the level of β cell apoptosis.

RESULTS

The level of glycemia and immunohistochemical data on day 31 is summarized in TABLE 1. The injection of 4 × 40 mg/kg body weight of streptozotocin did not have significant diabetogenic effects. Animals treated with IL-23 concomitant with diabetes induction developed delayed and sustained hyperglycemia accompanied by weight loss. The differences in these parameters reached statistical significance by day 18 and remained significant until the end of the experiment (day 31). The effect of IL-27 on diabetic induction was less pronounced and reached statistical significance only by day 31. It is

TABLE 1. Effect of IL-23 and IL-27 on the clinical and pathological signs of diabetes

	STZ only	STZ + IL-27	STZ + IL-27
Glycemia mmol/L	11.1 ± 0.45	17.1 ± 2.9 $P = 0.069$	$22.9 \pm 4.4^{**}$
Mononuclear cellular infiltration	24 ± 4.0	$80 \pm 5.0^{**}$	$83 \pm 6.0^{**}$
Percent insulin positivity	52.7 ± 1.4	$40 \pm 7.2^{*}$	$27.2 \pm 3.1^{**}$
Apoptotic cells	22 ± 6	$40 \pm 11.8^{**}$	52 ± 7
Percent weight gained	+5.1%	+3.4	-5.2^{*}

$^{*}P < 0.05$ in comparison to animals treated with STZ only.
$^{**}P < 0.005$ in comparison to animals treated with STZ only.

interesting to note the massive mononuclear cell infiltration induced by IL-27 despite its mild diabetogenic effect.

DISCUSSION

IL-23 and IL-27 appear to be required in the final effector phase of autoimmune inflammation in the CNS. To this, we now add the evidence that these cytokines may modulate MLD-STZ-induced diabetes. As has been observed in the CNS by Langrish *et al.*,[7] we have also recently demonstrated that the highly pathogenic, IL-23-dependent IL-17-producing cells are essential for the establishment of organ-specific inflammation in the pancreas[8] but unlike in EAE[1] and CIA,[7] our data indicate that the diabetogenic effect of IL-23 is accompanied by a dramatic increase in the expression of IFN-γ in the islets by day 16 after diabetes induction. It remains to be established whether INF-γ is a downregulating or disease-producing cytokine in this model. It is clear that despite milder effect on glycemia IL-27 induced significant influx of mononuclear cells in the islet similar or more pronounced than that induced by IL-23. However, the number of insulin- producing cells detected in IL-23-treated animals was lower that that seen after IL-27 treatment (TABLE 1) suggesting that IL-27 may induce downregulatory, in addition to pathogenic T cells infiltrating the islets.

ACKNOWLEDGMENT

This work was supported by UAE University Research Sector, grant No. 01-10-8-12/04 to MLL and FMHS research grant No. NP/24 to EPKMB.

REFERENCES

1. CUA, D.J., J. SHERLOCK, Y. CHEN, *et al.* 2003. Interleukin-23 rather than interleukin-12 is the critical cytokine for autoimmune inflammation of the brain. Nature **421:** 744–748.

2. GOLDBERG, R., Y. ZOHAR, G. WILDBAUM, *et al.* 2004. Suppression of ongoing experimental autoimmune encephalomyelitis by neutralizing the function of the p28 subunit of IL-27. J. Immunol. **173:** 6465–6471.
3. JOVANOVIC, D.V., J.A. DI BATTISTA, J. MARTERL-PELLETIER, *et al.* 1998. IL-17 stimulates the production and expression of proinflammatory cytokines, IL-beta and TNF-alpha, by human macrophages. J. Immunol. **160:** 3513–3521.
4. LUCAS, S., N. GHILARDI, J. LI, *et al.* 2003. IL-27 regulates responsiveness of naive CD4+ T cells through Stat1-dependent and -independent mechanisms. Proc. Natl. Acad. Sci. USA **100:** 15047–15052.
5. ELIA, S.D., H. PRIGOZIN, N. POLAK, *et al.* 1994. Autoimmune diabetes induced by the beta-cell toxin STZ. Immunity to the 60-kDa heat shock protein and to insulin. Diabetes **43:** 992–998.
6. LUKIC, M.L., E. MENSAH-BROWN, X. WEI, *et al.* 2003. Lack of the mediators of innate immunity attenuates the development of autoimmune diabetes in mice. J. Autoimmun. **21:** 239–246.
7. LANGRISH, C.L., Y. CHEN, W.M. BLUMENSCHEIN, *et al.* 2005. IL-23 drives a pathogenic T cell population that induces autoimmune inflammation. J. Exp. Med. **201:** 233–240.
8. MENSAH-BROWN, E.P.K., A. SHAHIN, M. AL-SHAMSI, *et al.* 2006. IL-23 leads to diabetes induction after subdiabetogenic treatment with multiple low doses of streptozotocin. Eur. J. Immunol. 216–223.

Glutamic Acid Decarboxylase-Specific CD4$^+$ Regulatory T Cells

CHIH-PIN LIU

Division of Immunology, Beckman Research Institute, City of Hope, Duarte, California 91010-3000, USA

ABSTRACT: It is known that CD4$^+$ regulatory T cells (Tr cells) play a central role in inducing immune tolerance in animals and humans. Compared to polyclonal Tr cells, autoantigen-specific Tr cells are more potent at blocking pathogenic immune responses. In order to better understand the role of Tr cells in controlling type 1 diabetes development and to help design effective antigen-specific cell-based therapeutic methods to treat the disease, it is necessary to: (*a*) determine the antigen specificity of Tr cells; (*b*) study how antigen-specific Tr cells behave *in vivo*; (*c*) investigate the interaction of Tr cells with pathogenic T cells (Tpath cells) and determine whether such interaction correlates with the progression or inhibition of diabetes; and (*d*) determine the cellular and molecular mechanisms underlying the regulation of diabetes by Tr cells. We have addressed these questions with a focus on the studies of glutamic acid decarboxylase (GAD)-specific T cells. Previous studies have suggested that GAD-specific T cells play a key role in type 1 diabetes. Treatment of NOD mice with GAD or its peptides can prevent the progression toward overt disease. The preventive effect could be due to either the deletion of antigen-specific pathogenic T cells or the induction of potent antigen-specific Tr cells. Using antigen-specific I-Ag7 tetramers we have isolated several populations of GAD peptide-specific T cells from diabetes-prone NOD and diabetes-resistant NOR mice. Herein, we summarize our studies on the role of these GAD peptide-specific T cells in type 1 diabetes. We present evidence that supports the hypothesis that the repertoire of T cells specific for these GAD peptides is biased toward Tr cells that inhibit diabetes rather than toward pathogenic T cells that induce diabetes.

KEYWORDS: glutamic acid decarboxylase (GAD65); NOD mice; NOR mice; diabetes; regulatory T cells; antigen-presenting cells; nitric oxide

INTRODUCTION

Type 1 diabetes, a very serious form of diabetes, is an autoimmune disease resulting from the selective destruction of islet β cells by T cells specific

Address for correspondence: Chih-Pin Liu, Beckman Research Institute, City of Hope, Division of Immunology, 1450E. Duarte, Duarte CA 91010. Voice: 626-359-8111; ext.: 62601; fax: 626-301-8186. e-mail: cliu@coh.org

Ann. N.Y. Acad. Sci. 1079: 161–170 (2006).
doi: 10.1196/annals.1375.025

for various autoantigens. The mechanisms regulating the development and activation of pathogenic T cells remain largely unclear. It is hypothesized that diabetes development in human and in non-obese diabetic (NOD) mice, an animal model for human type 1 diabetes, is dependent on the breakdown of self-tolerance to immunodominant epitopes of autoantigens. For example, regulatory mechanisms controlling pathogenic autoreactivity may not operate properly in at-risk humans and animals, such as NOD mice. As a result, an imbalanced population of autoantigen-specific pathogenic and regulatory T cells (Tr cells) or a change of cytokines secreted by these different types of T cells may contribute to the development of diabetes.[1,2] It is thus possible to prevent type 1 diabetes in mice and humans using autoantigens that can induce a shift in the T cells reactive to the administered antigen resulting in an expansion of Tr cells.[3] Nevertheless, antigen-based immunotherapy may induce unexpected harmful adverse effects, therefore, it is critical to understand the role of antigen-specific T cells induced in these antigen-based immunotherapy treatments in order to design an effective and safe therapy to treat the disease.

Many autoantigens have been identified as targets for T cell responses in type 1 diabetes patients and in spontaneous animal models, such as the NOD mice. Among these autoantigens, glutamic acid decarboxylase (GAD) has been proposed to play a key role in the pathogenesis of type 1 diabetes.[4,5] First, anti-GAD antibodies can be detected in the sera of a majority of diabetic and prediabetic patients.[6] Second, T cell responses against GAD65 can be detected in NOD mice by 3–4 weeks of age and in humans with type 1 diabetes.[5,6] Third, β cell-specific suppression of GAD expression in antisense GAD transgenic NOD mice leads to complete prevention of type 1 diabetes and blocks the generation of diabetogenic T cells.[7] Taken collectively, these findings suggest that the modulation of GAD autoimmunity can influence the development of type 1 diabetes in NOD mice. Indeed, treatment of NOD mice with GAD or its peptides via various routes can prevent the progression toward overt disease.[4,8–10]

However, despite these studies, the role of GAD in the actual pathogenesis of type 1 diabetes in NOD mice remains controversial. Only one diabetogenic GAD-specific clone has been identified and diabetes develops normally in GAD65 knockout NOD mice.[11,12] Additionally, it has been reported that transgenic NOD mice tolerant to GAD were not protected from diabetes and exhibited normal incidence and kinetics of type 1 diabetes onset.[13] Moreover, as demonstrated in previous reports on studies of GAD-specific T cells and on T cell receptor (TCR) transgenic mice, the disease protection observed in NOD mice pretreated with GAD or its peptides is associated with the induction of T cells with regulatory functions.[8–10,14,15] Therefore, the role of GAD and its peptides in the selection of T cells and in T cell-mediated β cell-autoimmunity remains to be further clarified.

In order to address these questions, it is necessary to identify and isolate GAD peptide-specific T cells from animals. However, it is a difficult task to isolate a

TABLE 1. Tetramers generated in our laboratory, their antigen specificity, and whether antigen-specific T cell lines were isolated from mice using these tetramers

Tetramers	Antigen specificity	T cell line
tetAg7/p206	GADp206-220	yes
tetAg7/p221	GADp221-235	yes
tetAg7/p286	GADp286-300	yes
tetAg7/p79	mimotope p79	yes
tetAg7/p17	mimotope p17	yes
tetAd/p206	GADp206-220	yes
tetAd/p221	GADp221-235	yes

sufficient number of autoantigen-specific T cells for further *in vitro* and *in vivo* studies. We have approached this question by isolating T cells specific for various GAD peptides using novel I-Ag7 tetramers specific for these peptides. Previous studies have identified several I-Ag7-binding GAD immunodominant epitopes.[16] We have generated I-Ag7 tetramers specific for different peptides (TABLE 1) and have isolated T cells from NOD mice and the disease-resistant congenic NOR mouse strain (NOR mice) using these tetramers (TABLE 2). The following sections briefly describe the results obtained from our studies on T cells specific for GAD p206-220 (p206) and p221-235 (p221) peptides that are isolated from NOD mice and NOR mice.

GAD p206- and p221-Specific T Cells Isolated from Peptide-Immunized NOD Mice Function as Regulatory T Cells

In order to understand the role of NOD mouse T cells specific for GAD p206 or p221 in type 1 diabetes, we have generated I-Ag7 tetramers containing the p206 or p221 peptide that specifically stains p206- or p221-specific T cells, respectively.[10,17] To our knowledge, these are the first I-Ag7 tetramers that can stain and identify autoantigen-specific T cells isolated from NOD mice. We have successfully used the tetAg7/p206 and the tetAg7/p221 tetramers to isolate p206-specific (N206 T cells) and p221-specific (N221 T cells) T cells from NOD mice, respectively.[10] We have characterized the *in vitro* function of these T cells and have determined whether they can cause or prevent diabetes

TABLE 2. GAD-specific T cell lines isolated using I-Ag7 tetramers and the summary of their *in vitro* functions and *in vivo* effect on diabetes

T cell line	Antigen	Mouse	*In vitro*	Effect on diabetes	Regulatory mechanism
N206	GADp206	NOD	Tr cell	inhibitory	IL-10-dependent
NR206	GADp206	NOR	Tr cell	inhibitory	IFN-γ/NO/cell contact-dependent
N221	GADp221	NOD	Tr cell	inhibitory	IL-10-dependent and Tr1 cells
naN221	GADp221	NOD	Tr cell	inhibitory	IL-10-dependent

in adoptive transfer experiments. Our results show that the N206 T cells are polarized T cells that secrete large quantities of interleukin-10 (IL-10) and IL-4. Interestingly, the N206 T cells possess regulatory functions and can inhibit the proliferation of other T cells, including the diabetogenic BDC2.5 T cells. The results of transwell assays show that N206 T cells can inhibit the proliferation of target cells independent of cell contact with the target cells. Further studies show that N206 T cells can exert their regulatory functions dependent on the secretion of IL-10 and not IL-4, because anti-IL-10 antibody but not anti-IL-4 antibody can abolish their regulatory function.

Additionally, the results from *in vivo* adoptive transfer experiments show that N206 T cells inhibit the development of insulitis and diabetes. One hypothesis explaining why N206 T cells can inhibit the development of insulitis is that they can prevent the migration of pathogenic T cells into the islets. In order to test this hypothesis, we have performed adoptive transfer experiments that determine whether the *in vivo* migration of the diabetogenic BDC2.5 T cells into lymph nodes is inhibited in the presence of N206 T cells. In these *in vivo* experiments, the BDC2.5 T cells are monitored using a novel I-Ag7 tetramer containing a previously identified synthetic mimic epitope, peptide 1040-79 (p79).[18] The p79 peptide is highly active in stimulating the BDC2.5 T cells.[18,19] Our results have demonstrated that the tetAg7/p79 tetramer can specifically stain BDC2.5 T cells and can be used as an excellent staining reagent to track these T cells *in vivo*.[18] Therefore, we have used this tetAg7/p79 tetramer to specifically monitor and identify the presence of BDC2.5 T cells in lymph nodes in the adoptive transfer experiments. Interestingly, our results obtained from the *in vivo* adoptive transfer experiments show that N206 T cells can effectively inhibit the migration of BDC2.5 T cells into lymph nodes when both of these two types of T cells are cotransferred into NOD/scid recipient animals. Therefore, these results are consistent with the hypothesis proposed above. Altogether, these studies have demonstrated that the N206 T cells are not pathogenic cells but are Tr cells, and that these potent IL-10-dependent N206 Tr cells can exert their regulatory function by suppressing the proliferation and/or migration of pathogenic T cells, such as the BDC2.5 T cells.

In our studies on p221-specific T cells isolated from p221-immunized NOD mice, our results from adoptive transfer experiments demonstrate that the N221 T cells can inhibit diabetes development.[10] Additional *in vitro* studies show that N221 T cells are also able to suppress the *in vitro* proliferation of other NOD mouse T cells, including the BDC2.5 T cells, without cell–cell contact. Our results show that N221 T cells probably perform their regulatory functions by secreting cytokines, and antibodies against these cytokines can block their suppressive effect. These studies show that treatment of NOD mice with p221 induces both IL-10-secreting Tr cells and interferon-γ (IFN-γ)(IL-10-secreting regulatory type 1 Tr (Tr1) cells. Further *in vivo* experiments show that N221 Tr cells can also block the migration of BDC2.5 T cells into lymph nodes. Therefore, treatment of NOD mice with p221 induce IL-10-dependent Tr cells and Tr1 cells that suppress the proliferation and/or block the migration of other T cells, including diabetogenic T cells, and inhibit diabetes development.

GAD Peptide-Specific Tr Cells are Present in Naïve NOD Mice

Although immunization of NOD mice with p221 can induce antigen-specific CD4$^+$ Tr cells, it is unclear whether these Tr cells acquire their regulatory capacity due to the immunization or whether they are constitutively harbored in unimmunized naïve mice. To address this question, we used tetAg7/p221 to isolate p221-specific T cells from naïve NOD mice (named herein as naN221 T cells) following peptide-specific *in vitro* expansion. The naN221 T cells produced IFN-γ and IL-10, but very little IL-4, in response to p221 stimulation.[15] Like the N221 T cells isolated from p221-immunized NOD mice, these naN221 T cells also function as Tr cells and inhibit *in vitro* proliferation of BDC2.5 T cells. Additional studies show that the regulatory function of naN221 T cells may involve IL-10 but not IFN-γ, and their suppressive activity is cell contact-independent and is abrogated by antibodies to IL-10 or IL-10 receptor. Interestingly, our studies also show that the IL-2 produced by other T cells present in the cell culture can induce nonactivated naN221 T cells to exhibit regulatory activities involving the production of IL-10. *In vivo*, naN221 T cells inhibited diabetes development when cotransferred with NOD splenocytes into NOD/scid mice. Altogether, these results demonstrate that p221-specific IL-10-dependent Tr cells are present in both naïve and peptide-immunized NOD mice. Therefore, the use of spontaneously arising populations of GAD peptide-specific Tr cells or the *in vivo* expansion of such Tr cells after antigen treatment may represent a promising immunotherapeutic approach for preventing type 1 diabetes.

GAD Peptide-Specific T Cells Isolated from NOR Mice also Function as Tr Cells

The susceptibility to type 1 diabetes is strongly determined by class II MHC genes.[20] It is known that the I-Ag7 genes must be present in both alleles in NOD mice for diabetes to develop, and expression of non-I-Ag7 class II MHC molecules protect NOD mice from diabetes.[21–23] Although the unique I-Ag7 molecule is necessary for diabetes development in NOD mice, other factors are also required for regulating the disease development. The mechanisms underlying the protection from diabetes by non-I-Ag7 molecules is unclear but it could be due to the selection of different TCR specificities, deletion of diabetogenic T cells, or the selection of regulatory T cells.[24–26] These questions may be partly addressed by studies using diabetes-resistant mouse strains, such as the NOR mice. NOR mice are a recombinant congenic strain that also express the I-Ag7 complex.[27] In addition to expressing I-Ag7, NOR mice share many features with NOD mice, such as peripheral T cell accumulation, reduced IL-1 secretion, and the defective peritoneal macrophage responses characteristic of NOD mice. However, unlike NOD mice, NOR mice may show more robust regulatory T cell functions than do NOD mice.[27] Therefore, it appears that the I-Ag7 molecules can select for not only autoantigen-specific pathogenic T cells, but also Tr cells. In support of these ideas, our studies have demonstrated that GAD peptide-specific $CD4^+$ Tr cells, such as those specific for the GAD p206 or p221 peptides, can be selected for by the I-Ag7 molecules and these T cells are present in NOD mice.

In addition to studying GAD peptide-specific T cells that were isolated from NOD mice, we also investigated the function of GAD peptide-specific T cells that were isolated from NOR mice. We did these experiments in order to further characterize GAD peptide-specific T cells isolated from diabetes-resistant mouse strains, and to compare them with NOD mouse T cells having the same antigen specificity. It is expected that these studies will help us evaluate whether T cells with the same antigen specificity that are isolated from NOD or NOR mice possess the same immune function. These studies should also help us to determine whether these different populations of T cells play the same role during the development of type 1 diabetes. We have used I-Ag7 tetramers specific for different GAD peptides to isolate antigen-specific T cells from NOR mice, including p206-specific T cells. We briefly describe below some of the results obtained from these studies. Our results on the studies of the NR206 T cells show that, like the N206 T cells isolated from NOD mice, the NR206 T cells also function as Tr cells and they can inhibit both insulitis and diabetes development. Interestingly, the results of these studies suggest that the underlying regulatory mechanism of the GAD peptide-specific Tr cells derived from these different strains of mice may not be the same.

GAD p206-Specific T Cells Isolated from NOR Mice

In order to understand the function of p206-specific T cells derived from NOR mice, we have used tetAg7/p206 to isolate p206-specific T cells from p206-immunized NOR mice. Our results show that the isolated p206-specific T cells (NR206 T cells) secrete IFN-γ ($\sim$10 ng/mL), very little IL-10 ($<$0.2 ng/mL), and no IL-4. Because NR206 T cells produce IFN-γ but not IL-4, we wanted to determine whether these cells express T-bet, a transcription factor that plays a critical role in the differentiation of Th1 cells.[28] Western blot analyses show that, unlike N206 T cells isolated from NOD mice, NR206 T cells express T-bet. Additional studies show that NR206 T cells probably acquired their phenotype and cytokine secretion profile *in vivo* rather than *in vitro* due to cell culture. The results from these studies show that freshly isolated splenocytes from naïve NOR mice exhibited a similar cytokine secretion profile in response to p206 stimulation prior to being cultured *in vitro*. However, surprisingly, rather than functioning as typical Th1 cells that induce diabetes, NR206 T cells function as Tr cells and can inhibit diabetes and insulitis development induced by either NOD mouse splenocytes or BDC2.5 T cells. In these studies, all of the NOD/scid mice receiving p79-activated BDC2.5 T cells develop diabetes within 10 days after cell transfer, but cotransfer of NR206 T cells with the BDC2.5 T cells inhibited diabetes development. Moreover, NR206 T cells can still inhibit diabetes development even when they are transferred into recipients 2 days after the transfer of BDC2.5 T cells. The timing of transferring NR206 T cells is critical for their inhibitory effect on diabetes, because NR206 T cells fail to inhibit diabetes when transferred into recipient animals on day 4 after the transfer of activated BDC2.5 T cells. In comparison, when NR206 T cells were adoptively transferred into NOD/scid recipient mice prior to the transfer of activated BDC2.5 T cells, none of the recipient animals developed diabetes.

In our studies to investigate the mechanisms underlying the regulatory function of NR206 Tr cells, we have found that NR206 Tr cells can suppress the *in vitro* proliferation of BDC2.5 T cells. Unlike the IL-10-dependent N206 Tr cells isolated from NOD mice, the regulatory function of NR206 T cells is dependent on IFN-γ. Our results show that their regulatory function can be abolished by a neutralizing anti-IFN-γ antibody but not by an anti-IL-10 antibody or by a soluble TNFRI recombinant protein that can block the function of tumor necrosis factor-α (TNF-α). Interestingly, although our RT-PCR results show that NR206 T cells do not express Foxp3, a transcription factor critical for the development and function of the $CD4^+CD25^+$ Tr cells,[29–31] their regulatory function is also cell contact dependent as demonstrated in transwell assays. In these transwell assays, the proliferation of BDC2.5 T cells was not suppressed when NR206 T cells were cultured in the transwell and were separated from BDC2.5 T cells cultured outside of the transwell. These results have raised the question as to why the regulatory function of NR206 T cells is dependent on both IFN-γ and cell contact. Our hypothesis is that NR206 T cells may require the presence of another cell population, and the interaction between NR206 T cells with these cells is necessary for them to exert their regulatory function. One such candidate cell population is the antigen-presenting cells (APCs). Therefore, we performed a panel of studies to evaluate whether the presence of APCs is required for NR206 T cells' regulatory function. Indeed, our results show that APCs are required for NR206 Tr cells to exert their regulatory function, suggesting that these Tr cells coordinate with APCs in suppressing other T cells. However, it is not clear how APCs mediate the suppressive effect on pathogenic T cells.

Previous studies have provided evidence that APCs can themselves function as regulatory cells, and the production of nitric oxide may contribute to their regulatory function.[32,33] In our additional mechanistic experiments, we have determined whether the regulatory function of NR206 T cells requires the production of NO. Our results have demonstrated that the regulatory function of NR206 T cells is also dependent on nitric oxide that is secreted by APCs. Addition of a NO inhibitor, N^G-monomethyl-L-arginine (L-NMMA), but not its inert analog control (D-NMMA) can restore the proliferation of BDC2.5 T cells in response to p79 stimulation. Moreover, the production of NO by APCs occurs only when APCs are cocultured with NR206 Tr cells. In addition, the mere presence of IFN-γ without NR206 Tr cells is not sufficient to induce NO production by APCs. Additional adoptive transfer experiments have shown that NO is required for NR206 Tr cells to inhibit diabetes. Therefore, NR206 Tr cells represent a novel population of Tr cells that mediate their IFN-γ- and cell contact-dependent regulatory function through immunosuppressive NO produced by APCs. These results demonstrate that, despite the same antigen specificity, NR206 Tr cells and N206 Tr cells isolated from NOD mice are not the same Tr cell population and they employ distinct mechanisms for their regulatory functions.

SUMMARY

In summary, our results have demonstrated that, although the I-Ag7 heterodimer is required for diabetes development, it can also select antigen-specific Tr cells with potent regulatory function that inhibit diabetes. Unlike the BDC2.5 T cells, all of the isolated GAD peptide-specific T cells in our studies are not pathogenic T cells but rather are Tr cells that can inhibit diabetes. Therefore, the results from these studies have provided strong evidence supporting the hypothesis that the GAD peptide-specific T cell repertoire of not only the diabetes-prone NOD mice but also diabetes-resistant NOR mice is biased toward Tr cells. Altogether, these results provide an explanation of why the treatment of NOD mice with GAD or its peptides can inhibit the development of diabetes. These studies suggest that induction of GAD-specific regulatory T cells rather than deletion of GAD-specific pathogenic T cells in the GAD or its peptide-treated NOD mice leads to the inhibition of diabetes. Moreover, our results also suggest that, although Tr cells specific for the same peptide are present not only in NOD mice but also in NOR mice, the underlying mechanisms responsible for their regulatory function may not be the same. Therefore, our results and those of others provide evidence that it is possible to identify and isolate GAD-specific Tr cells from at-risk humans or diabetic patients, and that these human Tr cells can be used as an effective treatment for type 1 diabetes.

ACKNOWLEDGMENTS

I want to thank all of the current and past members in my laboratory who have contributed to these studies. The work was supported by in part by grants from NIH.

REFERENCES

1. BACH, J.F. & L. CHATENOUD. 2001. Tolerance to islet autoantigens in type 1 diabetes. Annu. Rev. Immunol. **19:** 131–161.
2. FALCONE, M. & N. SARVETNICK. 1999. Cytokines that regulate autoimmune responses. Curr. Opin. Immunol. **11:** 670–676.
3. MCDEVITT, H. 2004. Specific antigen vaccination to treat autoimmune disease. Proc. Natl. Acad. Sci. USA **101**(Suppl 2): 14627–14630.
4. KAUFMAN, D.L., M. CARE-SALZLER, J. TIAN, *et al.* 1993. Spontaneous loss of T cell tolerance to glutamic acid decarboxylase in murine insulin-dependent diabetes. Nature **366:** 69–72.
5. TISCH, R., X.-D. YANG, S.M. SINGER, *et al.* 1993. Immune response to glutamic acid decarboxylase correlates with insulitis in non-obese diabetic mice. Nature **366:** 72–75.
6. ELLIS, T.M. & M.A. ATKINSON. 1996. The clinical significance of an autoimmune response against glutamic acid decarboxylase. Natl. Med. **2:** 148–153.
7. YOON, J.W., C.S. YOON, H.W. LIM, *et al.* 1999. Control of autoimmune diabetes in NOD mice by GAD expression or suppression in beta cells. Science **284:** 1183–1187.
8. TIAN, J., M. CLARE-SALZLER, A. HERSCHENFELD, *et al.* 1996. Modulating autoimmune responses to GAD inhibits disease progression and prolongs islet graft survival in diabetes-prone mice. Nat. Med. **2:** 1348–1353.
9. TISCH, R., B. WANG & D.V. SERREZE. 1999. Induction of glutamic acid decarboxylase 65-specific Th2 cells and suppression of autoimmune diabetes at late stages of disease is epitope dependent. J. Immunol. **163:** 1178–1187.
10. CHEN, C., W.-H. LEE, P. YUN, *et al.* 2003. Induction of autoantigen-specific Th2 and Tr1 regulatory T cells and modulation of autoimmune diabetes. J. Immunol. **171:** 733–744.
11. ZEKZER, D., F.S. WONG, O. AYALON, *et al.* 1998. GAD-reactive CD4+ Th1 cells induce diabetes in NOD/scid mice. J. Clin. Invest. **101:** 68–73.
12. KASH, S.F., B.G. CONDIE & S. BAEKKESKOV. 1999. Glutamate decarboxylase and GABA in pancreatic islets: lessons from knock-out mice. Hormone Metab. Res. **31:** 340–344.
13. JAECKEL, E., L. KLEIN, N. MARTIN-OROZCO, *et al.* 2003. Normal incidence of diabetes in NOD mice tolerant to glutamic acid decarboxylase. J. Exp. Med. **197:** 1635–1644.
14. MCDEVITT, H. 2003. The T cell response to glutamic acid decarboxylase 65 in T cell receptor transgenic NOD mice. Ann. N. Y. Acad. Sci. **1005:** 75–81.
15. YOU, S., C. CHEN, W.H. LEE, *et al.* 2004. Presence of diabetes-inhibiting, glutamic acid decarboxylase-specific, IL-10-dependent, regulatory T cells in naive nonobese diabetic mice. J. Immunol. **173:** 6777–6785.
16. CHAO, C.C. & H.O. MCDEVITT. 1997. Identification of immunogenic epitopes of GAD 65 presented by Ag7 in non-obese diabetic mice. Immunogenetics **46:** 29–34.
17. LIU, C.P., K. JIANG, C.H. WU, *et al.* 2000. Detection of glutamic acid decarboxylase-activated T cells with I-Ag7 tetramers. Proc. Natl. Acad. Sci. USA **97:** 14596–14601.
18. YOU, Y., C. CHEN, W.H. LEE, *et al.* 2003. Detection and characterization of T cells specific for BDC2.5 T cell-stimulating peptides. J. Immunol. **170:** 4011–4020.

19. JUDKOWSKI, V., C. PINILLA, K. SCHRODER, *et al.* 2001. Identification of MHC class II-restricted peptide ligands, including a glutamic acid decarboxylase 65 sequence, that stimulate diabetogenic T cells from transgenic BDC2.5 nonobese diabetic mice. J. Immunol. **166:** 908–917.
20. TODD, J.A. & L.S. WICKER. 2001. Genetic protection from the inflammatory disease type 1 diabetes in humans and animal models. Immunity **15:** 387–395.
21. MIYAZAKI, T., M. UNO, M. UEHIRA, *et al.* 1990. Direct evidence for the contribution of the unique I-Anod to the development of insulitis in non-obese diabetic mice. Nature **345:** 722–724.
22. LUND, T., L. O'REILLY, P. HUTCHINGS, *et al.* 1990. Prevention of insulin-dependent diabetes mellitus in non-obese diabetic mice by transgenes encoding modified I-A b chain or normal I-E a chain. Nature **345:** 727–729.
23. SLATTERY, R.M., L. KJER-NIELSEN, J. ALLISON, *et al.* 1990. Prevention of diabetes in non-obese diabetic I-Ak transgenic mice. Nature **345:** 724–726.
24. SCHMIDT, D., J. VERDAGUER, N. AVERILL, *et al.* 1997. A mechanism for the major histocompatibility complex-linked resistance to autoimmunity. J. Exp. Med. **186:** 1059–1075.
25. LUHDER, F., J. KATZ, C. BENOIST, *et al.* 1998. Major histocompatibility complex class II molecules can protect from diabetes by positively selecting T cells with additional specificities. J. Exp. Med. **187:** 379–387.
26. VERDAGUER, J., A. AMRANI, B. ANDERSON, *et al.* 1999. Two mechanisms for the non-MHC-linked resistance to spontaneous autoimmunity. J. Immunol. **162:** 4614–4626.
27. PROCHAZKA, M., D.V. SERREZE, W.N. FRANKEL, *et al.* 1992. NOR/Lt mice: MHC-matched diabetes-resistant control strain for NOD mice. Diabetes **41:** 98–106.
28. SZABO, S.J., S.T. KIM, G.L. COSTA, *et al.* 2000. A novel transcription factor, T-bet, directs Th1 lineage commitment. Cell **100:** 655–669.
29. HORI, S., T. TAKAHASHI & S. SAKAGUCHI. 2003. Control of autoimmunity by naturally arising regulatory CD4+ T cells. Adv. Immunol. **81:** 331–371.
30. FONTENOT, J.D., M.A. GAVIN & A.Y. RUDENSKY. 2003. Foxp3 programs the development and function of CD4+CD25+ regulatory T cells. Nat. Immunol. **4:** 330–336.
31. KHATTRI, R., T. COX, S.A. YASAYKO, *et al.* 2003. An essential role for Scurfin in CD4+CD25+ T regulatory cells. Nat. Immunol. **4:** 337–342.
32. HUANG, F.P., W. NIEDBALA, X.Q. WEI, *et al.* 1998. Nitric oxide regulates Th1 cell development through the inhibition of IL-12 synthase by macrophages. Eur. J. Immunol. **28:** 4062–4070.
33. ZHANG, M., H. TANG, Z. GUO, *et al.* 2004. Splenic stroma drives mature dendritic cells to differentiate into regulatory dendritic cells. Nat. Immunol. **5:** 1124–1133.

Metabolism Genes Are among the Differentially Expressed Ones Observed in Lymphomononuclear Cells of Recently Diagnosed Type 1 Diabetes Mellitus Patients

DIANE M. RASSI,[a,b] CRISTINA M. JUNTA,[b] ANA LÚCIA FACHIN,[b] PAULA SANDRIN-GARCIA,[b] STEFANO MELLO,[b] MÁRCIA M.C. MARQUES,[b] ANA PAULA M. FERNANDES,[c] MARIA CRISTINA FOSS-FREITAS,[d] MILTON C. FOSS,[d,e] ELZA T. SAKAMOTO-HOJO,[b] GERALDO A.S. PASSOS,[b] AND EDUARDO A. DONADI[a,b,e]

[a]Immunology Program, [b]Molecular Immunogenetics Group, [c]General and Specialized Nursing, [d]Division of Endocrinology, and [e]Division Clinical Immunology, Faculty of Medicine of Ribeirão Preto, Ribeirão Preto, University of São Paulo, SP, Brazil - 14049-900

ABSTRACT: The large-scale differential gene expression in lymphomononuclear cells of six patients with recently diagnosed type), and six normal individuals matched to patients for sex and age were studied. Glass slides containing 4608 cDNAs from the IMAGE library were spotted using robotic technology. Statistical analysis was carried out by the SAM program, and gene function assessed by the FATIGO program. Thirty differentially expressed genes (21 induced and 9 repressed) were disclosed when DM-1 patients were compared with controls. Although presenting with distinct biological function, most of the induced or repressed genes were related with protein, phosphate, DNA, RNA, carboxylic acid, and fatty acid metabolism. Although some of these genes have been previously associated with the pathogenesis of T1DM, many other genes were identified for further studies.

KEYWORDS: type 1 diabetes mellitus; gene expression; microarrays; metabolism genes

INTRODUCTION

The breakdown in T cell tolerance against pancreatic autoantigens results in infiltration of the insulin-producing β cells by a cohort of lymphoid and other

Address for correspondence: Dr. Eduardo A. Donadi, Divisão de Clínica Médica, Faculdade de Medicina de Ribeirão Preto, Universidade de São Paulo, USP, 14049-900, S.P., Brasil. Voice: +55-16-3602-2566; fax: +55-16-3633-6695.
e-mail: eadonadi@fmrp.usp.br

Ann. N.Y. Acad. Sci. 1079: 171–176 (2006).
doi: 10.1196/annals.1375.026

inflammatory cells, where T cells play a critical role in islet destruction, giving rise to clinical type 1 diabetes mellitus (T1DM).[1] Although pathogenetic mechanisms have not been completely elucidated, T ($CD4^+$ and $CD8^+$) cells, B cells, and antigen-presenting cells are the most frequently involved. Since insulin plays a major role in glucose metabolism and protein synthesis regulation in a number of tissues and culture systems,[2] and since recently diagnosed T1DM patients represent the end stage of pancreatic β cell destruction, in this article we evaluated the differential large-scale gene expression in total peripheral blood mononuclear cells obtained from recently diagnosed T1DM patients.

MATERIALS AND METHODS

Subjects

Six prepuberty recently diagnosed (<6 months) T1DM patients age 3 to 13 years (median = 8), from the Outpatient Clinics of the Division of Endocrinology, Department of Medicine, Faculty of Medicine of Ribeirão Preto, University of São Paulo, Brazil, and six normal individuals presenting no family history of T1DM and matched to patients in terms of sex and age were studied. All subjects were submitted to complete anamnesis and physical examination, and presented no infectious diseases. Patients were selected only after adequate insulin treatment achieving metabolic control of the disease, that is, normalization of glucose and glycate hemoglobin levels. Informed written consent was obtained from all individuals, and the local ethics committee approved the protocol of the study (Process 7945/99).

Total RNA Extraction

Total peripheral blood mononuclear cells were isolated by gradient density using Ficoll-Hypaque (Sigma, St. Louis, MO). Total RNA was extracted using Trizol® (Invitrogen, Carlsbad, CA) according to the manufacturer's instructions. The integrity of RNA samples was evaluated by denaturing agarose gel electrophoresis under standard conditions and Northern blot analysis using an oligonucleotide probe that recognizes the 28S rRNA fraction (data not shown).

cDNA Microarrays

The gene expression of healthy or patient lymphomononuclear cells was assessed using glass slide cDNA microarrays, containing 4608 sequences (in replicates) from the human-expressed sequence tags (ESTs) cDNA library

(IMAGE Consortium, http://image.llnl.gov). The microarrays were prepared on the basis of published protocols using 0.75- to 1.0-kb PCR product from the cDNA clones.[3]

Data Analysis

Data normalization and centralization were applied to minimize differences between distinct hybridization events. Statistical analysis was performed by the significance analysis of microarrays (SAM) using three to four pair wise experimental duplicates to determine genes displaying significant differential expression. The data regarding gene location and biological function were obtained at SOURCE (http://genome-www5.stanford.edu/cgi-bin/SMD/source/source), NCBI (http://www.ncbi.nlm.nih.gov/), and FATIGO (http://fatigo.bioinfo.cipf.es) program.

RESULTS

Thirty differentially expressed genes, 9 repressed and 21 induced, were observed when patients were compared to healthy controls. According to the major biological process attributed to these genes, those involved with protein, phosphate, DNA, RNA, carboxylic acid, and fatty acid metabolism were among the differentially expressed ones. Other processes involved in induced genes include transport, response to DNA damage stimulus, cell organization and biogenesis, cell proliferation, response to wounding, oxidative stress and defense, and cell-surface receptor-linked signal transduction. Other processes involved in repressed genes include response to hormone stimulus and intracellular signaling cascade. TABLE 1 shows some features of these genes.

DISCUSSION

Although presenting with distinct biological function, differentially expressed genes were related with protein and phosphate metabolism (induced, repressed, or both), and DNA (induced), RNA, carboxylic acid, and fatty acid (repressed) metabolism.

Many of the differentially expressed genes may potentially be associated with DM-1 pathogenesis; however, only those considered to be of more interest to disease pathogenesis were pinpointed to be discussed. Among induced genes, the bromodomain gene has been associated with the autoimmune polyendocrine syndromes type 1 and 2 (APS-1 and APS-2), caused by mutation in an autoimmune regulator gene, mapped in chromosome 21, which share

TABLE 1. Differentially expressed genes (21 induced and 9 repressed) with patients versus controls

Gene	Function	Chromosome	UniGene
Insulinoma-associated 1	Transformation of neuroendocrine cells	20p11.2	NM-002196
HMG-box transcription factor 1	Regulation of transcription, DNA-dependent	7q22-q31	NM-12257
RAB14, member RAS oncogene family	GTP binding, GTPase activity	9q32-q34.11	AL162081
Ubiquitin-conjugating enzyme E2G2	Ligase activity, ubiquitin-conjugating enzyme activity	21q22.3	AK122700
Peroxiredoxin 5	Oxireductase activity, transporter electron, peroxidase activity	11q13	BU734349
UL16-binding protein 2	Stimulated lipid degradation in adipocytes	6q25	BC034689
Pre-mRNA	Component of pre-mRNA cleavage complex ii	11Q13	BC0655384
Putative translation initiation factor	Probably involved in translation	17q21.2	AL0550005
Bromodomain	Possible transcription activator	3p26-p25	NM-001003694
Core 1 UDP galactosidase	Transferase activity	7p14-p13	AK023557
Protein kinase	Protein kinase	7-p22	AL833563
Cyclin M1	Fatty acid biosynthesis	10q24.2	NM-020348
Spermatogenesis-associated 13	Regulated synaptic differentiation	13q12.12	BX648244
Phosphatidylinositol glycan, class O	Hydrolase activity	9p13.3	AL833956
Aldehyde dehydrogenase 3	Detoxification of aldehydes generated by alcohol metabolism and lipid peroxidation	17p11.2	U46689
Basic leucine zipper	Transcription factor activity	1q24	U79751
PDZ domain contain 10	Signaling pathways involved in cell motility, proliferation, and apoptosis	Xp22.2	XM-045712
Kinase suppressor of Ras	Transduction of mitogenic signals from the cell membrane to the nucleus	17q11.2	XM-290793
Chromosome 6 open reading frame 154	Chromosome 6 open reading frame 154	6p21.1	XM-168060
Protein kinase	Protein kinase	8q11	NM-006904
Insulin-like growth factor binding protein 4	*Insulin-like growth factor binding*	*17q12-q21.1*	*NM-001552*
RNA polymerase I	*RNA polymerase I*	*9p13.2*	*AK125471*
Protein inhibitor of activated STAT 2	*Regulation of transcription DNA-dependent, transcription*	*18q21.1*	*CR749597*
Arrestin domain	*Transduction of signals*	*9q34.3*	*CR627251*

Six genes with no defined biological function are not shown. Repressed genes are shown in italics.

with T1DM the HLA-DR3 and HLA-DR4 allele group susceptibility.[4] The cyclin M1 gene is highly expressed on pancreas islets and regulates cell cycle. Although M cyclins have not been associated with T1DM, D1 and D2 cyclins are essential for the expansion of β cells in adult mice, suggesting that cyclins regulate the activity of β pancreatic cells, and may serve as a tool to prevent or even cure diabetes.[5] Protein 2 ligand of UL16 gene mapped on the chromosome 6q25 natural killer (NK) cluster is involved with the activation of NK cells for receptors NKG2D. Daily treatment of NOD mice with NKG2D monoclonal antibody during the prediabetic stage, completely abrogates disease development and functioning of autoreactive T $CD8^+$ cells.[6] The polymorphism of the aldehyde dehydrogenase gene has been associated with susceptibility to T1DM. These patients primarily have the (62.2%) ALDH2*1/ALDH2*1 genotype, followed by the ALDH2*1/ALDH2*2 (30.9%), and ALDH2*2/ALDH2*2 (7.0%) genotypes.[7] Among repressed genes, the inhibitory protein of activated STAT2 (PIAS2) gene is involved in signaling of the proinflammatory cytokines INF-γ, TNF-α and IL-1, which are important in the initial process of insulitis. The RNA polymerase I-associated factor 53 gene (PAF53) has been described to be modulated by insulin. Decreased synthesis of PAF53 has been associated with insulin deprivation in culture hepatocytes, which is restored after insulin treatment.[8]

In the present study, several genes were differentially expressed in recently diagnosed T1DM patients, which may potentially be associated with disease pathogenesis. How much the glycation mechanisms induced in the prediabetes/diabetes stage or how much immunological alterations seen in the end stage of beta cell destruction are responsible for such findings are questions that need further studies.

ACKNOWLEDGMENT

This work was financially supported by Fapesp—Fundação de Amparo a Pesquisa do Estado de São Paulo (Grant: 01/04101-9 and 99/12135-9).

REFERENCES

1. SERREZE, D.V. & E.H. LEITER. 2001. Genes and cellular requirements for autoimmune diabetes susceptibility in nonobese diabetic mice. Curr. Dir. Autoimmun. **4:** 31–67.
2. HANNAN, K.M., L.I. ROTHBLUM & L.S. JEFFERSON. 1998. Regulation of ribosomal DNA transcription by insulin. Am. J. Physiol. **275**(1 Pt 1): C130–C138.
3. HEDGE, P.O.L.K., C. ABERNATHY, S. GAY, *et al.* 2000. Concise guide to cDNA microarray analysis. Biotechniques **29:** 548–562.
4. REDONDO, M.J. & G.S. EISENBARTH. 2002. Genetic control of autoimmunity in type 1 diabetes and associated disorders. Diabectologia **45:** 605–622.

5. KUSHNER, J.A., M.A. CIEMERYCH, E. SICINSKA, *et al.* 2005. Cyclins D2 and D1 are essential for postnatal pancreatic beta-cell growth. Mol. Cell Biol. **25:** 3752–3762.
6. OGASAWARA, K., J.A. HAMERMAN, L.R. EHRLICH, *et al.* 2004. NKG2D blockade prevents autoimmune diabetes in NOD mice. Immunity **20:** 757–767.
7. SUZUKI, Y., N. MATSUURA, S. SUZUKI, *et al.* 2003. Aldehyde dehydrogenase 2 genotype in type 1 diabetes mellitus. Diabetes Res. Clin. Pract. **60:** 139–141.
8. KIMBALL, S.R., T.C. VARY & L.S. JEFFERSON. 1994. Regulation of protein synthesis by insulin. Annu. Rev. Physiol. **56:** 321–348.

In Vitro TNF-α and IL-6 Production by Adherent Peripheral Blood Mononuclear Cells Obtained from Type 1 and Type 2 Diabetic Patients Evaluated according to the Metabolic Control

MARIA CRISTINA FOSS-FREITAS,[a] NORMA TIRABOSCHI FOSS,[b] EDUARDO ANTONIO DONADI,[c] AND MILTON CESAR FOSS[a]

[a]*Divisions of Endocrinology and Metabolism, Department of Medicine, Ribeirão Preto Medical School, São Paulo University, Ribeirão Preto, Brazil 14049-900*

[b]*Division of Dermatology, Department of Medicine, Ribeirão Preto Medical School, São Paulo University, Ribeirão Preto, Brazil 14049-900*

[c]*Division of Clinical Immunology, Department of Medicine, Ribeirão Preto Medical School, São Paulo University, Ribeirão Preto, Brazil 14049-900*

ABSTRACT: Tumor necrosis factor-α (TNF-α) and interleukin-6 (IL-6) levels were evaluated in lipopolysaccharide (LPS)-stimulated cell cultured monocytes obtained from 24 type 1 and type 2 diabetic patients presenting inadequate (IN) or adequate (AD) metabolic control, and in 21 healthy individuals paired to patients for sex and age. The TNF-α levels in stimulated cultures of diabetic patients were similar to healthy individuals, and type 1 diabetic patients showed increased IL-6 supernatant levels. The tendency toward increased TNF-α and IL-6 levels was observed with metabolic control of type 1 and type 2 diabetic patients, suggesting that the control of diabetes improves the capacity of activation and maintenance of the proinflammatory immune response.

KEYWORDS: type 1 diabetes mellitus; type 2 diabetes mellitus; TNF-α; interleukin-6; metabolic control

INTRODUCTION

Cytokines have been implicated in the development of many chronic complications of diabetes mellitus patients, including neurological and vascular lesions.[1] Besides, the increased susceptibility to infection may be caused by

Address for correspondence: Milton C. Foss, Department of Medicine, Ribeirão Preto Medical School, University of São Paulo, Av. Bandeirantes, 3900, Monte Alegre, Ribeirão Preto (SP), Brazil, 14049-900. Voice: + 55-16-602-2467; fax: + 55-16-633-6695.
e-mail: mcfoss@fmrp.usp.br

Ann. N.Y. Acad. Sci. 1079: 177–180 (2006).
doi: 10.1196/annals.1375.027

acquired immunological system defects.[2] Interleukin-6 (IL-6) is a major mediator of acute-phase response that has many diabetogenic actions including adrenocorticotropic hormone (ACTH) stimulation.[3] Tumor necrosis factor-α (TNF-α) also acts as an acute-phase reactant, contributing to insulin resistance by inhibiting the insulin receptor tyrosine kinase activity and producing down-regulation of glucose transporter genes.[4] Controversial results regarding TNF-α and IL-6 concentration in monocyte-simulated cultures have been reported; however, few studies have been conducted on the influence of metabolic control in diabetic patients. In the present article we evaluated the *in vitro* IL-6 and TNF-α production by adherent peripheral blood mononuclear cells obtained from type 1 or type 2 diabetic patients, evaluated before and after adequate (AD) metabolic control.

SUBJECTS AND METHODS

Twenty-four patients (11 with type 1 and 13 with type 2 diabetes) seen at the Outpatient Clinics of the University Hospital of the Medical School of Ribeirão Preto-USP, Brazil, and 21 healthy individuals paired to patients for sex, age, and body mass index for type 1 (C1) and type 2 (C2) diabetic patients, were studied. Patients were evaluated before and after metabolic control, and did not present chronic macro/microvascular and neurological complications. Inadequate (IN) metabolic control was defined when fasting glucose was $\geq$200 mg/dL and glycated hemoglobin $\geq$ 11%. Patients did not present infectious disease and were not taking drugs that might interfere with the results. Patients were hospitalized for 2–3 weeks to obtain AD metabolic control with regular daily capillary blood glucose measurements at 7 AM, 11 AM, 17 PM, and 23 PM, and after regular insulin administration. The study protocol was approved by the local ethics committee, and all subjects gave informed written consent to participate in the study. Blood samples for cytokine measurements were obtained on the first and last day of hospitalization. Mononuclear cells were isolated by gradient density using Ficoll-Hypaque® (Sigma, St. Louis, MO).[5] A total of 1.5×10^6 plastic adherent cells/mL were cultivated during 24 h in the presence or absence of lipopolysaccharide (LPS). IL-6 and TNF-α were assayed in cell culture supernatants using ELISA. Statistical analyses were performed by the Kruskal–Wallis and Wilcoxon signed rank tests using the GraphPad Prism program (San Diego, CA). A P value < 0.05 was considered to be significant.

RESULTS

The four groups studied, that is, type 1 and type 2 diabetic patients and healthy individuals paired for type 1 and type 2 diabetes patients, did not differ significantly in terms of age, sex, and body mass index. Metabolic control evaluated by the daily mean glycemic profile during the hospitalization period showed a significant improvement with treatment between the first and last day of hospitalization in type 1 and type 2 diabetic patients ($P = 0.0002$ and $P = 0.0001$, respectively). Comparisons between median TNF-α levels observed before (IN) and after (AD) the metabolic control, in type 1 (IN: 1541.5 and AD: 1556.2 pg/mL) and type 2 (IN: 796.3 and AD: 1018.9 pg/mL) patients were higher than the normal control group (C1: 1073.6 and C2: 557.9 pg/mL). Although significant differences were not observed, a clear trend toward increased TNF-α levels was observed in patients presenting an AD metabolic control.

Median IL-6 levels observed before and after metabolic control in type 1 (IN: 16,278.5 and AD: 16,571.2 pg/mL) patients were increased in relation to those observed for respective controls (C1:11,917.5 pg/mL), yielding P values < 0.001. However, in type 2 diabetic patients before and after metabolic control, the IL-6 levels (IN: 4643.3 and AD: 6289.0 pg/mL) were reduced compared to the normal controls (C2 = 5375 pg/mL), yielding P values 0.03 and 0.02, respectively. Median IL-6 levels in type 1 diabetic patients were higher than type 2 levels, yielding P values < 0.0002.

DISCUSSION

Little attention has been devoted to the role of metabolic control on cytokine levels, a fact that may be important to cope with infections, a well-known complication, particularly for type 2 patients. TNF and IL-6 are highly involved with macrophage activation and increased levels of these cytokines have been observed in insulin resistance stages and diabetes mellitus development.[6] In this study, TNF-α levels produced by monocytes of diabetic patients were closely similar to those observed in control groups, as previously described.[7] Notwithstanding, there was a tendency of increase in TNF-α levels with the AD metabolic control. The IL-6 data suggest that type 1 diabetic patients present a pattern of acute inflammatory response, independently of the metabolic control. The IL-6 and TNF-α increased levels in type 2 diabetic patients after insulin treatment suggest that the metabolic control improves the capacity of activation and maintenance of the proinflammatory immune response, possibly contributing to decrease the susceptibility to infections.

REFERENCES

1. SHANMUGAM, N. *et al.* 2003. High glucose-induced expression of pro-inflammatory cytokine and chemokine genes in monocytic cells. Diabetes **52:** 1256–1264.
2. GEERLINGS, S.E. & A.I.M. HOEPELMAN. 1999. Immune dysfunction in patients with diabetes mellitus (DM). FESM Immunol. Med. Microbiol. **26:** 259–265.

3. AKIRA, T. *et al.* 1993. Interleukin-6 in biology and medicine. Adv. Immunol. **54:** 1–78.
4. HOTAMISLIGIL, G.S. & B.M. SPIEGELMAN. 1994. Tumor necrosis factor alpha: a key of the obesity-diabetes link. Diabetes **43:** 1271–1278.
5. FOSS, N.T. *et al.* 1993. Correlation between TNF production, increase of plasma C reactive protein level and suppression of T lymphocyte response to concanavalin A during erythema nodosum leprosum. Intl. J. Lepr. **61:** 218–226.
6. PICKUP, J.C. *et al.* 2000. Plasma interleukin-6, tumor necrosis factor α and blood cytokine production in type 2 diabetes. Life Sci. **67:** 291–300.
7. GEELINGS, S.E. *et al.* 2000. Cytokine secretion is impaired in women with diabetes mellitus. Eur. J. Clin. Invest. **30:** 995–1001.

T Cell Immunity to Glutamic Acid Decarboxylase in Fulminant Type 1 Diabetes without Significant Elevation of Serum Amylase

KANEMI AOKI,[a] MATSUO TANIYAMA,[a] CHIEKO NAGAYAMA,[a] YOICHI OIKAWA,[b] AND AKIRA SHIMADA[b]

[a]*Department of Internal Medicine, Division of Endocrinology and Metabolism, Showa University Fujigaoka Hospital, Fujigaoka, Aoba, Yokohama, Kanagawa, Japan 227-8501*

[b]*Department of Internal Medicine, Keio University School of Medicine, Tokyo, Japan*

ABSTRACT: We encountered three patients with fulminant type 1 diabetes whose serum amylase levels were not elevated and evaluated their immunological characteristics. Although all three patients had no antibodies to islet antigens including glutamic acid decarboxylase (GAD), GAD-reactive T lymphocytes were detected in two patients. Combined with the findings that human leukocyte antigen (HLA) class II haplotype associated with fulminant type 1 diabetes is the same as that of autoimmune type 1 diabetes, an immune process similar to autoimmune type 1 diabetes may be involved in at least a part of fulminant type 1 diabetes.

KEYWORDS: fulminant type 1 diabetes; T cell immunity; glutamic acid decarboxylase; amylase

Type 1 diabetes is generally thought to be caused by autoimmune destruction of pancreatic β cells. Some diabetic patients with total loss of β cells function are negative for antibodies to islet antigens, and their diabetes is classified as non-immune idiopathic type 1 diabetes (or type 1B). Fulminant type 1 diabetes, that is characterized by the abrupt onset with low initial HbA1c levels and the absence of the islet-associated autoantibodies, was recently identified by Imagawa *et al.* as a subtype of idiopathic type 1 diabetes.[1] Another characteristic of this type of diabetes is the elevation of serum pancreatic exocrine enzymes. Histological examination reveals the absence of insulitis, and

Address for correspondence: Matsuo Taniyama, M.D., Department of Internal Medicine, Division of Endocrinology and Metabolism, Showa University Fujigaoka Hospital, 1-30 Fujigaoka, Aoba, Yokohama, Kanagawa, Japan 227-8501. Voice: +81-45-971-1151; fax: +81-45-973-1019.
e-mail: taniyama@showa-university-fujigaoka.gr.jp

Ann. N.Y. Acad. Sci. 1079: 181–185 (2006). © 2006 New York Academy of Sciences.
doi: 10.1196/annals.1375.028

mononuclear cell infiltration to exocrine pancreas is observed. The etiology of fulminant type 1 diabetes is controversial. Imagawa *et al*. speculated that β cell destruction in this type of diabetes is not mediated by an autoimmune process because the autoantibodies to islet antigens or insulitis are absent. Tanaka *et al*., however, reported that $CD8^+$ lymphocytes infiltrated into the pancreatic islets in a patient who died of fulminant type 1 diabetes.[2] Furthermore, peripheral glutamic acid decarboxylase (GAD)-reactive interferon (INF)-γ-producing $CD4^+$ lymphocytes were detected in a 33-year-old man with fulminant type 1 diabetes.[3] These findings suggest that T cell-mediated immunity may be involved in this type of diabetes. We have seen three patients with abrupt-onset sero-negative type 1 diabetes whose clinical characteristics were similar to fulminant type 1 diabetes except for the absence of significant elevation of serum amylase. We evaluated the immunological characteristics of these patients including human leukocyte antigen (HLA) and GAD-reactive INF-γ-producing $CD4^+$ lymphocytes, to clarify whether the immune process of islet antigens is involved in fulminant type 1 diabetes.

PATIENTS AND METHODS

Patients

Three patients (2 men and 1 woman, aged 36–56 years) with abrupt onset of insulin-dependent diabetes characterized by the absence of islet-related autoantibodies (anti-GAD antibodies and islet cell antibodies) whose initial HbA1c levels were low (5.0–6.0%) were studied. Symptoms of marked hyperglycemia appeared only a few days before the development of ketoacidosis. Two patients had symptoms of upper respiratory infection shortly before the onset of diabetes. Patients did not show significant elevation of serum amylase levels (one patient showed marginal elevation without symptoms). Diabetes of these patients was classified as type 1 because β cells were completely lost. (TABLE 1).

METHODS

HLA class I and class II were determined by Terasaki's standard plates. GAD-specific responses of peripheral INF-γ-producing $CD4^+$ T lymphocytes were analyzed at 1–3 years after the onset of diabetes by intracellular cytokine assay (FastImmune Cytokine System, Becton Dickinson Immunocytometry Systems, San Jose, CA) as previously reported by Shimada *et al*.[4] In brief, peripheral whole blood was incubated at 37°C in a 5% CO_2 atmosphere in the presence of recombinant GAD65 and CD28 antibodies for 68 h and then treated with Brefeldin A for 4 h. After the surface marker was labeled with CD4-PC5 antibodies, the mononuclear cells were isolated and were reacted

TABLE 1. Clinical features of patients

Patient	1	2	3
Age (years)	36	43	56
Sex	M	F	M
Duration[a] (day)	1	3	3
Plasma glucose (mg/dL)	1,760	348	913
HbA1c (%)	5.0	6.0	5.6
Arterial pH	6.977	7.275	7.007
Serum amylase[b]	1.7	0.4	0.8
Glucagon stimulated serum CPR (ng/mL)	0.1	< 0.2	0.3
Urinary CPR (g/day)	< 0.3	< 0.3	3.7
Anti-GAD antibodies	Negative	Negative	Negative
Islet cell antibodies	Negative	Not done	Negative
HLA typing	A2 A24 B54 B61 Cw1 Cw3 DR4 DR8	A24 A26 B54 B59 Cw1 DR4	A24 A33 B44 B61 DR4 DR9
GAD-reactive $CD4^+$ T cells (/50,000 $CD4^+$ T cells)	560	240	0

[a]Duration refers to the length of hyperglycemic symptoms before diagnosis.
[b]Values expressed by multiples of upper limit of normal values.

with fluorescence-labeled INF-γ antibodies following to permeabilization of the cell membrane. The $CD4^+$ cells positive for intracellular INF-γ were then counted by flow cytometry.

RESULTS

All had DR4, which is related to autoimmune type 1 diabetes in the Japanese population. GAD-reactive INF-γ-producing $CD4^+$ cells were detected in 1 patient at 560 and in another patient at 240 per 50,000 $CD4^+$ cells (TABLE 1). (The mean value in type 2 diabetic patients without anti-GAD antibodies is 0.3 per 50,000 $CD4^+$ cells).

DISCUSSION

The present three patients had characteristics of fulminant type 1 diabetes except for the absence of significant elevation of serum amylase. Despite the absence of islet-associated autoantibodies, these patients' diabetes is classified as type 1 because β cell function was completely lost. Destruction of the β cells must have been very rapid because HbA1c levels at diagnosis were almost normal. Abrupt onset and the absence of autoantibodies to pancreatic β cell antigens lead to the diagnosis of fulminant type 1 diabetes even though these patients did not show significant elevation of serum amylase. We only examined amylase, not other exocrine pancreatic enzymes, such as lipase and elastase 1. Therefore, we cannot exclude the involvement of the exocrine pancreas. Imagawa *et al.* reported about a nationwide survey in Japan of fulminant type 1 diabetes.[5] In some patients serum amylase levels were not elevated but either lipase or elastase 1 level was elevated in most of these patients. Thus, some patients show elevation of lipase or elastase 1 only. There is still a possibility of the existence of fulminant type 1 diabetes without elevation of exocrine pancreatic enzymes. Yamazaki *et al.* reported a case of rapid-onset sero-negative type 1 diabetes in which exocrine pancreas was not involved.[6] Idiopathic type 1 diabetes, including the fulminant type 1 diabetes was characterized by the absence of antibodies to islet-related antigens. However, in autoimmune type 1 diabetes, T cell-mediated autoimmunity plays an important role in the destruction of β cells and lack of humoral immunity to β cells does not mean the absence of cellular immunity to β cells. The findings of positive GAD-reactive T lymphocytes in peripheral blood in the present two patients, as well as in the case reported by Shimada *et al.* may indicate that immune process is involved in at least a part of the sero-negative abrupt-onset type 1 diabetes with or without exocrine pancreatic enzyme elevation. GAD-reactive T lymphocytes were also demonstrated in fulminant type 1 diabetes by the Elispot assay.[7] Furthermore, all three presented patients had HLA DR4, which is associated with autoimmune type 1 diabetes in the Japanese population. The initial report and further investigations[8] revealed that HLA class II haplotype associated with autoimmune type 1 diabetes is also strongly associated with fulminant type 1 diabetes. Thus, immunogenetic features and the presence of peripheral GAD-reactive T lymphocytes in our patients suggest that at least a part of fulminant type 1 diabetes is associated with autoimmunity to the islet. GAD-reactive T lymphocytes were not detected in one patient in the present study, however, this may suggest that there is still the possibility of the existence of type 1 diabetes not being associated with an immune process.

REFERENCES

1. Imagawa, A., T. Hanafusa, J. Miyagawa, *et al.* 2000. A novel subtype of type 1 diabetes mellitus characterized by a rapid onset and an absence of diabetes-related antibodies. N. Engl. J. Med. **342:** 301–307.
2. Tanaka, S., T. Kobayashi & T. Momotsu. 2000. A novel subtype of type 1 diabetes mellitus. N. Engl. J. Med. **342:** 1835–1837.
3. Shimada, A., J. Morimoto, K. Kodama, *et al.* 2002. T-cell-mediated autoimmunity may be involved in fulminant type 1 diabetes. Diabetes Care **25:** 635–636.
4. Shimada, A., K. Kodama & J. Morimoto. 2003. Detection of GAD-reactive CD4+ cells in so-called "type 1B" diabetes. Ann. N. Y. Acad. Sci. **1005:** 378–386.
5. Imagawa, A., T. Hanafusa, Y. Uchigata, *et al.* 2003. Fulminant type 1 diabetes. Diabetes Care **26:** 2345–2352.
6. Yamazaki, M. & T. Hayashi. 2002. Rapid-onset type 1 diabetes mellitus without pancreatic exocrine dysfunction. Ann. Intern. Med. **137:** 145–146.

7. KOTANI, R., M. NAGATA, A. IMAGAWA, *et al.* 2004. T lymphocyte response against pancreatic beta cell antigens in fulminant type 1 diabetes. Diabetologia **47:** 1285–1291.
8. TANAKA, S., T. KOBAYASHI, K. NAKANISHI, *et al.* 2002. Association of HLA-DQ genotype in autoantibody-negative and rapid-onset type 1 diabetes. Diabetes Care **25:** 2302–2307.

Expression Levels of CXC Chemokine Receptors 3 Are Associated with Clinical Phenotype of Type 1 Diabetes

SATORU YAMADA,[a] YOICHI OIKAWA,[b] GEN SAKAI,[b]
YOSHIHITO ATSUMI,[c] TARO MARUYAMA,[d] AND AKIRA SHIMADA[b]

[a]*Department of Internal Medicine, Kitasato Institute Hospital, Tokyo 108-8642, Japan*

[b]*Department of Internal Medicine, Keio University School of Medicine, Tokyo 160-8582, Japan*

[c]*Department of Internal Medicine, Saiseikai Central Hospital, Tokyo 108-0073, Japan*

[d]*Department of Internal Medicine, Saitama Social Insurance Hospital, Saitama 330-0074, Japan*

ABSTRACT: Type 1 diabetes is recognized as one of T helper 1 cell (Th1)-mediated diseases. The purpose of this article was to investigate the expression levels of CXC chemokine receptor 3 (CXCR3) and CC chemokine receptor 5 (CCR5) on CD4 T cells as Th1 markers in Japanese patients with type 1 diabetes and control subjects. A total of 72 patients with type 1 diabetes and 24 healthy subjects were enrolled. Their peripheral mononuclear cells were obtained and stained with anti-CXCR3, anti-CCR5, and anti-CD4 monoclonal antibodies. Flow-cytometric analysis was performed and patients were classified according to their onset pattern as fulminant, typical, or slow onset. Statistical analysis was performed using ANOVA. CXCR3 expression on CD4 T cells in patients with a fulminant pattern of onset was significantly lower than that in the other groups, and that in patients with a typical pattern of onset was significantly higher than that in the other groups. CCR5 expression on CD4 T cells was not different among the three clinical phenotypes. CXCR3 expression level is associated with the onset pattern of type 1 diabetes. Further studies are needed to clarify the role of chemokines in type 1 diabetes.

KEYWORDS: CXCR3; CCR5; chemokine; diabetes

Address for correspondence: Satoru Yamada, M.D., Ph.D., 5-9-1 Shirokane, Minato-ku, Tokyo 108-8642, Japan. Voice: +81-3-3444-6161; fax: +81-3-3448-0553.
e-mail: yamada-s@kitasato.or.jp

**Ann. N.Y. Acad. Sci. 1079: 186–189 (2006). © 2006 New York Academy of Sciences.
doi: 10.1196/annals.1375.029**

BACKGROUND

Type 1 diabetes mellitus is recognized as an autoimmune disease related to cell-mediated immunity. However, there is no appropriate way to examine cell-mediated immunity. CXC chemokine receptor 3 (CXCR3) and CC chemokine receptor 5 (CCR5), which are expressed on T helper 1 cells (Th1) have been hypothesized to associate with type 1 diabetes.[1] Therefore, we evaluated the expression of CXCR3 and CCR5 in peripheral T cells in Japanese type 1 diabetic patients and classified them according to their pattern of onset of diabetes into fulminant,[2] typical, and slow type.[3]

RESEARCH DESIGN AND METHODS

A total of 72 Japanese patients with type 1 diabetes, from Kitasato Institute Hospital, Keio University Hospital, Saitama Social Insurance Hospital, and Saiseikai Central Hospital, were included in this study. The mean age of the patients was 44.6 ± 14.3 years (range 21–73 years). Among them, 10 patients satisfied Imagawa's criteria for fulminant type 1 diabetes[2] (group A; present age was 46.8 ± 12.1 [mean ± SD] years, onset age was 43.6 ± 10.8 years, 9 male, 1 female); 42 patients were found to have typical type 1 diabetes that is ketoacidosis prone and within 6 months from diagnosis to insulin dependency (group B; present age was 41.5 ± 14.5 years, onset age was 32.3 ± 16.2 years, 21 male, 21 female); and 20 patients had slow onset type 1 diabetes (group C; present age was 50.3 ± 14.9 years, onset age was 40.1 ± 12.4 years, 15 male, 5 female). Patients in group C had been originally diagnosed as having type 2 diabetes and were autoantibodies to glutamic acid decarboxylase (GAD) and/or Insulinoma-associated antigen 2 (IA-2) positive. In addition, we registered 24 unrelated healthy Japanese subjects as controls (age was 30.2 ± 17.1 years, $n = 24$, 16 male, 8 female).

All probands gave their informed consent before their inclusion in the study. This study was approved by the institutional ethical board, and all investigations were performed according to the principles of the appropriate version of the Declaration of Helsinki.

Blood samples were drawn to isolate peripheral blood mononuclear cells (PBMC). PBMC were isolated by Ficoll-Paque density gradient centrifugation (Amersham Biosciences Corp., Piscataway, NJ) and immediately used for fluorescence-activated cell sorter (FACS) staining. PBMC of the patients and control subjects were examined for the expression of chemokine receptors by two-colored direct immunofluorescence and flowcytometry using a FACScan (Becton Dickinson, Franklin Lakes, NJ). Cells were immunostained with monoclonal antibody (mAb) to CD4 conjugated with fluorescein isothiocyanate (FITC) and phycoethrin (PE)-conjugated mAb to CXCR3 or CCR5 (PharMingen, San Diego, CA).

Comparison between a patient group and control subjects was performed by ANOVA and Scheffe's correction for *post hoc* test. Data were analyzed with STATA (version 8 Stata Co., College Station, TX). $P < 0.05$ was regarded as statistically significant.

RESULTS

There was no significant difference in the Th1-associated chemokine receptors CXCR3 and CCR5 on CD4 T cells between type 1 diabetics and control subjects. However, group A (fulminant type) patients showed significantly lower expression of CXCR3 than control subjects and group B patients. Group B (typical type) patients showed higher expression of CXCR3 than control subjects and group C patients as well as group A (FIG. 1). CCR5 expression on CD4 T cells in group C patients (11.6 ± 4.8%) tended to be higher than that in control subjects (6.4 ± 3.6%), group A (7.7 ± 3.6%), or group B (8.7 ± 7.3%), but the difference was not significant. This difference in CXCR3 was not affected by GAD antibody or IA-2 antibody positivity and titer. Sex, disease duration, and present age did not affect CXCR3 or CCR5 expression in this study.

DISCUSSION

In our study, CXCR3 expression differed according to the onset pattern. The highly expressed CXCR3 in typical type 1 diabetes suggests that CXCR3 is a

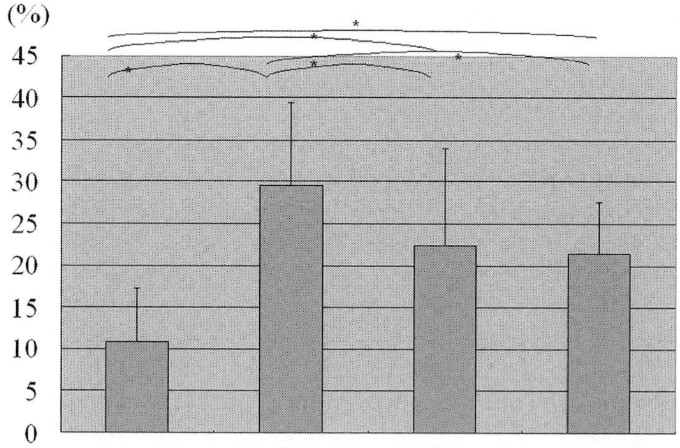

FIGURE 1. Expression level of CXCR3 on CD4 cells patients within 6 months after diabetic ketoacidosis (DKA) onset were excluded. n = 10 (group A), 42 (group B), 20 (group C), and 24 (control), respectively. * < 0.05

stable Th1 marker and that typical type 1 diabetes is a Th1 disease. Although the reason CXCR3 expression level was low in fulminant type is unknown, it should be associated with pathogenesis. Nationwide survey in Japan revealed that 71.7% of fulminant type 1 diabetes had flu-like symptoms[2] and Imagawa *et al.* reported high titers of IgA antibodies to enterovirus was observed in fulminant type 1 diabetes.[4] Therefore, we hypothesize that CXCR3-positive cells which were activated by viral infection may accumulate in pancreatic lymph nodes, resulting in β cell destruction in fulminant type 1 diabetes.

CCR5 expression did not differ among the three clinical phenotypes. But this result does not necessarily deny the association of CCR5 in the pathogenesis of type 1 diabetes, because we recently experienced the case of a patient in whom CCR5 expression was diminished only at the onset of fulminant type 1 diabetes (unpublished data). Whether CXCR3 positive cells or CCR5 positive cells are preferably induced in Th1 autoimmune disease models may depend on whether the immunogens are external or intrinsic self antigens.[5] Therefore, this case might show the association of autoimmunity in fulminant type 1 diabetes.

Further studies are needed to clarify the role of chemokines in the onset of type 1 diabetes. Especially, we should focus on the relationship between chemokine receptors expression on peripheral T cells and serum chemokines, such as CXCL-10.[6,7]

REFERENCES

1. LOHMANN, T., S. LAUE, U. NIETZSCHMANN, *et al.* 2002. Reduced expression of Th1-associated chemokine receptors on peripheral blood lymphocytes at diagnosis of type 1 diabetes. Diabetes **51:** 2474–2480.
2. IMAGAWA, A., T. HANAFUSA, Y. UCHIGATA, *et al.* 2003. Fulminant type 1 diabetes. A nationwide survey in Japan. Diabetes Care **26:** 2345–2352.
3. KOBAYASHI, T., T. TAMEMOTO, K. NAKANISHI, *et al.* 1993. Immunogenetic and clinical characterization of slowly progressive IDDM. Diabetes Care **16:** 780–788.
4. IMAGAWA, A., T. HANAFUSA, H. MAKINO, *et al.* 2005. High titres of IgA antibodies to enterovirus in fulminant type 1 diabetes. Diabetologia **48:** 290–293.
5. MORIMOTO, J., H. YONEYAMA, A. SHIMADA, *et al.* 2004. CXC chemokine ligand 10 neutralization suppresses the occurrence of diabetes in nonobese diabetic mice through enhanced beta cell proliferation without affecting insulitis. J. Immunol. **173:** 7017–7024.
6. SHIGIHARA, T., Y. OIKAWA, Y. KANAZAWA, *et al.* 2006. Significance of serum CXCL10/IP-10 level in type 1 diabetes. J. Autoimmun. **26:** 66–71.
7. SHIMADA, A., J. MORIMOTO, K. KODAMA, *et al.* 2001. Elevated serum IP-10 levels observed in type 1 diabetes. Diabetes Care **24:** 510–515.

HLA Class I Epitope Discovery in Type 1 Diabetes

PETER VAN ENDERT,[a,b] YOUSRA HASSAINYA,[a,b] VIVIAN LINDO,[c] JEAN-MARIE BACH,[d] PHILIPPE BLANCOU,[d] FRANÇOIS LEMONNIER,[e] AND ROBERTO MALLONE[a,b]

[a]*INSERM U580, Hôpital Necker, 75015 Paris, France*

[b]*Université René Descartes Paris 5, 75015 Paris, France*

[c]*M-SCAN, Wokingham RG 41 2TZ, UK*

[d]*Immuno-Endocrinology Unit, ENVN/INRA/University, 44307 Nantes, France*

[e]*Department of Immunology, Institut Pasteur, 75015 Paris, France*

ABSTRACT: Type 1 diabetes mellitus (T1DM) results from the destruction of β cells by autoantigen-specific T cells. In the non-obese diabetic (NOD) mouse model, CD8$^+$ T cells play an essential role in both the initial triggering of insulitis and its destructive phase, and proinsulin (PI) is one of the dominant target antigens (Ags). However, little is known about the beta cell epitopes presented by HLA class I molecules and recognized by human CD8$^+$ T cells. We and other groups recently applied reverse immunology approaches to identify HLA class I-restricted PI epitopes. To establish an inventory of potential naturally processed epitopes, whole human PI or the transitional region between the B-chain and C-peptide were digested with purified proteasome complexes. By combining proteasome digestion data with epitope prediction algorithms, candidate epitopes restricted by HLA-A2.1 and other HLA class I molecules were identified. We validated immunogenicity and natural processing of the identified PI epitopes in HLA-A2.1-transgenic mice, while others demonstrated recognition of multiple PI epitopes by CD8$^+$ T cells from T1DM and healthy subjects in the context of different HLA class I molecules. These results demonstrate the power of reverse immunology strategies for epitope discovery. DNA vaccination of HLA-transgenic mice may be another rapid and efficient reverse immunology approach to map additional epitopes derived from other T1DM Ags, such as IA-2 and glutamic acid decarboxylase 65 (GAD 65). Transfer of this information to Elispot- and MHC tetramer-based assay formats should allow to reliably detect and characterize autoreactive CD8$^+$ T cell responses in T1DM, and may open new avenues for early T1DM diagnosis and immune intervention.

Address for correspondence: Peter van Endert, INSERM U580, Hôpital Necker, 161 rue de Sèvres, 75015 Paris, France. Voice: +33-1-4449-2563; fax: +33-1-4449-5382.
e-mail: vanendert@necker.fr

Ann. N.Y. Acad. Sci. 1079: 190–197 (2006).
doi: 10.1196/annals.1375.030

KEYWORDS: **CD8$^+$ T cell; proteasome; proinsulin; Elispot; tetramer; DNA vaccination**

INTRODUCTION

T cell responses in type 1 diabetes mellitus (T1DM) are actively investigated in the quest for immune surrogate markers capable of predicting T1DM development and response to immune interventions. Accumulating evidence shows that, in the non-obese diabetic (NOD) mouse model, CD8$^+$ T lymphocytes have a prominent, and possibly an initiating role in beta cell destruction.[1–3] This new emphasis on CD8$^+$ T cells has also expanded the list of relevant beta cell antigens (Ags) beyond the "classical" trio of proinsulin (PI), IA-2, and glutamic acid decarboxylase 65 (GAD65). Islet-specific glucose-6-phosphatase catalytic subunit-related protein (IGRP)[2], glial fibrillary acidic protein,[4] and dystrophia myotonica kinase[5] are among the most promising new candidates. This makes CD8$^+$ T cell responses an appealing new field of research for immune monitoring strategies in human T1DM.

However, several technical difficulties make the transfer of this knowledge from mouse to man a challenging task. On one hand, the only human biological material routinely available is peripheral blood, where self Ag-reactive CD8$^+$ and CD4$^+$ T cells are very rare (1 in 10^4–10^6) and possibly of average lower avidity.[6,7] On the other hand, information about the epitopes presented by HLA class I molecules and recognized by human autoreactive CD8$^+$ T cells is anecdotic at best.[8–10]

Among the T cell target Ags of T1DM, the primary importance of PI is supported by four strong lines of evidence: (*a*) NOD mice knocked out for the PI 1 (islet isoform) gene display diabetes protection,[11] while (*b*) NOD mice defective for the PI 2 (thymic isoform) gene show accelerated diabetes, likely related to defective deletion of insulin-reactive T cells in the thymus[12]; (*c*) an insulin $B_{15–23}$ epitope is the target of both a highly diabetogenic CD8$^+$ T cell clone[13] and of an early subpopulation of islet-infiltrating CD8$^+$ T cells.[14] This epitope and/or the overlapping MHC class II-restricted epitope $B_{9–23}$ seem of primary importance since (*d*) PI 1/PI 2 double knockout NOD mice carrying a PI transgene mutated at position B16 do not develop insulitis or diabetes.[15]

We have therefore started to fill up the gap in CD8$^+$ T cell epitope information by identifying human PI-derived naturally processed epitopes restricted by the common HLA-A2.1 allele using a reverse immunology approach.[16]

MATERIALS AND METHODS

Proteasome Digestions

Proteasome complexes were purified from lymphoblastoid cell lines by immunoaffinity chromatography using monoclonal antibody MCP21. Fractions were monitored for proteasome content using the fluorogenic substrate Suc-LLVY-amido-methylcoumarin (Bachem, Weil am Rhein, Germany). Recombinant PI was provided by Eli Lilly (Indianapolis, IN). Before digestion, PI cysteines were carboxymethylated by incubation with 10 mmol/L dithiothreitol (DTT) for 60 min followed by incubation with 20 mmol/L iodoacetic acid for 20 min. Carboxymethylated PI thus obtained (40 μg) was digested at 37°C for various periods with 2 μg purified proteasome. Digestions were stopped by adding 8% acetonitrile and fractionated by reversed-phase chromatography (uRPC C2/C18 column; Amersham, Orsay, France). To identify digestion products, fractions were analyzed by matrix-associated laser desorption ionization/time of flight mass spectrometry with a Voyager STR spectrometer coupled with delayed extraction (Applied Biosystems, Warrington, UK). Mass accuracy was 20–40 ppm. Sequences were confirmed by tandem mass spectrometry analysis on a Micromass Q-TOF instrument (Waters, Elstree, UK).

HLA-A2.1 binding affinities were predicted using both the SYFPEITHI (http://www.syfpeithi.de) and BIMAS (http://bimas.cit.nih.gov) algorithms. HLA-A2 and transporter associated with Ag processing binding affinities were experimentally determined using previously described competitive binding assays.[17,18]

Murine Cytotoxic T Cell Lines

Cytotoxic T lymphocyte (CTL) lines were generated by immunization of HLA-A2.1-transgenic HHD mice.[19] Five HHD mice per PI peptide were immunized subcutaneously at the base of the tail with 100 μg of PI peptide and 140 μg of the MHC class II-restricted helper peptide TPPAYRPPNAPIL emulsified in incomplete Freund's adjuvant (Difco, Detroit, MI). Twelve days later, spleens were removed and splenocytes restimulated using irradiated HHD splenocytes previously pulsed for 2 h with 10 ug/mL of peptide. Restimulated cells were tested 6 days later in ^{51}Cr release assays using peptide-pulsed HeLa S3 or TAP-deficient RMA-S cells transfected with the previously described HHD construct conferring G418 resistance.[19] CTL lines showing specific target cell lysis were cultured in RPMI with 10% fetal calf serum, 10% T cell growth factor, and 0.1 mmol/L 2-mercaptoethanol and maintained by weekly restimulation with peptide-pulsed HHD splenocytes.

Recombinant Vaccinia Virus Expressing Pre-PI

The human pre-PI coding sequence was amplified from human pancreas cDNA (PCR-ready cDNA; Ambion, Huntington, UK) using a high-fidelity thermostable DNA polymerase (Advantage HF kit; Invitrogen, Cergy Pontoise,

France) and the primers 5′ TTAGATCTACCATGGCCCTGTGGATGC (sense) and 5′ AAGGTACCTACTAGTTGCAGTAGTTCTCCA (antisense). The PCR product was cloned in pCR Blunt (Invitrogen), sequenced to confirm the absence of errors, and subcloned into the vaccinia virus transfer vector pSC65. The resulting plasmid and purified wild-type vaccinia DNA were cotransfected into CV-1 cells that were simultaneously infected with strain WR wild-type vaccinia virus (ATCC, Manassas, VA). Recombinant viruses were selected in plaque assays with blue/white selection. HeLa S3 target cells were infected with recombinant or wild-type vaccinia virus and tested against PI-specific CTL lines in ^{51}Cr release assays as above.

RESULTS

Since most or all HLA class I-presented epitope sequences carry a proteasome cleavage site at the C terminus, we began identification of HLA-A2.1-restricted PI epitopes by digesting PI with purified proteasome complexes. A map of the proteasome cleavage sites, corresponding to the C terminus of candidate epitopes, was thus obtained. Surprisingly, most observed cleavage sites were in the C-peptide. Biochemical analysis suggested that this is due to reoxidation of PI, which, despite pretreatment with 10 mM DTT, shows a strong tendency to reform its disulfide bridges, thus inhibiting proteasome digestion (Y. Hassainya *et al.*, manuscript in preparation).

The digestion map was then compared with the PI epitopes predicted by the BIMAS and SYFPEITHI algorithms to identify 9- and 10-mer peptides carrying a C-terminal proteasome cleavage site. Ten peptides were thus selected, and their HLA-A2.1 and TAP binding affinity experimentally determined.

The immunogenicity of these 10 selected peptides was subsequently tested by immunizing HHD mice. These mice express the HHD single-chain HLA-A2.1/β_2 microglobulin construct as the only MHC class Ia molecule, so that all their $CD8^+$ T cells are HLA-A2.1 restricted. Seven of the 10 epitopes were found to be immunogenic.

Immunogenicity documents the presence of a T cell repertoire specific for a given epitope and sufficient MHC binding affinity, but does not clarify whether the epitope is naturally processed, that is, produced and presented by a cell expressing the source protein. A recombinant vaccinia virus encoding human pre-PI was therefore produced to introduce this Ag into the endogenous processing pathway of Ag-presenting cells, which were then used as targets in CTL assays. By these means, natural processing was tested in 6 of the 7 immunogenic peptides, and was confirmed in all cases. Two of these 6 PI epitopes ($B_{9–18}$ and $B_{10–18}$) were later found to be recognized by the same T cells. A prospect of the 5 final epitopes thus selected is shown in TABLE 1 and FIGURE 1.

TABLE 1. Summary of the HLA-A2.1-restricted PI epitopes identified

Peptide	Sequence	A2.1 affinity	C-terminal proteasome cleavage	Immunogenicity	Natural processing	Identity human–mouse
$PI_{B10–18}$ $PPI_{34–42}$	HLVEALYLV	+++	++	++	+	PI1–PI2
$PI_{C20–28}$ $PPI_{76–84}$	SLQPLALEG	+	++	++	++	no
$PI_{C29–A5}$ $PPI_{85–94}$	SLQKRGIVEQ	+	++	++	++	no
$PI_{A1–10}$ $PPI_{90–99}$	GIVEQCCTSI	+++	+	++	++	no
$PI_{A12–20}$ $PPI_{101–109}$	SLYQLENYC	+++	–	+	++	PI1–PI2

Peptide numbering refers to both $PI_{B1–A21}$ and $PPI_{1–110}$ sequence nomenclature. Binding affinity for HLA-A2.1 was measured by competitive assay as previously described.[18] Immunogenicity refers to the efficiency of CTL induction upon peptide immunization of HHD mice. Natural processing refers to peptide presentation by vaccinia/pre-PI-infected CTL targets. Scores are given on an arbitrary +/++/+++ scale. – = no cleavage.

DISCUSSION

Epitope identification traditionally relies on prediction models and experimental measurements of the HLA binding affinity. The panel of candidate peptides is then validated by testing recognition by T cells following a variety of strategies. Epitope identification based exclusively on HLA class I binding

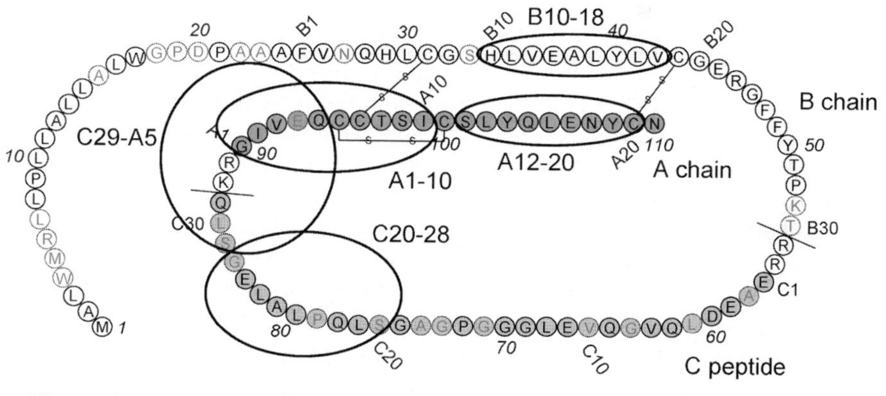

Figure 1. HLA-A2.1-restricted human PI epitopes identified. Epitopes, written in large characters, are circled in the sequence of human pre-PI. Amino acid numbering is given both with respect to the complete pre-PI sequence (aa 1–110) and to the sequence of the three PI components B chain, C-peptide, and A chain. Sites of C-peptide cleavage giving rise to mature insulin are indicated by cross lines. Amino acid positions differing between human and mouse pre-PI are printed in light characters.

affinity has, however, two drawbacks: (*a*) epitopes with low affinity, which may be of particular interest in autoimmunity,[20,21] are likely to be missed; and (*b*) most peptides with high binding affinity are actually not natural epitopes, due to filters in Ag processing and/or T cell repertoires.[22]

These problems can partly be addressed by using a "reverse" immunology approach, in which emphasis is given not only to the epitope selection imposed by MHC class I molecules but also to that by processing steps preceding peptide binding to class I. Digestion of source Ags by the proteasome, probably the most selective step in MHC class I Ag processing, is therefore taken into account for epitope identification. Besides accuracy, this method dramatically reduces the number of candidate epitopes to test for T cell recognition, as compared to strategies based solely on MHC class I binding affinity.

This approach allowed us to identify several naturally processed HLA-A2.1-restricted PI epitopes. A similar strategy was recently reproduced by Toma *et al.*, who focused on the pre-PI region 28–64 ($PI_{B4–C8}$) to identify PI epitopes restricted for several HLA class I alleles. For the A2.1 allele, these investigators confirmed the identification of our $PI_{B10–18}$ (preproinsulin$[PPI]_{34–42}$) epitope, while proposing a second $PI_{B18–27}$ ($PPI_{42–51}$) epitope, which was not immunogenic in our study, perhaps due to its identity between mouse and human. Recognition of these PI epitopes by $CD8^+$ T cells of T1DM patients and, to a lesser extent, of healthy subjects was also documented by IFN-γ Elispot.[23]

Besides *in vitro* proteasome digestion, another powerful reverse immunology approach relies on gene gun immunization of HLA-transgenic mice with plasmid-DNA encoding either the Ag of interest or an irrelevant protein as control. With this approach, the Ag is endogenously synthesized and directly processed into epitopes rather than being exogenously administered as a peptide preparation. Subsequent *in vitro* CTL and/or recall assays therefore allow for simultaneous evaluation of both immunogenicity and natural processing of a given epitope.[24,25] Our preliminary results suggest that DNA immunization of HLA-A2.1-transgenic mice may be another rapid and efficient system to further map epitopes derived from other T1DM islet Ags, such as IA-2 and GAD65, which are less amenable to proteasome digestion because of their higher molecular weight.

Recent emphasis on the role of $CD8^+$ T cells in T1DM and the identification of new beta cell Ags targeted by these lymphocytes in the NOD mouse prompts for a systematic human $CD8^+$ T cell epitope exploration. Reverse immunology strategies should prove valuable in focusing these $CD8^+$ T cell studies on a restricted panel of robust HLA class I-restricted candidate epitopes.

REFERENCES

1. AMRANI, A., J. VERDAGUER, P. SERRA, *et al.* 2000. Progression of autoimmune diabetes driven by avidity maturation of a T-cell population. Nature **406:** 739–742.

2. HAN, B., P. SERRA, A. AMRANI, *et al.* 2005. Prevention of diabetes by manipulation of anti-IGRP autoimmunity: high efficiency of a low-affinity peptide. Nat. Med. **11:** 645–652.
3. LIBLAU, R.S., F.S. WONG, L.T. MARS, *et al.* 2002. Autoreactive CD8 T cells in organ-specific autoimmunity: emerging targets for therapeutic intervention. Immunity **17:** 1–6.
4. WINER, S., H. TSUI, A. LAU, *et al.* 2003. Autoimmune islet destruction in spontaneous type 1 diabetes is not beta-cell exclusive. Nat. Med. **9:** 198–205.
5. LIEBERMAN, S.M., T. TAKAKI, B. HAN, *et al.* 2004. Individual nonobese diabetic mice exhibit unique patterns of CD8+ T cell reactivity to three islet antigens, including the newly identified widely expressed dystrophia myotonica kinase. J. Immunol. **173:** 6727–6734.
6. MALLONE, R. & G.T. NEPOM. 2004. MHC class II tetramers and the pursuit of antigen-specific T cells: define, deviate, delete. Clin. Immunol. **110:** 232–242.
7. MALLONE, R. & G.T. NEPOM. 2005. Targeting T lymphocytes for immune monitoring and intervention in autoimmune diabetes. Am. J. Ther. **12:** 534–550.
8. PANINA-BORDIGNON, P., R. LANG, P.M. VAN ENDERT, *et al.* 1995. Cytotoxic T cells specific for glutamic acid decarboxylase in autoimmune diabetes. J. Exp. Med. **181:** 1923–1927.
9. TAKAHASHI, K., M.C. HONEYMAN & L.C. HARRISON. 2001. Cytotoxic T cells to an epitope in the islet autoantigen IA-2 are not disease-specific. Clin. Immunol. **99:** 360–364.
10. PANAGIOTOPOULOS, C., H. QIN, R. TAN, *et al.* 2003. Identification of a beta-cell-specific HLA class I restricted epitope in type 1 diabetes. Diabetes **52:** 2647–2651.
11. MORIYAMA, H., N. ABIRU, J. PARONEN, *et al.* 2003. Evidence for a primary islet autoantigen (preproinsulin 1) for insulitis and diabetes in the nonobese diabetic mouse. Proc. Natl. Acad. Sci. USA **100:** 10376–10381.
12. THEBAULT-BAUMONT, K., D. DUBOIS-LAFORGUE, P. KRIEF, *et al.* 2003. Acceleration of type 1 diabetes mellitus in proinsulin 2-deficient NOD mice. J. Clin. Invest. **111:** 851–857.
13. WONG, F.S., I. VISINTIN, L. WEN, *et al.* 1996. CD8 T cell clones from young nonobese diabetic (NOD) islets can transfer rapid onset of diabetes in NOD mice in the absence of CD4 cells. J. Exp. Med. **183:** 67–76.
14. WONG, F.S., J. KARTTUNEN, C. DUMONT, *et al.* 1999. Identification of an MHC class I-restricted autoantigen in type 1 diabetes by screening an organ-specific cDNA library. Nat. Med. **5:** 1026–1031.
15. NAKAYAMA, M., N. ABIRU, H. MORIYAMA, *et al.* 2005. Prime role for an insulin epitope in the development of type 1 diabetes in NOD mice. Nature **435:** 220–223.
16. HASSAINYA, Y., F. GARCIA-PONS, R. KRATZER, *et al.* 2005. Identification of naturally processed HLA-A2 restricted proinsulin epitopes by reverse immunology. Diabetes **54:** 2053–2059.
17. VAN ENDERT, P.M., D. RIGANELLI, G. GRECO, *et al.* 1995. The peptide-binding motif for the human transporter associated with antigen processing. J. Exp. Med. **182:** 1883–1895.
18. CULINA, S., G. LAUVAU, B. GUBLER, *et al.* 2004. Calreticulin promotes folding of functional human leukocyte antigen class I molecules in vitro. J. Biol. Chem. **279:** 54210–54215.

19. PASCOLO, S., N. BERVAS, J.M. URE, *et al.* 1997. HLA-A2.1-restricted education and cytolytic activity of CD8(+) T lymphocytes from beta2 microglobulin (beta2m) HLA-A2.1 monochain transgenic H-2Db beta2m double knockout mice. J. Exp. Med. **185:** 2043–2051.
20. GAMMON, G. & E. SERCARZ. 1989. How some T cells escape tolerance induction. Nature **342:** 183–185.
21. RIDGWAY, W.M., M. FASSO & C.G. FATHMAN. 1999. A new look at MHC and autoimmune disease. Science **284:** 749–751.
22. YEWDELL, J.W. & J.R. BENNINK. 1999. Immunodominance in major histocompatibility complex class I-restricted T lymphocyte responses. Annu. Rev Immunol. **17:** 51–88.
23. TOMA, A., S. HADDOUK, J.P. BRIAND, *et al.* 2005. Recognition of a subregion of human proinsulin by class I-restricted T cells in type 1 diabetic patients. Proc. Natl. Acad. Sci. USA **102:** 10581–10586.
24. GAUVRIT, A., M. DEBAILLEUL, A.T. VU, *et al.* 2004. DNA vaccination encoding glutamic acid decarboxylase can enhance insulitis and diabetes in correlation with a specific Th2/3 CD4 T cell response in non-obese diabetic mice. Clin. Exp. Immunol. **137:** 253–262.
25. JOUSSEMET, B., A.T. VU, P. SAI, *et al.* 2005. Gene-gun biolistic immunization encoding glutamic acid decarboxylase: a model for studying Langerhans cell abnormalities and mimicry in the nonobese diabetic mouse. Ann. N. Y. Acad. Sci. **1051:** 613–625.

Upregulation of Foxp3 Expression in Mouse and Human Treg Is IL-2/STAT5 Dependent

Implications for the NOD STAT5B Mutation in Diabetes Pathogenesis

MATTHEW R. MURAWSKI, SALLY A. LITHERLAND, MICHAEL J. CLARE-SALZLER, AND ABDOREZA DAVOODI-SEMIROMI

Department of Pathology, Immunology and Laboratory Medicine, College of Medicine, University of Florida, Gainesville, Florida 32610, USA

ABSTRACT: Regulatory T cells (Treg), characterized as $CD4^+/CD25^{+hi}$ T cells, are critical for sustaining and promoting immune tolerance. Treg are highly dependent on IL-2 and IL-2 signaling to maintain their numbers and function and interruption of this pathway promotes autoimmunity. The transcription factor, Foxp3, is also required for Treg function as defective Foxp3 promotos autoimmunity in both mice and humans. We previously reported a point mutation in the DNA-binding domain of the NOD STAT5B gene that limits DNA binding when compared to wild-type STAT5 mice. Based on the presence of five STAT5B consensus sequences in the Foxp3 promotor, we hypothesized a critical linkage between IL-2 signaling/STAT5B and Foxp3 expression in Treg. Our data show IL-2 activates long-form (LF) STAT5 and sustains Foxp3 expression in Treg. In contrast, $CD4^+/CD25^-$ T cells do not active LF STAT5 and do not express Foxp3 under the same conditions. In addition, blocking LF STAT5 activation with a Jak inhibitor (AG-490) significantly reduced Foxp3 expression in Treg. Examination of human Treg using flow cytometry and intracellular staining for Foxp3 expression likewise demonstrates that IL-2 maintains Foxp3 expression through LF STAT5 signaling. These studies reveal a critical link between IL-2 mediated JAK-STAT5 signaling and the maintenance of Foxp3 expression in Treg of mice and humans.

KEYWORDS: natural regulatory T cell; Foxp3; STAT5; IL-2; CD25

Address for correspondence: Michael J. Clare-Salzler, M.D., Department of Pathology, Immunology and Laboratory Medicine, College of Medicine, University of Florida, 1600 SW Archer Road, Gainesville, FL 32610, USA. Voice: 352-392-9886; fax: 352-392-5393.
e-mail: salzler@ufl.edu

Ann. N.Y. Acad. Sci. 1079: 198–204 (2006). © 2006 New York Academy of Sciences.
doi: 10.1196/annals.1375.031

INTRODUCTION

Natural regulatory T cells (Treg) ($CD4^+/CD25^{+hi}$) are generated in both the thymus and the periphery and are essential for the promotion of immune tolerance while preventing the onset of autoimmune disease.[1–3] Treg express the alpha chain of interleukin (IL)-2 receptor (CD25) and are vitally dependent on exogenous IL-2 secreted from naïve and effector T cells (Teff) for maintenance in the periphery.[4] This notion is supported by experiments that demonstrate depletion of IL-2 (IL-2KO) or the IL-2 receptor-signaling pathway (IL2α−/−, IL-2β−/−) ablates Treg in mice and leads to the development of autoimmune disease.[5] Treatment of these mice with IL-2 restores Treg number and function.[5] It is also known that the transcription factor, Foxp3, is critical for suppressor activity of Treg because mice lacking Foxp3 succumb to severe lymphoproliferative and autoimmune disease.[6] Interestingly, Van Parijs and colleagues reported that STAT5 KO mice exhibited a loss of Treg and over expression of STAT5 in IL-2 KO mice restores Treg numbers *in vivo.*[7] These findings demonstrate that Jak/STAT5 signaling is an essential component of murine Treg. We recently reported a novel point mutation in the DNA-binding domain in the STAT5B gene in NOD mice and demonstrated that mutated STAT5B has a weaker DNA-binding affinity when compared with normal C57BL/J6 mice.[8] We hypothesize that this mutation may affect the maintenance of Foxp3 in murine Treg. Our data show the Jak/STAT5-signaling pathway is utilized to maintain Foxp3 expression and blockage of this pathway completely inhibited activation of STAT5 while significantly reducing Foxp3 expression in both mouse and human natural Treg.

MATERIALS AND METHODS

Mice

C57BL/6J (B6) mice were purchased from Jackson Laboratories and housed in our mouse colony facilities in the Department of Pathology, Immunology, and Laboratory Medicine, University of Florida. All mice used in these experiments were maintained in a specific pathogen-free environment and in accordance with the University of Florida institutional animal care and use committee (IACUC). All experiments were conducted on 4- to 6-week-old female mice.

Treg Purification

Murine $CD4^+/CD25^+$ T cells were purified from the spleens of three mice. Cell suspensions were made by passing tissue through a metal mesh grid followed by a passage through a 70-μM cell strainer (BD Biosciences, Bedford,

MA). The cells were pelleted, resuspended in 30 mL of RPMI-1640, counted using a hemocytometer, and assessed for viability (viability >95% as judged by Trypan Blue staining). The $CD4^+/CD25^+$ T cells were separated using mouse $CD4^+/CD25^+$ Treg cell purification kit (Miltenyi Biotech, Auburn, CA) with an AutoMACS instrument according to manufacture's instructions (Miltenyi Biotech).

Cell Culture

The purified $CD4^+/CD25^+$ Treg were cultured in RPMI-1640 plus 10% FBS (Mediatech, Inc., Herndon, VA) and PSN antibiotics (Invitrogen Co., Carlsbad, CA). For Western blotting, at the end of culture, cells were washed twice in cold PBS, pelleted, and kept frozen at $-80°C$ until analysis.

Western Blotting

A total number of 2.0×10^5 $CD4^+/CD25^+$ T cells were cultured in the presence or absence of cytokines and inhibitor and then lysed in Laemmli sample buffer (Biorad Laboratories, Hercules, CA). The protein was denatured for 5 min in boiling water and loaded onto a 10% Tris-HCl acrylamide gel (Biorad) followed by a 1 h transfer to polyvinylidene fluoride (PVFD) membrane (Amersham Biosciences Corp., Piscataway, NJ). Tyrosine-phosphorylated STAT5 was detected using anti-STAT5A/B antibody (Cat #05-495, Upstate) and pan-STAT5A/B antibody (Cat #SC-835 and #SC-836, Santa Cruz Biotech, Santa Cruz, CA). Mouse IL-2 (Cat #1271164, Roche Applied Sciences, Indianapolis, IN) was used to stimulate T cells at a concentration range of 5–100 U/mL. Anti-mouse Foxp3 antisera was a generous gift from Dr. Alexander Rudensky (Department of Medicine, Division of Rheumatology, University of Washington, Seattle, WA). AG490 (Calbiochem, La Jolla, CA) was preincubated with cell cultures for 30 min prior to lysis at 100 μM (lane 6–7) concentration.

PBMC Isolation

Whole blood was collected from healthy controls under Institutional Review Board (IRB) approval in our lab using venupuncture. Peripheral blood mononuclear cells (PBMC) were isolated from whole blood using Ficoll Paque (Amersham Biosciences Corp., Piscataway, NJ, USA) according to manufacturer protocol. PBMC were stained with anti-CD4 and anti-CD25 antibodies (BD Biosciences) in PBS with 2% FBS and sodium azide. After surface staining, cells were intracellular stained for Foxp3 using anti-Foxp3 monoclonal antibody (E-biosciences, clone #PCH101, San Diego, CA) according to manufacturer protocol. Cells were analyzed using four-color cytometric analysis

(FacsCaliber™, BD Biosciences). Appropriate isotype controls were included for all antibodies. PBMC were cultured for 24 h in RPMI-1640 plus glutamine (Mediatech, Inc.) and PSN antibiotics (Invitrogen Co.). A 2% autologous serum was added at the beginning of culture. AG-490 was diluted in DMSO as per manufacturer specifications and added to cultures 30 min prior to IL-2 stimulation. A DMSO control was included and did not affect results (data not shown).

RESULTS

TABLE 1 shows the position of the STAT5 consensus-binding sequences located within the first three kilobases of the murine Foxp3 promotor region. Each site has been tested for binding activity using electromobility gel shift assays and all were found to be active in binding STAT5 in Treg (data not shown). In agreement with our previous observations, mutated STAT5B in NOD Treg had a threefold weaker DNA binding when compared with normal B6 Treg (ADS and MCS manuscript in preparation). This suggests IL-2/STAT5 signaling may directly regulate Foxp3 expression in Treg.

In FIGURE 1 A, we tested the hypothesis that IL-2/STAT5 signaling is important to maintain Foxp3 expression in murine Treg. In lane 1, freshly isolated Treg express Foxp3 and lack phosphorylated STAT5. In the absence of IL-2 for 24 h, Foxp3 expression is lost, suggesting that IL-2 is required for the maintenance of this transcription factor (lane 2). Culturing Treg in the presence of IL-2 not only maintains expression of Foxp3 but also promotes phosphorylation of LF-STAT5 (lane 3). In lanes 3–5, we demonstrate that increasing concentrations of IL-2 sustains Foxp3 expression and activates STAT5. However, culturing Treg in the presence of a selective Jak2/3 inhibitor (AG-490) and IL-2 abrogates STAT5 activation and substantially diminished the expression of Foxp3 in Treg (FIG. 1 A, lanes 6–7). We observed similar results in human Treg. As shown in FIGURE 1 B, freshly isolated human Treg express Foxp3

TABLE 1. The murine Foxp3 promotor contains five STAT5B consensus binding sequences

Position	Consensus sequence	Strand
810–828	tttcgTTCcgaGAAgtggc	Negative
1007–1025	actgtTTCttaGAAgctgt	Negative
1124–1142	cctctTTCtgaGAAtgtac	Positive
1530–1548	cacggTTCtagGAAgccag	Positive
1717–1735	gtagcTTCtgaGAAcagcc	Negative

NOTE: A 3-kb region of the Foxp3 promotor from the initiation of the translation codon (ATG) was searched for the presence of STAT5B consensus sequences using Genomatics software (www.genomatix.de). The positions are listed and the conserved binding domain, TTC(N)^{3}GAA, in the genomic DNA is shown for each position. Negative Strand = antisense strand; Positive strand = sense strand.

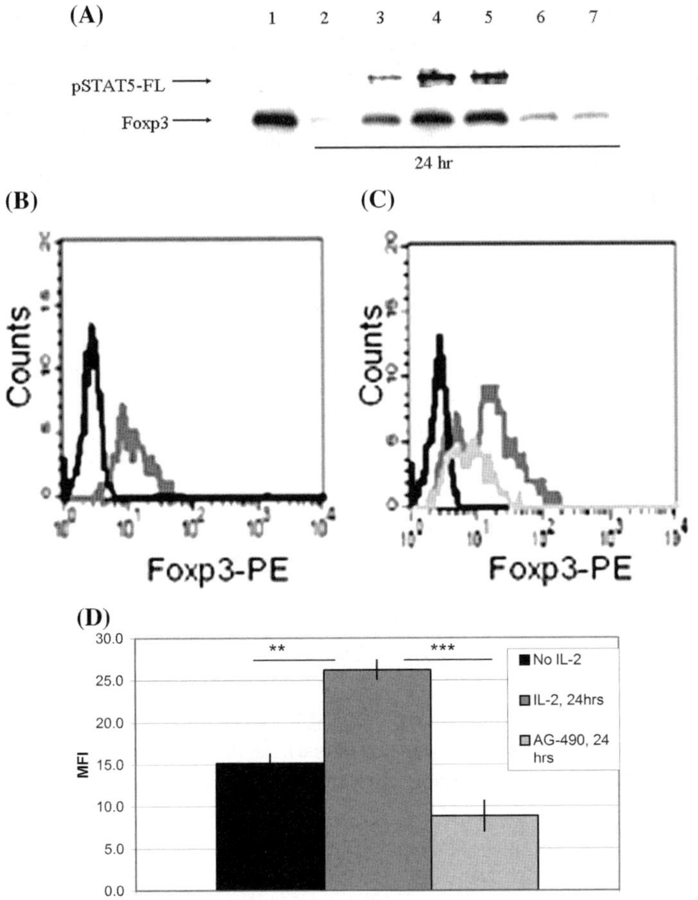

FIGURE 1. (**A**) Murine regulatory T cells were examined via Western blot for expression of Foxp3 and FL-pSTAT5. Lane 1: freshly isolated cells without IL-2. Lane 2: cultured Treg without IL-2. Lanes 3–5: cultured Treg with different concentrations of IL-2 ranging from 5 to 100 U/mL. Lanes 6 and 7: Treg cultured with AG-490 (100 μM) in the presence of IL-2 (100 U/mL). This represents one of at least three independent experiments. (**B**) Human TREG were examined via flow cytometry for expression of Foxp3 using a PE-labeled monoclonal antibody. The isotype is shown in black and Foxp3 expression of freshly isolated Treg is shown in dark gray. This represents one of three independent experiments. (**C**) Human TREG examined via flow cytometry for expression of Foxp3 after 24 h in culture. The isotype is shown in black. Foxp3 expression after 24 h of IL-2 (1000 U/mL) stimulation is shown in dark gray. Foxp3 expression after 24 h of IL-2 (1000 U/mL) stimulation and AG-490 pretreatment (100 μM) is shown in light gray. This represents one of three independent experiments (**D**) Statistical significance of mean fluorescence intensity from **B** and **C** above. Error bars represent ± SD.

(dark gray histogram). In FIGURE 1 C, Foxp3 expression is upregulated by IL-2 stimulation (1000 U/mL) after 24 h, (dark gray histogram) and downregulated with the addition of AG-490 (100 μM) (light gray histogram). The isotype control for Foxp3 is shown in black for both histograms. FIGURE 1 D shows the statistical significance among groups ($P = 0.002$) using the ANOVA repeated measures ($n = 3$). *Post hoc t*-tests were used to assess significance between the groups ($^{**} = 0.001$, $^{***} = 0.0001$).

DISCUSSION

In this study, we attempt to identify how the IL-2 signaling pathway contributes to the maintenance of natural Treg. IL-2 has been shown to initiate a multitude of cellular events, specifically, augmentation and suppression of cytokine secretion by T lymphocytes and proliferation of naïve T cells.[9] Recently, two independent studies demonstrate IL-2 is not directly required for Treg function, differentiation, or expansion of suppressor Treg in the thymus, but is required for the survival of mature Foxp3$^+$ Treg.[10,11] Our data support these findings and suggest that IL-2 signaling maintains Foxp3 expression in both murine and human Treg through the Jak/STAT5 pathway. We also demonstrate that blockade of the Jak/STAT5 pathway via AG-490, which selectively blocks Jak2/3, abrogates STAT5 activation and severely diminished Foxp3 expression. Thus, IL-2 binding to the high-affinity IL-2 receptor CD25 initiates a signaling cascade by which Foxp3 is maintained in Treg. Without IL-2, this signaling pathway is not activated and Foxp3 expression is lost, perhaps altering the suppressive capabilities of both murine and human Treg. We theorize that CD25 expression maintains Treg function even in environments of low IL-2 concentration, for example, immune homeostasis. Thus, Treg maintain Foxp3 in response to a wide spectrum of IL-2 concentrations, promoting suppression, and limiting the ability of Teff to proliferate in response to IL-2.

ACKNOWLEDGMENTS

This study was supported by a research grant awarded to MCS (JDF 1-2004-690) and a transitional grant awarded to ADS (JDF10-2001-589) from the Juvenile Diabetes Research Foundation International (JDRFI).

REFERENCES

1. SAKAGUCHI, S. *et al.* 1995. Immunologic self-tolerance maintained by activated T cells expressing IL-2 receptor alpha-chains (CD25). Breakdown of a single mechanism of self-tolerance causes various autoimmune diseases. J. Immunol. **155:** 1151–1164.

2. Asano, M. *et al.* 1996. Autoimmune disease as a consequence of developmental abnormality of a T cell population. J. Exp. Med. **184:** 387–396.
3. Itoh, M. *et al.* 1999. Thymus and autoimmunity: production of CD25+CD4+ naturally anergic and suppressive T cells as a key function of the thymus in maintaining immunologic self-tolerance. J. Immunol. **162:** 5317–5326.
4. Thornton, A.M. & E.M. Shevach. 1998. CD4+CD25+ immunoregulatory T cells suppress polyclonal T cell activation in vitro by inhibiting interleukin 2 production. J. Exp. Med. **188:** 287–296.
5. Malek, T.R. *et al.* 2002. CD4 regulatory T cells prevent lethal autoimmunity in IL-2Rβ-deficient mice. Implications for nonredundant function of IL-2. Immunity **17:** 167–178.
6. Fontenot, J.D. *et al.* 2003. Foxp3 programs the development and function of CD4+CD25+ T regulatory cells. Nat. Immunol. **4:** 330–336.
7. Van Parijs, L. *et al.* 2003. Essential role for STAT5 in CD25+CD4+ regulatory T cell homeostasis and the maintenance of self-tolerance. J. Immunol. **171:** 3435–3441.
8. Davoodi-Semiromi, A. *et al.* 2004. A mutant Stat5b with weaker DNA binding affinity defines a key defective pathway in nonobese diabetic mice. J. Biol. Chem. **12:** 11553–11561.
9. Malek, T.R. 2004. Tolerance, not immunity, crucially depends on IL-2. Nat. Rev. Immunol. **4:** 665–674.
10. Fontenot, J.D. *et al.* 2005. A function for interleukin 2 in Foxp3-expressing regulatory T cells. Nature Immunol. **11:** 1142–1151.
11. D'Cruz, L.M. 2005. Development and function of agonist-induced $CD25^+$ $Foxp3^+$ regulatory T cells in the absence of interleukin 2 signaling. Nature Immunol. **11:** 1152–1159.

Normal T Cell Development in the Absence of Thymic Insulin Expression

MARIA CARLSÉN[a] AND CORRADO M. CILIO[a,b]

[a]*Cellular Autoimmunity Unit, Department of Clinical Sciences, Malmö University Hospital, Lund University, 205 02 Malmö, Sweden*

[b]*Department of Pediatrics, Malmö University Hospital, Lund University, 205 02 Malmö, Sweden*

ABSTRACT: Ectopic expression of insulin in thymus has been suggested to be involved in tolerance induction against pancreatic β cells and in type 1 diabetes (T1D) pathogenesis. However, it is not known whether thymic insulin expression would also influence thymocyte maturation and differentiation. To address these questions, we have used mice that are insulin deficient. Early fetal thymi were cultured in fetal thymic organ cultures (FTOCs) and the development of thymocytes was studied by flow cytometry. The results revealed no significant difference in thymocyte maturation in the absence of thymic insulin. Taken together, these data do not support a role for thymic insulin in thymocyte differentiation and growth.

KEYWORDS: type 1 diabetes; insulin; thymus; autoantigen

INTRODUCTION

Genes with organ-specific expression, such as the type 1 diabetes (T1D) autoantigens insulin, glutamic acid decarboxylase (GAD), and the tyrosine-phosphatase-like protein IA-2 (or ICA512) have now been recognized to be ectopically expressed in the thymus.[1–3] However, it has not been fully established whether or not they serve as antigens involved in negative selection of T cells and whether they are also important for the maturation and differentiation of thymocytes. Insulin is a hormone widely known for its growth promoting effects. Therefore, insulin expression in the thymus could also function as an important growth factor for the maturation of thymocytes. This has been shown to be true for insulin-like growth factor (IGF) 1 and 2 as well as for growth hormone (GH).[4,5]

Address for correspondence: Corrado M. Cilio, Cellular Autoimmunity Unit, Department of Clinical Sciences, CRC, entrance 72, Malmö University Hospital, Lund University, 20502 Malmö, Sweden. Voice: +4640332395; fax: +4640337042.
e-mail: corrado.cilio@med.lu.se

Ann. N.Y. Acad. Sci. 1079: 205–212 (2006).
doi: 10.1196/annals.1375.032

We have investigated the impact of thymic insulin on the development of thymocytes by using insulin deficient mice. Mice have two insulin genes (*ins1 and ins2*), but whether or not both genes are expressed in the thymus is still controversial.[3,6,7] In order to eliminate any effect of residual insulin expression, we used fetal thymic organ culture (FTOC) technique to investigate thymocyte development in the presence or absence of thymic insulin. Our results suggest that thymocytes do develop normally in the absence of insulin. Moreover, we were able to show that there was no difference in the development of $CD4^{+}CD25^{+}$ thymic regulatory T cell subset. Therefore, the expression of insulin in the thymus is not essential for the maturation of thymocytes.

MATERIALS AND METHODS

Mice

The two mouse strains deficient in *Ins1* and *Ins2*[8] were obtained from Dr. J. Jamie (Institute Cochin, Paris, France) and kept under standard conditions at Malmö University Hospital animal facility. Mice were first intercrossed to generate $Ins1^{-/+}Ins2^{+/-}$ and $Ins1^{-/-}Ins2^{+/-}$, which were further intercrossed in order to generate double knockout embryos.

Genotyping

Fetal tail DNA was used to genotype $Ins1^{-/-}Ins2^{+/+}$, $Ins1^{-/-}Ins2^{+/-}$, and $Ins1^{-/-}Ins2^{-/-}$ embryos. DNA was prepared by hot sodium hydroxide and tris preparation as described previously.[9] $Ins1^{-/-}Ins2^{+/-}$ mice were screened on the presence of the *LacZ* gene according to the vector construct.[8] The primers used were the following (5′-3′): *Ins1* wt sense TCAGTGCTG-CACCAGCATCT, antisense TCCAGATACTTGAATTATTCCT, *Ins2* wt sense TGCTCAGCTACTCCTGACTG, antisense GTGCAGCACTGATCTACAAT, *LacZ* sense TTCACTGGCCGTCGTTTTACAACGTCGTGA, antisense AT-GTGAGCGAGTAACAACCCGTCGGATTCT. The polymerase chain reaction (PCR) was run under standard conditions (for *Ins* primers: an initial denaturing phase at 92°C for 1 min followed by 35 cycles of 92°C for 45 s, 55°C for 45 s, 74°C for 1 min and 30 s, and a final extension step at 74°C for 10 min. For *LacZ* primers: an initial denaturing phase at 94°C for 1 min followed by 30 cycles of 94°C for 1 min and 72°C for 2 min, and a final extension step at 72°C for 10 min). The PCR product was visualized on a 2% agarose gel with ethidium bromide.

RNA Isolation and RT-PCR

RNA was extracted from thymocytes using TRIZOL® reagent (Invitrogen Life Technologies, Carlsbad, CA). RNA was reverse transcribed to cDNA in a 20 μL reaction containing 1 μL of 50 ng/μL random hexamer primers (Invitrogen Life Technologies) and 1 μL of 10 mM dNTP (Amersham Pharmacia Biotech, Uppsala, Sweden). The mixture was incubated for 5 min at 65°C and for 1 min at 4°C, after which 4 μL of 5X first strand buffer (Invitrogen Life Technologies), 1 μL of Ribolock™ Ribonuclease inhibitor (Fermentas Life Sciences GmBH, St. Leon-Rot, Germany), 2 μL of 0.1 M DTT (Invitrogen Life Technologies), and 1 μL of RevertAid™ H Minus M-MuLV Reverse Transcriptase (Fermentas Life Sciences) were added. The samples were then incubated for 10 min at 25°C, for 2 h at 42°C and for 30 min at 70°C. Ten percent or 20% of the cDNA product were used for subsequent PCR for *Ins1*, *Ins2,* and β-*actin* as house keeping gene. The primers used were the following (5′-3′): *Ins1:* sense AGTGACCAGCTATAATCAGAG, antisense ATGCTGGTGCAGCACTGATC; *Ins2:* sense GCTCTTCCTCTGGGAGTCCCAC antisense ATGCTGGTGCAGCACTGATC; β-*actin:* sense GGTGGGAATGGGTCAGAAGGACT antisense CCACGCTCGGTCAGGATCTTCAT. The PCR was run under standard conditions (an initial denaturing phase at 94°C for 3 min followed by 38 cycles of 94°C for 30 s, 60°C for 30 s, 72°C for 1 min, and a final extension step at 72°C for 10 min) and the product was visualized on a 2% agarose gel with ethidium bromide.

Fetal Thymic Organ Culture

Fetal thymic lobes were prepared from $Ins1^{-/-}Ins2^{+/-}$ females on embryonic day 14.5. Fetal thymic lobes were placed on 25 mm/8 μm pore Nucleopore Track-Etch Membranes (Whatman, Clifton, NJ, USA), which floated in Iscoves-modified Dulbecco medium (IMDM; Invitrogen Life Technologies) supplemented with 10% fetal calf serum (FCS; Sigma-Aldrich, St. Louis, MO), 100 μg/mL penicillin and 100 μg/mL streptomycin, 0.05 mM 2-β-mercaptoethanol, 1 mM sodium pyruvate and 1% of modified essential medium (MEM) nonessential amino acids (Invitrogen Life Technologies) or in Aim V serum-free media (Invitrogen Life Technologies) supplemented as described above without FCS. The lobes were cultured for 7 days in 37°C and 5% CO_2. Cell suspension was prepared by flushing the lobes first with a 23G 06*0.25 mm needle and then with a 27G 0.4*19 mm needle in phosphate buffered saline (PBS) supplemented with 2 mM EDTA and 0.5% bovine serum albumin (BSA).

Antibodies and Flow Cytometry

The following antibodies were used for flow cytometry: PercP-conjugated anti-CD3, PercP-conjugated anti-CD4, PercP-conjugated anti-CD8, phycoerythrin (PE)-conjugated anti-CD8, fluorescein isothiocyanate

(FITC)-conjugated anti-CD25, and PE-conjugated anti-CD44 (all from BDPharmingen^{TM}; BD Biosciences-Pharmingen, San Jose, CA). If not stated otherwise, thymocytes were added to 96 round bottom well plates, blocked with Fc-block for 15 min on ice, washed and stained with directly conjugated antibodies for 15 min on ice. For the analysis of CD44 and CD25 expression in early T cell precursors, $CD3^+CD4^+CD8^+$ cells were gated out (damp channel) based on PercP fluorescence. All samples were acquired using a FACSCalibur and analyzed by CellQuest software (both from Becton Dickinson, San Jose, CA).

Statistical Analysis

The data was analyzed using Student's *t*-test, $P < 0.05$ was accepted as significant. Data are expressed as the mean $\pm$ SEM.

RESULTS AND DISCUSSION

The expression of organ-specific antigens in the thymus, such as insulin, has been speculated to be important for negative selection of developing thymocytes.[10–12] However, the question of insulin as growth factor for thymocytes has not been fully addressed yet. In order to study the impact of thymic insulin expression on thymocyte growth and development, we generated insulin deficient mice by crossing *Ins1* and *Ins2* deficient mice into $Ins1^{+/-}Ins2^{+/-}$ that were intercrossed to obtain $Ins1^{-/-}Ins2^{+/-}$ mice, which were again intercrossed to generate $Ins1^{-/-}Ins2^{-/-}$ embryos. Tail DNA was used to screen the presence or absence of *Ins1* and *Ins2* genes and $Ins1^{-/-}Ins2^{+/-}$ and $Ins1^{-/-}Ins2^{+/+}$ were identified based on the presence or absence of the *LacZ* reporter gene for the *Ins2* knockout construct. PCR on fetal tail DNA is shown in FIGURE 1 A. $Ins1^{-/-}Ins2^{-/-}$ embryos showed no insulin bands and both $Ins1^{-/-}Ins2^{-/-}$ and $Ins1^{-/-}Ins2^{+/-}$ embryos presented the *LacZ* knockout reporter band whereas the $Ins1^{-/-}Ins2^{+/+}$ display only the *Ins2* band confirming that the *Ins1* and *Ins2* genes were disrupted in $Ins1^{-/-}Ins2^{-/-}$. In order to verify that insulin expression was lacking in the $Ins1^{-/-}Ins2^{-/-}$ fetal thymi, RNA was extracted from $Ins1^{-/-}Ins2^{+/-}$ and $Ins1^{-/-}Ins2^{-/-}$ FTOC thymocytes. The reverse transcriptase PCR (RT-PCR) shows that $Ins1^{-/-}Ins2^{+/-}$ lack *Ins1* and express *Ins2*, but no insulin expression was detected in the $Ins1^{-/-}Ins2^{-/-}$ thymocytes (FIG. 1 B). These results demonstrate that we were able to obtain $Ins1^{-/-}Ins2^{-/-}$ thymi.

Because $Ins1^{-/-}Ins2^{-/-}$ mice die due to acute hyperglycemia,[8] we used FTOC technique to study thymocyte development. Embryonic thymi from $Ins1^{-/-}Ins2^{+/-}$ pregnant females were dissected at embryonic day 14.5 and cultured in FTOC for 7 days after which thymocytes were prepared, stained for

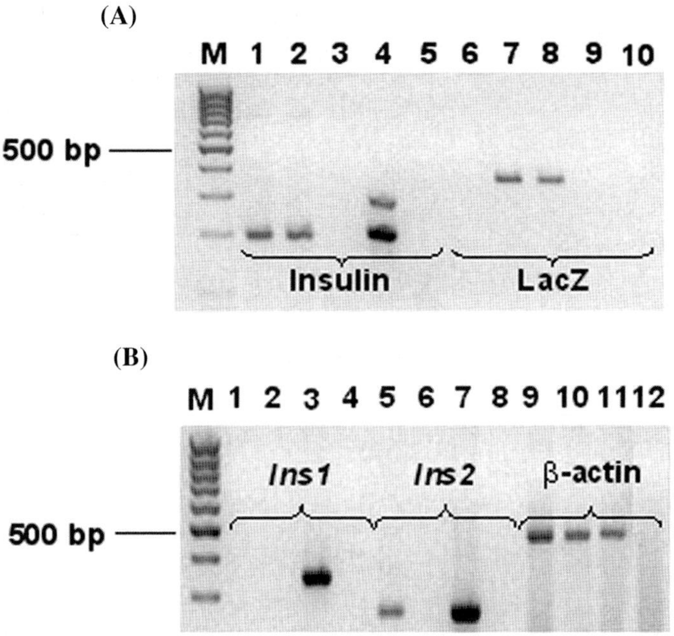

FIGURE 1. Genotyping and thymic insulin expression in insulin deficient mice. (**A**) PCR from fetal tail DNA. M = marker, lanes 1 and 2 show the presence of only *Ins2* in $Ins1^{-/-}Ins2^{+/+}$ and $Ins1^{-/-}Ins2^{+/-}$ embryos, respectively lane 3 shows $Ins1^{-/-}Ins2^{-/-}$ embryo lacking the insulin genes lane 4 is a wt control with both insulin genes lane 5 is the negative control lane 6 shows that $Ins1^{-/-}Ins2^{+/+}$ lacks the *LacZ* knockout reporter gene lanes 7 and 8 are the presence of *LacZ* reporter gene in $Ins1^{-/-}Ins2^{+/-}$ and $Ins1^{-/-}Ins2^{-/-}$ embryos, respectively, lane 9 is a wt control, and lane 10 the negative control. (**B**) RT-PCR showing insulin expression in thymus from the different genotypes. Lanes 1–5 contain samples with *Ins1* primers, lanes 5–8 with *Ins2* primers and lanes 9–12 with the endogenous control β-actin primers. M = marker, lanes 1, 5, and 9 = $Ins1^{-/-}Ins2^{+/-}$, lanes 2, 6, and 10 = $Ins1^{-/-}Ins2^{-/-}$, lanes 3, 7, and 11 = wt pancreas control, lanes 4, 8, and 12 = negative control.

cell surface markers to differentiate stages of maturation and analyzed by flow cytometry. The analysis included the earliest CD4 and CD8 double negative (DN) T cell precursors that were further characterized by the expression of CD25 and CD44 in four different maturation stages (DN 1–4), double positive thymocytes in later stages of differentiation expressing both CD4 and CD8 (DP), single positive (SP) CD4 or CD8 mature thymocytes as well as the frequency of thymic $CD4^{+}CD25^{+}$ regulatory T cells (FIG. 2 A). There was no significant difference in any of the DN stages (FIG. 2 B) or in DP and SP thymocytes (FIG. 2 C) between the different embryos. Moreover, there was no significant difference in the frequency of $CD4^{+}CD25^{+}$ thymocytes between the different genotypes (FIG. 2 C). To address the possibility that trace of

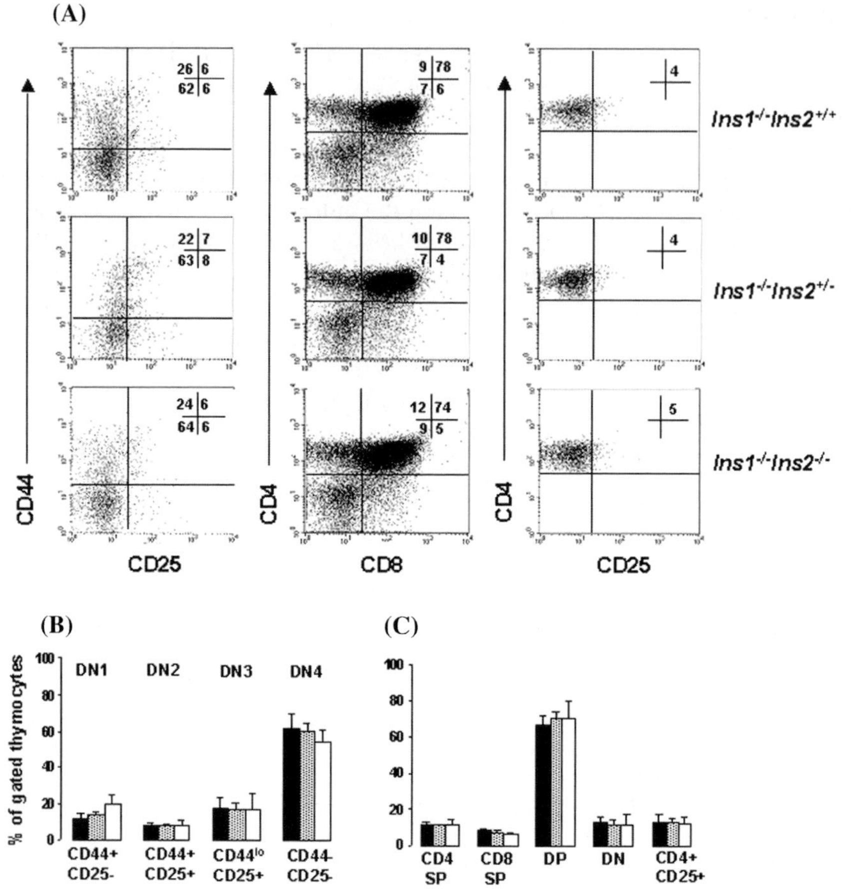

FIGURE 2. Flow cytometric analysis of thymocytes subsets from 7 days FTOCs. (**A**) Left panel shows representative dot plots for CD44 and CD25 staining among CD3, CD4, and CD8 negative thymocytes (DN), the middle panel shows expression of CD4 and CD8 on total thymocytes, and the right panel displays thymocytes gated on SP CD4$^+$ cells expressing CD25 (thymic regulatory T cells). The percentage of each subset is indicated. Lymphocytes were gated based on forward and side scatter parameters. (**B**) Cumulative analysis of CD44 and CD25 expression in DN thymocytes defining early stages of maturation (DN1, DN2, DN3, and DN4). (**C**) Cumulative analysis of CD4 and CD8 SP, DP and total DN thymocytes as well as CD4$^+$CD25$^+$ mature thymic regulatory T cells. Open bars = *Ins1*$^{-/-}$*Ins2*$^{+/+}$ (n = 4), shaded bars = *Ins1*$^{-/-}$*Ins2*$^{+/-}$ (n = 13), and filled bars = *Ins1*$^{-/-}$*Ins2*$^{-/-}$ (n = 6). The results are based on three independent experiments. Mean percentage values ± SEM are shown.

active bovine insulin in serum could affect the results, the experiments were also performed in serum-free conditions with similar results (data not shown).

IGF-1 and GH have been shown to influence the thymic environment in mouse and human and also to enhance the interaction between thymocytes and thymic epithelial cells.[13] Furthermore, thymocytes have been shown to express receptors for IGF-1, -2, and GH and in FTOCs treated with antibodies against IGF-1 and -2 the DN and DP cells decreased while the CD4^{+} cells were increased.[4,14–17] Moreover, IGF-2 transgenic mice demonstrate increased thymic cellularity and an amplified generation of the CD4^{+} population.[18,19] Among the pancreatic hormones, glucagon and somatostatin have been shown to be expressed in the thymus[7,20–24] and the latter also to enhance thymocyte development.[22] Thus, the expression of hormones in the thymus has a direct impact on thymocyte development. In the present study, we investigated the effect of thymic insulin expression on T cell development by using double-insulin deficient mice and demonstrated for the first time that absolute lack of thymic insulin do not affect T cell development at any stage of differentiation (DN1-4, DP, and SP) as well as the development of CD4^{+}CD25^{+} thymic regulatory T cells.

Since our data prove that lack of thymic insulin does not interfere with normal T cell development and therefore cannot hinder the outcome of functional studies, this mouse model will allow investigating whether thymic insulin expression does influence either negative selection of developing thymocytes, selection of CD4^{+}CD25^{+} regulatory T cells, or both.

REFERENCES

1. Sospedra, M. *et al.* 1998. Transcription of a broad range of self-antigens in human thymus suggests a role for central mechanisms in tolerance toward peripheral antigens. J. Immunol. **161:** 5918–5929.
2. Heath, V.L. *et al.* 1998. Intrathymic expression of genes involved in organ specific autoimmune disease. J. Autoimmun. **11:** 309–318.
3. Pleau, J.M. *et al.* 2001. Pancreatic hormone and glutamic acid decarboxylase expression in the mouse thymus: a real-time PCR study. Biochem. Biophys. Res. Commun. **283:** 843–848.
4. Kecha, O. *et al.* 2000. Involvement of insulin-like growth factors in early T cell development: a study using fetal thymic organ cultures. Endocrinology **141:** 1209–1217.
5. Murphy, W.J., S.K. Durum & D.L. Longo. 1993. Differential effects of growth hormone and prolactin on murine T cell development and function. J. Exp. Med. **178:** 231–236.
6. Deltour, L. *et al.* 1993. Differential expression of the two nonallelic proinsulin genes in the developing mouse embryo. Proc. Natl. Acad. Sci. USA **90:** 527–531.
7. Throsby, M. *et al.* 1998. Pancreatic hormone expression in the murine thymus: localization in dendritic cells and macrophages. Endocrinology **139:** 2399–2406.
8. Duvillie, B. *et al.* 1997. Phenotypic alterations in insulin-deficient mutant mice. Proc. Natl. Acad. Sci. USA **94:** 5137–5140.
9. Truett, G.E. *et al.* 2000. Preparation of PCR-quality mouse genomic DNA with hot sodium hydroxide and tris (HotSHOT). Biotechniques **29:** 52–54.

10. PUGLIESE, A. *et al.* 2001. Self-antigen-presenting cells expressing diabetes-associated autoantigens exist in both thymus and peripheral lymphoid organs. J. Clin. Invest. **107:** 555–564.
11. CHENTOUFI, A.A. & C. POLYCHRONAKOS. 2002. Insulin expression levels in the thymus modulate insulin-specific autoreactive T-cell tolerance: the mechanism by which the IDDM2 locus may predispose to diabetes. Diabetes **51:** 1383–1390.
12. THEBAULT-BAUMONT, K. *et al.* 2003. Acceleration of type 1 diabetes mellitus in proinsulin 2-deficient NOD mice. J. Clin. Invest. **111:** 851–857.
13. DE MELLO-COELHO, V. *et al.* 1997. Pituitary hormones modulate cell-cell interactions between thymocytes and thymic epithelial cells. J. Neuroimmunol. **76:** 39–49.
14. DE MELLO-COELHO, V. *et al.* 1998. Growth hormone and its receptor are expressed in human thymic cells. Endocrinology **139:** 3837–3842.
15. GAGNERAULT, M.C., M.C. POSTEL-VINAY & M. DARDENNE. 1996. Expression of growth hormone receptors in murine lymphoid cells analyzed by flow cytofluorometry. Endocrinology **137:** 1719–1726.
16. KOOIJMAN, R. *et al.* 1995. Type I insulin-like growth factor receptor expression in different developmental stages of human thymocytes. J. Endocrinol. **147:** 203–209.
17. VERLAND, S. & S. GAMMELTOFT. 1989. Functional receptors for insulin-like growth factors I and II in rat thymocytes and mouse thymoma cells. Mol. Cell. Endocrinol. **67:** 207–216.
18. KOOIJMAN, R. *et al.* 1995. T cell development in insulin-like growth factor-II transgenic mice. J. Immunol. **154:** 5736–5745.
19. SAVINO, W. *et al.* 2005. Abnormal thymic microenvironment in insulin-like growth factor-II transgenic mice. Neuroimmunomodulation **12:** 100–112.
20. AGUILA, M.C. *et al.* 1991. Evidence that somatostatin is localized and synthesized in lymphoid organs. Proc. Natl. Acad. Sci. USA **88:** 11485–11489.
21. FERONE, D. *et al.* 1999. *In vitro* characterization of somatostatin receptors in the human thymus and effects of somatostatin and octreotide on cultured thymic epithelial cells. Endocrinology **140:** 373–380.
22. SOLOMOU, K., M.A. RITTER & D.B. PALMER. 2002. Somatostatin is expressed in the murine thymus and enhances thymocyte development. Eur. J. Immunol. **32:** 1550–1559.
23. HANSEN, L.H., N. ABRAHAMSEN & E. NISHIMURA. 1995. Glucagon receptor mRNA distribution in rat tissues. Peptides **16:** 1163–1166.
24. KOH, W.S. *et al.* 1996. Expression of functional glucagon receptors on lymphoid cells. Life. Sci. **58:** 741–751.

Antigenic Determinants to GAD Autoantibodies in Patients With Type 1 Diabetes With and Without Autoimmune Thyroid Disease

HYEWON PARK,[a] LIPING YU,[b] TAEWHA KIM,[a] BOYOUN CHO,[c] JUNGOO KANG,[a] AND YONGSOO PARK[a]

[a]*Department of Internal Medicine and Bioengineering, Hanyang University College of Medicine and Engineering, 471-020 Seoul, South Korea*

[b]*Barbara Davis Center for Childhood Diabetes, University of Colorado Health Sciences Center, Denver, Colorado 80262, USA*

[c]*Department of Internal Medicine, Seoul National University College of Medicine, Seoul, South Korea*

ABSTRACT: Type 1 diabetes (T1D) is frequently associated with other autoimmune diseases. Most T1D patients' sera contain two distinct glutamic acid decarboxylase (GAD) antibody specificities, of which one targets an epitope region in the middle-third of GAD65 (amino acids 221–359) and the other targets the carboxy-third of GAD65 (amino acids 453–569). Using five chimeric GAD65/GAD67 proteins to maintain conformation-dependent epitopes of GAD65, we compared the humoral repertoire of antibodies from 127 T1D patients with and without autoimmune thyroid diseases (ATD). Thirty-one patients with T1D (24%) expressed antithyroid autoantibodies ATA and 22 patients (17%) had ATD in comparison to 6% of age-matched controls having ATA. GAD65-antibody-positive patients much more often (28% versus 5%, $P < 0.0004$) had ATD. Of 66 GAD65-autoantibody-positive T1D patients, 34 had autoantibodies reacting with both middle and carboxy epitopes. Autoantibodies of the other 32 reacted with middle, carboxy, or other epitopes but not with both middle- and carboxy-third. Those with GAD65 autoantibodies reacting with both middle- and carboxy-third had less ATD. Of 22 (23%) patients with ATD, 5 compared to 29 of 47 (62%) T1D patients without ATD had GAD65 autoantibodies reacting with both middle- and carboxy-third (relative risk = 0.2, $P < 0.01$). These results indicate that there are both similarities and differences in the humoral response to GAD65 in ATD and T1D, and expression of antibodies to middle- and carboxy-third at the same time is a feature specific to T1D.

Address for correspondence: Yongsoo Park, M.D., Department of Internal Medicine, Hanyang University Hospital, 249-1 Kyomun-dong, Kuri, Kyunggi-do, 471-020 Seoul, South Korea. Voice: 82-31-560-2239; fax: 82-31-553-7369.
e-mail: parkys@hanyang.ac.kr

Ann. N.Y. Acad. Sci. 1079: 213–219 (2006).
doi: 10.1196/annals.1375.033

KEYWORDS: **type 1 diabetes mellitus; autoimmune thyroid disease; GAD epitopes**

INTRODUCTION

Type 1 diabetes (T1D) is frequently associated with other organ-specific autoimmune diseases, including autoimmune thyroid diseases (ATD).[1] There have also been reports indicating that ATD patients have a high prevalence of autoantibodies specific for T1D.[2] The glutamic acid decarboxylase 65 (GAD65) autoantibodies occur in 60–80% of recent-onset T1D patients, while autoantibodies to the GAD67 occur in only 15–20% of T1D patients.[3] In most cases, epitopes are shared between the two GAD isoforms.[3] In most sera from recent-onset patients with T1D, GAD autoantibodies react with two conformation-dependent epitopes between amino acids 221–359 (middle-third, IDDM-E1) and 453–569 (carboxy-third, IDDM-E2) of the GAD65 protein, whereas in Stiff-man syndrome, GAD autoantibodies recognize at least three GAD65 epitopes located between amino acids 1–16, 188–442, and 442–563 in addition to two conformation-dependent epitopes located in the middle and the C terminus of the protein.[4]

Those whose insulin secretion has been stable for over 10 years also frequently express GAD antibodies. These individuals might express a particular subset of GAD autoantibodies other than the typical two conformation-dependent epitopes of T1D. In Asia, the T1D patients with ATD usually have higher age at onset and slow onset compared with sex-matched and disease-duration-matched patients without ATD.[2] The autoimmune pancreatic β cell damage in slow-onset patients tends to be more slowly progressive than that observed in the abrupt-onset group.[5] In Caucasians with GAD autoantibodies, DQB1*0602-positive patients had stable insulin secretion for over 10 years and expressed a particular subset of GAD autoantibodies recognizing a major epitope comprised of amino acids 421–442 and a minor epitope between amino acids 1–195.[6] In this study, we compared the humoral repertoire of antibodies from T1D patients with and without ATD using five chimeric GAD65/GAD67 proteins to maintain conformation-dependent epitopes of GAD65.

METHODS

For this investigation, 127 cases of T1D patients were selected randomly from the Korean Seoul Registry.[7] Their mean age at diagnosis was 7.9 ± 4.1 years with the mean diabetes duration of 4.5 ± 3.1 years. Thirty-six nondiabetic control subjects, with no family history of diabetes, matched by sex and age, were selected from the same geographical area. Their mean current age was 13.4 years (range 1.4–20 years). All of the patients and control subjects gave their informed consent to the study.

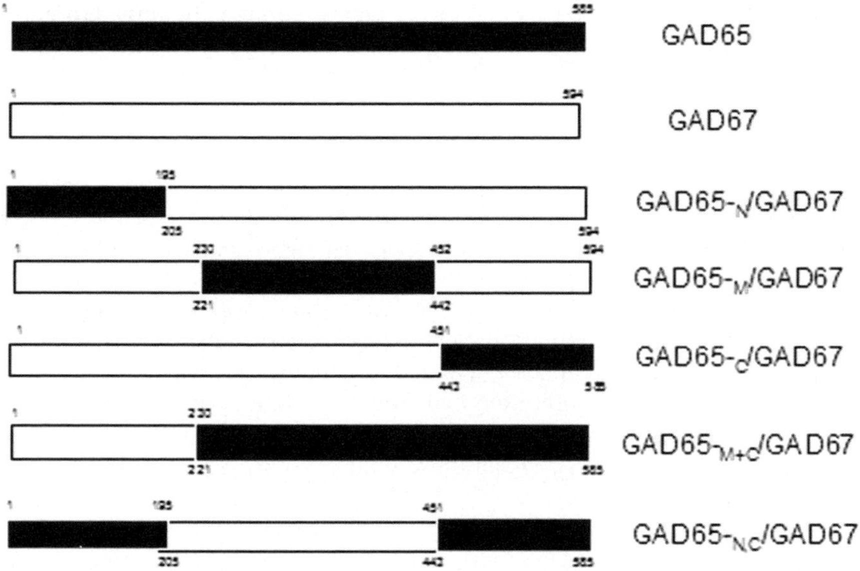

FIGURE 1. Schematic presentation of the different chimeric GAD proteins used in the epitope determination in comparison with GAD65 and GAD67.

The presence of ATD was being assessed by high titers (>0.3 ng/mL) of thyroid peroxidase or thyroglobulin antibodies, the level of TSH, and a positive medical history and/or physical exam. Thyroid peroxidase antibodies and thyroglobulin antibodies were measured by radioimmunoassay using commercial kits developed by RSR Limited (Cardiff, UK).

Five constructs of GAD65/GAD67 cDNAs created in the lab of Dr. Alvin C. Powers as described previously[3] were used for the GAD epitope mapping (FIG. 1). Human and rat GAD65, human GAD67, and five GAD chimeric molecules were produced using the TNT-coupled rabbit reticulocyte lysate *in vitro* translation system. Autoantibodies against to these molecules were detected in duplicate using *in-vitro*-transcribed/*in-vitro*-translated [S^{35}]-methionine-labeled (1000 Ci/mmol) recombinant antigen as described previously.[8] As for the chimeric GAD65/GAD67 proteins, "positive" for the assays were also based on the 99th percentile of sera from 110 healthy control subjects. For competition of autoantibody binding to *in-vitro*-translated ^{35}S-labeled proteins, unlabeled full-length rat GAD65, human GAD67, and chimeric GAD65/GAD67 proteins were prepared as described previously and used for blocking.[8]

Molecular typing of the generic typing of HLA DRB1 and DQB1 alleles was done by PCR-SSOP method as described previously.[7] Difference in the HLA genotype distributions was determined using the χ^2 test with Yates' correction (two-tailed). All other data are presented in the form of mean ± SD. Comparisons between the groups were made by unpaired parametric test (Student's *t*-test) and nonparametric test (Mann-Whitney *U* test).

RESULTS

Thirty-one patients with T1D (24%) were antithyroid autoantibodies (ATA)(+) [relative risk (RR) = 5.5 versus controls, $P < 0.05$], but only 22 patients (17%) of T1D were found to have ATD, whereas 2 of 36 (5.6%) of age-matched controls were ATA(+). The T1D patients with ATD had a longer duration of T1D and were mainly composed of the females (TABLE 1). Fifty-two percent of T1D patients (66/127) had antibodies to GAD65. Those with GAD65 autoantibodies more often had ATA ($P = 0.06$) and coexisting ATD ($P < 0.001$). There was no difference in the titer of anti-GAD65 between the patients with and without ATD, but those with anti-GAD65 autoantibody had more ATD ($P < 0.001$).

Using five chimeric GAD65/GAD67 proteins to maintain conformation-dependent epitopes of GAD65, we compared the humoral repertoire of antibodies from these T1D patients with and without ATD. Of 66 anti-GAD65-autoantibody-positive T1D patients, 34 reacted with both IDDM-E1 and IDDM-E2 and the other 32 reacted with IDDM-E1 ($n = 18$), IDDM-E2 ($n = 12$), or other epitopes ($n = 2$; one with N-terminal epitope and the other without any significant binding activity to chimeric constructs). Those with GAD65 epitopes IDDM-E1 and IDDM-E2 together less often had coexisting ATD than those with other GAD65 epitopes. Of 34 (15%) anti-GAD65-positive T1D patients with GAD65 epitopes IDDM-E1 and IDDM-E2 together, 5 had ATD, whereas 14 of 32 (44%) anti-GAD65-positive patients with other epitopes had ATD (RR = 0.2, $P < 0.05$) (TABLE 2). Of 22 (23%) T1D patients with ATD, 5 had IDDM-E1 and IDDM-E2 at the same time, while 29 of 105 (28%) T1D patients without ATD had both. We did not find a difference in the frequency distribution of HLA DR3/4-DQ8 genotypes between those with

TABLE 1. Comparison of the clinical characteristics between T1D patients with and without ATD

	ATD (+)	ATD (−)	*P* value
Number	22	105	
Sex (M:F)	4:18	56:49	<0.01
Duration (years)	5.9 ± 3.8	4.2 ± 3.2	<0.05
Age (years)	13.1 ± 3.9	11.9 ± 5.4	NS
Age at diagnosis (years)	7.4 ± 3.3	7.7 ± 4.4	NS
History of DKA, *n* (%)	8 (36)	42 (40)	NS
Family history of type 1 diabetes, *n* (%)	6 (27)	31 (30)	NS
HLA DR3/4-DQ8, *n* (%)	0 (0)	13 (12)	NS
GAD65 autoantibody (index)	0.26 ± 0.40	0.17 ± 0.31	NS

TABLE 2. Comparison of the clinical characteristics between T1D patients with and without typical T1D GAD65 antigenic epitopes, IDDM-E1 (amino acids 221–359), and IDDM-E2 (amino acids 453–569) together

	IDDM-E1 and IDDM-E2	Other epitope patterns*	*P* value
Number	34	32	
Sex (M:F)	19:15	14:18	NS
Duration (years)	4.2 ± 3.2	4.5 ± 3.4	NS
Age (years)	11.6 ± 4.6	12.1 ± 4.5	NS
Age at diagnosis (years)	7.4 ± 3.7	7.7 ± 3.7	NS
History of DKA, *n* (%)	14 (41)	10 (31)	NS
Family history of type 1 diabetes, *n* (%)	7 (21)	9 (28)	NS
HLA DR3/4-DQ8, *n* (%)	6 (18)	4 (13)	NS
Autoimmune thyroid disease prevalence, *n* (%)	5 (15)	14 (44)	<0.05

*The other 32 had IDDM-E1 ($n = 18$), IDDM-E2 ($n = 12$), or other epitopes ($n = 2$; one with N-terminal epitope and the other without any significant binding activity).

and without ATD or between those with and without sera reacting without IDDM-E1 and IDDM-E2 (TABLE 2).

DISCUSSION

The broad concept of polyendocrinopathies takes into consideration that patients affected by at least one endocrine disease may also possess a positive serologic reactivity against other endocrine cell targets.[1] Although we did not find a difference in the levels of GAD65 autoantibodies for positive patients, T1D patients with ATD had a higher prevalence of GAD65 autoantibodies. In contrast to the typical high-titer autoantibodies to GAD presumed to be a premonitory marker for the future development of diabetes, GAD antibodies are also present in some individuals with a low risk. A number of individuals whose insulin secretion has been stable for over 10 years express GAD autoantibodies: some of these individuals also express the DQB1*0602 allele and therefore are very unlikely to progress to diabetes.[6] Although the majority of these individuals were reported to express a particular subset of GAD autoantibodies recognizing a major epitope comprised of amino acids 421–442 and a minor epitope between amino acids 1–195, the antibody repertoire to GAD in T1D patients with ATD, who frequently develop at higher age and manifest more slowly progressive phenotype, has not been studied yet.

Since the GAD67 isoform is highly homologous to GAD65 but is usually not a target of the GAD autoantibodies in T1D sera, we applied five GAD65/GAD67 chimeric proteins to maintain the overall GAD protein conformation and used these chimeric proteins to map conformation-dependent epitopes of GAD65 targeted by T1D sera. We find that the GAD binding present in half of the T1D sera ($n = 66$ of 127) is mainly comprised of two distinct GAD antibody specificities that target different conformation-dependent regions of the GAD65 protein, IDDM-E1 and IDDM-E2. Of 66 GAD65 positive sera, 34 reacted with both IDDM-E1 and IDDM-E2. We confirmed these epitopes by competition studies. Binding was blocked completely by concomitant incubation of GAD67 (1–230)/GAD65 (221–585) or abrogated partially by incubation of either GAD67 (1–451)/GAD65 (443–585) or GAD67 (1–230)/GAD65 (221–442)/GAD67 (452–594). One T1D serum ($n = 1$ of 127) bound the GAD65 (1–195)/GAD67 (231–451)/GAD65 (443–585) protein, but the binding was not completely abolished by the incubation of either GAD67 (1–451)/GAD65 (443–585) or GAD65 (1–195)/GAD67 (205–594). The other T1D serum ($n = 1$ of 127) did not bind any chimeric proteins though it reacted with intact GAD65.

In our study, we found an increased prevalence of ATD in childhood-onset T1D patients compared with controls. Interestingly, none of the DR3/4-DQ8 patients had concomitant ATD. However, we did not find a significant difference in the frequency distribution of HLA DR3/4-DQ8 genotypes between those with and without ATD. It may be feasible that more frequent screening of thyroid function test irrespective of their HLA may facilitate the identification of the individuals who are at risk for the development of ATD. The observation that T1D is associated with ATD suggests a similar pathogenesis for these entities. It may well be that each disease has same separate genetic determinants and a common organ-specific defect in immunoregulation. Our results indicate that there are both similarities and differences in the humoral response to GAD65 in ATD and T1D and expression of antibodies to middle- and carboxy-third at the same time is a feature specific to T1D.

ACKNOWLEDGMENTS

This work was supported by the grants from Korea Science and Engineering Foundation (R01-2001-00177 and R01-2005-10075) and a grant from the Korea Health 21 R&D Project, Ministry of Health and Welfare, South Korea (A05-0463-B50704-05N1-00030B).

REFERENCES

1. Bottazzo, G.F. & D. Doniach. 1985. Polyendocrine autoimmunity: an extended concept. *In* Autoimmunity and Endocrine Disease. R. Volpe, Ed.: 375–404. Marcel Dekker. New York.
2. Kawasaki, E. *et al.* 1994. Autoantibodies to glutamic acid decarboxylase in patients with IDDM and autoimmune thyroid disease. Diabetes **43:** 80–86.

3. HAGOPIAN, W.A. *et al.* 1993. Autoantibodies in IDDM primarily recognize the 65,000-Mr rather than the 67,000-Mr isoform of glutamic acid decarboxylase. Diabetes **42:** 631–636.
4. DAW, K. *et al.* 1996. Glutamic acid decarboxylase autoantibodies in Stiff-man syndrome and insulin-dependent diabetes mellitus exhibit similarities and differences in epitope recognition. J. Immunol. **156:** 818–825.
5. PARK, Y. *et al.* 1996. The low prevalence of immunogenetic markers in Korean adult-onset IDDM patients. Diabetes Care **19:** 241–245.
6. UJIHARA, N. *et al.* 1994. Identification of glutamic acid decarboxylase autoantibody heterogeneity and epitope regions in type I diabetes. Diabetes **43:** 968–975.
7. PARK, Y. *et al.* 1998. Combinations of HLA DR and DQ molecules determine the susceptibility to insulin-dependent diabetes mellitus in Koreans. Hum. Immunol. **59:** 794–801.
8. PARK, Y. *et al.* 2000. Humoral autoreactivity to an alternatively spliced variant of ICA512/IA-2 in type 1 diabetes. Diabetologia **43:** 1293–1301.

TSH Receptor Antibodies in Subjects with Type 1 Diabetes Mellitus

AMBIKA G. UNNIKRISHNAN,[a] VELAYUTHAM KUMARAVEL,[a] VASANTHA NAIR,[a] ANANTH RAO,[b] ROHINI V. JAYAKUMAR,[a] HARISH KUMAR,[a] AND CARANI B. SANJEEVI[c]

[a]*Department of Endocrinology and the* [b]*Department of Biochemistry, Amrita Institute of Medical Sciences Cochin, Kerala 682026, India*

[c]*Department of Molecular Medicine, Karolinska Hospital Campus, Karolinska Institute, S-17176 Stockholm, Sweden*

ABSTRACT: The research was undertaken to study the prevalence of TSH receptor antibody positivity in patients with type 1 diabetes. A total of 74 subjects with type 1 diabetes were enrolled in this cross-sectional study. Thyroid function test and assessment of thyroid autoimmunity with anti-TPO and TSH receptor antibody were done in all patients. A total of 33 males and 41 females with type 1 diabetes were studied. The prevalence of TSH receptor antibody positivity alone was 18%. The prevalence of thyroid autoimmunity with anti-TPO as a marker was 28%; the prevalence increased to 43% when TSH receptor antibody was also measured. Majority of the subjects with antithyroid antibody positivity were also positive for GAD65 antibodies. As a significant proportion of type 1 diabetic subjects have positivity to TSH receptor antibody, we suggest that larger studies should be conducted to study the benefits of TSH receptor antibody-based screening for thyroid dysfunction in type 1 diabetic subjects. As the TSH receptor antibodies could be of the stimulating or of the blocking type, subjects with antibody positivity could be at risk of developing hyperthyroidism or hypothyroidism.

KEYWORDS: Graves' disease; autoimmune thyroiditis; type 1 diabetes; TSH receptor antibody; hypothyroidism

INTRODUCTION

Autoimmune thyroid disease (AITD) is the most prevalent autoimmune disorder associated with type 1 diabetes mellitus.[1] AITD may present as hypothyroidism, a euthyroid state with positivity to antithyroid antibodies, or rarely, as hyperthyroidism (i.e., Graves' disease). Conventionally, only measurements

Address for correspondence: Dr. C.B. Sanjeevi, Karolinska Institute, Department of Molecular Medicine, Karolinska Hospital Campus, CMM L5:01, S-17176, Stockholm, Sweden. Voice: +46-8-51776254; fax: + 46-8-51776179.
e-mail: Sanjeevi.Carani@ki.se

Ann. N.Y. Acad. Sci. 1079: 220–225 (2006).
doi: 10.1196/annals.1375.034

of T4, T3, thyroid stimulating hormone (TSH) and antibodies to thyroid peroxidase (anti-TPO), and antithyroglobulin have been used to evaluate AITD in type 1 diabetes mellitus. It has been reported that the positivity to anti-TPO antibodies in euthyroid subjects with type1 diabetes predicts the progression to eventual hypothyroidism.[2]

The association between Graves' disease and type 1 diabetes mellitus is well known.[3] Graves' disease is due to the presence of antibodies directed against the TSH receptor. These antibodies are usually stimulatory to the TSH receptor on the thyroid cells; chronic unopposed stimulation of the TSH receptor leads to hyperthyroidism. Sometimes, however, TSH receptor-blocking antibodies are produced, and these cause hypothyroidism: TSH receptor-blocking antibodies have reportedly been detectable in about half or more of subjects with chronic autoimmune thyroiditis.[4,5]

We report the results of a pilot study assessing the prevalence of TSH receptor antibodies among subjects with type 1 diabetes mellitus, and also screened the subjects for current evidence of thyroid dysfunction. We hypothesized that the detection of TSH receptor antibody could be a useful test for three reasons.[6,7] First, TSH receptor antibodies are disease specific, unlike other thyroid antibodies (antithyroglobulin or anti-TPO). Second, TSH receptor antibody has been detected in subjects with Graves' disease as well as those with chronic autoimmune thyroiditis, and could potentially identify subjects at risk of either hypothyroidism or hyperthyroidism. Finally, the newer assays for TSH receptor antibody are advantageous because they are easy-to-perform, inexpensive, faster, and efficacious.

SUBJECTS, MATERIALS, AND METHODS

Seventy-four type 1 diabetic subjects attending the outpatient wing of the Endocrinology Department were prospectively enrolled in this study. Type 1 diabetic subjects were enrolled only if the disease onset was before 18 years of age. All these patients required insulin to maintain their blood sugar in the euglycemic range. The institution's Research Ethics Committee approval was obtained prior to study enrollment. Informed consent was obtained in all cases.

The basic clinical examination was performed in all subjects and the presence of goiter, hypo- or hyperthyroid symptoms were noted. All patients underwent testing for FT4, TSH, anti-TPO, TSH receptor antibody, and glutamic acid decarboxylase 65 (GAD65) antibody. Anti-TPO antibodies were measured by chemiluminescence assays and GAD65 antibodies were measured by ELISA. TSH receptor antibody was measured by ELISA (Kronus Inc., Boise, ID) employing a kit used for routine clinical care. The assay specificity was reported to be 98% and the analytical sensitivity was 0.5 U/L. The intra-assay and the interassay coefficients of variation at TSH binding inhibitory levels of about 3 U/L were 3.9% and 10%, respectively. The assay does not cross-react with high values of TSH, luteinizing hormone (LH), or follicle stimulating hormone (FSH). The assay was carried as per the instructions in the booklet supplied with the commercial kit, but the procedure can be briefly summarized as follows: TSH receptor antibody in the patients serum is allowed to bind to TSH receptors coated on to ELISA well plates and the amount of binding is assessed by addition of streptavidin peroxidase and the peroxidase substrate tetramethyl benzidine. The values were then read off a standard curve. A value of 1.5 U/L or more was taken as positive. A patient was defined as hypothyroid if the TSH was more than 5 μIU/ml and/or if the patient had been on thyroxine therapy on the basis of raised TSH values documented earlier. Subclinical hypothyroidism was defined as a normal free T4 in association with a raised TSH in subjects not on thyroxine therapy. Fisher's exact test was used to compare frequencies.

RESULTS

Baseline characteristics of the study subjects were as follows (mean ± SD): mean age at study enrollment was 16.8 ± 7.4 years, and the mean age at diagnosis had been 9.4 ± 5.4 years. Thirty-three out of the 74 were males (45%).

Thirteen of the 74 subjects (18%) had antibodies to the TSH receptor. Among them, 2 subjects were positive for both anti-TPO as well as TSH receptor antibody. A total of 21 subjects (28%) had positivity for anti-TPO antibodies. While 9 out of the 13 subjects with TSH receptor antibody positivity were males, only 9 out of the 21 subjects with anti-TPO positivity were males. This gender difference between the two antibodies was not significant ($P = 0.17$).

Details of the subjects who were positive for the TSH receptor antibody are given in TABLE 1. Seven out of the 13 subjects positive for TSH receptor antibody had evidence of thyroid dysfunction, as compared to 8 out of the 21 positive for anti-TPO antibodies ($P = 0.48$).

Among the 42 subjects in whom both antibodies were negative, 3 subjects had abnormal thyroid function. Among the 32 subjects who were positive for at least 1 antibody, 14 had thyroid dysfunction. When compared with subjects without antibody positivity (see table), there was a significantly higher prevalence of thyroid dysfunction among subjects with TSH receptor antibody

TABLE 1. Prevalence of thyroid dysfunction among the antibody positive and negative subjects

Variable	TRAb +ve $n = 11$ (15%)	Anti-TPO +ve $n = 19$ (25%)	Both +ve $n = 2$ (3%)	Both −ve $n = 42$ (57%)
Hypothyroidism (22%)	5	7	1	3
Hyperthyroidism (1%)	1	0	0	0
Euthyroid state (77%)	5	12	1	39

NOTE: TRAb-TSH receptor antibody; +ve = positive; −ve = negative.

positivity ($P = 0.0007$), those with anti-TPO positivity ($P = 0.0042$) and among subjects with at least one antithyroid antibody positivity ($P = 0.0005$).

Among the 7 TSH antibody positive subjects with thyroid dysfunction, 1 subject had subclinical hyperthyroidism (TSH $< 0.001\,\mu$IU/ml and a normal free T4), and 6 subjects had overt primary hypothyroidism (TSH$>$ 10 μIU/ml and a low free T4). Among the 8 anti-TPO positive subjects with thyroid dysfunction, 6 had overt primary hypothyroidism, while 2 subjects had subclinical hypothyroidism.

Sixty-six (89%) of the 74 subjects were positive for GAD65 antibodies. The prevalence of GAD65 was not significant ($P = 0.25$) among the anti-TPO positive subjects, the value being 81% (17/21) when compared with a prevalence of 62% (8/13) among the TSH receptor positive subjects. The prevalence of GAD65 antibody positivity was higher among the subjects negative for antithyroid antibodies (41/42) as compared with the subjects positive for antithyroid antibodies (25/32; $P = 0.018$)

DISCUSSION

The results of the pilot study show that a significant proportion (18%) of subjects with type 1 diabetes mellitus are positive for TSH receptor antibodies. Majority (7/13) of these subjects with TSH receptor antibodies have current evidence of thyroid dysfunction. Fifteen percent of the 74 subjects were positive for TSH receptor antibodies but negative for anti-TPO antibodies. This suggests that TSH receptor antibody measurements could pick up cases of AIID (of the euthyroid, hypothyroid, and hyperthyroid forms) among type 1 diabetic subjects, which could be missed by performing anti-TPO alone. As TSH receptor antibodies are disease specific and not significantly found in the normal population,[7–9] it is likely that even the euthyroid subjects with TSH receptor antibody positivity will eventually develop some thyroid dysfunction, but this needs confirmation by longitudinal studies.

A potential disadvantage of the assay we have used is its inability to differentiate between TSH receptor stimulating and blocking antibodies. In other words, the assay detects only TSH receptor binding inhibiting immunoglobulin, which can cause blocking (and thus hypothyroidism) or stimulation (and thus hyperthyroidism) of the receptor. However, this makes it a useful test for screening, because of its ability to detect both the potential for autoimmune hypothyroidism as well as hyperthyroidism, with high specificity and sensitivity.[7] One small Indian study measured TSH receptor antibody in Graves' disease patient and controls and showed undetectable TSH receptor antibody in all controls while 87% positivity in patients with Graves' disease. This is the only study, which has measured TSH receptor antibody levels in healthy Indian subjects, but the number is too small ($n = 14$) for any significant conclusion.[8] In another study in 282 Caucasian volunteers the prevalence of TSH receptor antibodies (measured by three different techniques) were found to be very low, that is, less than 0.4%.[9]

The prevalence of thyroid autoimmunity with anti-TPO as a marker was 28%; the prevalence increased to 43% when TSH receptor antibody was also measured. Only two among the 32 antibody positive subjects had positivity to both TSH receptor and TPO antibodies, and this suggests that there is not much overlap between anti-TPO and TSH receptor antibodies. Thus the two antibodies could potentially detect two different subgroups of type 1 diabetes mellitus potentially at risk for AITD. This is an important area for further studies, which needs to focus on the use of both thyroid antibodies together for screening purposes. We did not study antithyroglobulin antibodies as they have a very low specificity.

Two small previous studies have looked at the prevalence of TSH receptor antibodies in type 1 diabetes mellitus. One study by Bliddal *et al.* on 46 subjects concluded that 22% had positivity based on radioreceptor assays, while 33% had positivity on cAMP-based stimulation assays.[10] Another study found that the prevalence was 4.8% among 63 children.[11] Certainly, the results of these studies show that TSH receptor antibody positivity is not uncommon in type 1 diabetes. Though cost-effectiveness remains an issue to be studied further, the use of newer immunoassays for TSH receptor antibodies has made the test relatively inexpensive when compared to previous radioreceptor as well as cAMP-based assays.

One limitation of our study is the small sample size. The higher prevalence of GAD65 positivity in thyroid antibody negative subjects is quite intriguing; as antibodies to the beta cell and thyroid have been shown to cluster together.[12] This could be a chance finding due to the small sample size.

No recommendations can be made on the basis of this small pilot study. However, this study definitely makes a case for larger studies on the issue of TSH receptor antibody-based screening for thyroid autoimmunity in type 1 diabetic subjects, and with a follow-up arm to assess the predictive value of these antibodies in *euthyroid* subjects with antithyroid antibody positivity.

ACKNOWLEDGMENTS

We thank Ms. Parvathi and Ms. Sabitha for helping us out in carrying the TSH receptor antibody assay. We also thank Mr. Jithesh for helping us in collecting and compiling the patient data, and the Kerala Chapter of the Research Society for the Study of Diabetes in India for funding this project.

REFERENCES

1. JAEGER, C., E. HATZIAGELAKI, R. PETZOLDT & R.G. BRETZEL. 2001. Comparative analysis of organ-specific autoantibodies and celiac disease–associated

antibodies in type 1 diabetic patients, their first-degree relatives, and healthy control subjects. Diabetes Care **24:** 27–32.

2. UMPIERREZ, G.E., K.A. LATIF, M.B. MURPHY, *et al.* 2003. Thyroid dysfunction in patients with type 1 diabetes: a longitudinal study. Diabetes Care **26:** 1181–1185.
3. LEONG, K.S., M. WALLYMAHMED, J. WILDING & I. MACFARLANE. 1999. Clinical presentation of thyroid dysfunction and Addison's disease in young adults with type 1 diabetes. Postgrad. Med. J. **75:** 467–470.
4. CHO, B.Y., W.B. KIM, J.H. CHUNG, *et al.* 1995. High prevalence and little change in TSH receptor blocking antibody titres with thyroxine and antithyroid drug therapy in patients with non-goitrous autoimmune thyroiditis. Clin. Endocrinol. (Oxf.) **43:** 465–471.
5. BRYANT, W.P., E.R. BERGERT & J.C. MORRIS. 1995. Identification of thyroid blocking antibodies and receptor epitopes in autoimmune hypothyroidism by affinity purification using synthetic TSH receptor peptides. Autoimmunity **22:** 69–79.
6. MICHELANGELI, V., C. POON, J. TAFT, *et al.* 1998. The prognostic value of thyrotropin receptor antibody measurement in the early stages of treatment of Graves' disease with antithyroid drugs. Thyroid **8:** 119–124.
7. KAMIJO, K. 2003. TSH-receptor antibody measurement in patients with various thyrotoxicosis and Hashimoto's thyroiditis: a comparison of two two-step assays, coated plate ELISA using porcine TSH-receptor and coated tube radioassay using human recombinant TSH-receptor. Endocr. J. **50:** 113–116.
8. VADIVELU, N., D.C. STEPHEN, A.S. KANAGASABAPATHY & M.S. SESHADRI. 1990. Thyroid stimulating hormone receptor antibody in thyroid diseases. Indian J. Med. Res. **92:** 220–223.
9. COSTAGLIOLA, S., N.G. MORGENTHALER, R. HOERMANN, *et al.* 1999. Second generation assay for thyrotropin receptor antibodies has superior diagnostic sensitivity for Graves' disease. J. Clin. Endocrinol. Metab. **84:** 90–97.
10. BLIDDAL, H., K. BECH, K. JOHANSEN & J. NERUP. 1984. Thyroid-stimulating immunoglobulins in insulin-dependent diabetes mellitus. Eur. J. Clin. Invest. **14:** 474–478.
11. LOPEZ MEDINA, J.A., R. LOPEZ-JURADO ROMERO DE LA CRUZ, A. DELGADO GARCIA, *et al.* 2004. Beta-cell, thyroid and coeliac autoimmunity in children with type 1 diabetes. An. Pediatr. (Barc.) **61:** 320.
12. MAUGENDRE, D., E. SONNET, C. DERRIEN, *et al.* 1999. Combined analysis of long-term anti-beta-cell humoral reactivity in type 1 diabetes with and without thyroid disease. Diabetes Metab. **25:** 28–33.

Time-Resolved Fluorescence Imaging of Islet Cell Autoantibodies

PAULI VUORINEN,[a,b] MARIS RULLI,[a,b] ARI KUUSISTO,[e] SATU SIMELL,[a,b] TUULA SIMELL[a,b] TERO VAHLBERG,[d] JORMA ILONEN,[a,e] HEIKKI HYÖTY,[a,f,g] MIKAEL KNIP,[a,h,i] AND OLLI SIMELL[a,b]

[a]*The JDRF Center for the Prevention of Type 1 Diabetes in Finland*

[b]*Department of Pediatrics,* [c]*Biostatistics,* [d]*Virology, University of Turku, 20014 Turku, Finland*

[e]*PerkinElmer Life Sciences, 20101 Turku, Finland*

[f]*Department of Virology, University of Tampere, 33014 Tampere, Finland*

[g]*Department of Clinical Microbiology, Centre for Laboratory Medicine, Pirkanmaa Hospital District, 33521 Tampere, Finland*

[h]*Department of Pediatrics, Tampere University Hospital, 33521 Tampere, Finland*

[i]*Hospital for Children and Adolescents, University of Helsinki, 00029 HUS Helsinki, Finland*

ABSTRACT: Time-resolved fluorescence of lanthanide chelates has been widely used in bioanalytical assays. Long fluorescence time, large Stokes shift, and minute fading out of the fluorescence over years are major advantages of the lanthanides over the conventional fluorescent dyes. We have now applied time-resolved fluorescence imaging (TRFI) also for measurement of type 1 diabetes mellitus (T1DM)-related islet cell autoantibodies (ICA). Retaining the accuracy of conventional ICA, TRFI has over 10 times better signal-to-noise ratio than the conventional fluorochromes. The technology allows objective determination of fluorescence intensity with the camera and computer software, and serial dilutions for obtaining the antibody titer in autoantibody-positive samples are unnecessary. We now describe the TRFI as a method and its application for measurement of ICA.

KEYWORDS: type 1 diabetes; children; islet cell autoantibodies; time-resolved fluorescence imaging; lanthanides

Address for correspondence: Pauli Vuorinen, BM, Research Fellow, University of Turku, Department of Pediatrics, Lemminkaisenkatu 14-18 A 5.krs, 20520 Turku, Finland. Voice: +358-2-313-3488; fax: +358-2-313-3491.
e-mail: pauli.vuorinen@utu.fi

**Ann. N.Y. Acad. Sci. 1079: 226–228 (2006). © 2006 New York Academy of Sciences.
doi: 10.1196/annals.1375.035**

INTRODUCTION

Assessing the risk of a child to progress to overt type 1 diabetes mellitus (T1DM) is currently based on genetic screening for certain HLA-alleles and measurement of T1DM-related autoantibodies, such as autoantibodies against islet cells (ICA), glutamate decarboxylase (GADA), insulin (IAA), and tyrosine phosphatase-like antigen (IA-2A). Despite intensive work toward standardization of the indirect immunofluorescence assay of ICA, the assay still has the shortcomings of dependency on pancreatic substrates and the need of international standard serum. Furthermore, serial dilutions of autoantibody positive samples are needed for the measurement of the autoantibody concentration and determination of fluorescence intensity is based on subjective visual estimation. Use of fluorescein-isothiocyanate (FITC) as a fluorescent limits the assay accuracy because the specific fluorescence is disturbed by the natural autofluorescence of the pancreatic tissue, and FITC fluorescence bleaches rapidly if exposed to light, limiting the microscopy time to a few minutes. To overcome some of these problems we have used time-resolved fluorescence imaging (TRFI) to measure islet cell autoantibodies.

MEASUREMENT OF ICA WITH TRFI[1]

Cryosectioned, 8 μm thick pancreatic slices on a microscope slide are incubated with 15 μL of serum for 30 min. After three times 5-min washing Eu^{3+}-labeled goat anti-human IgG (PerkinElmer Life and Analytical Sciences, Turku, Finland) is then added for 30 min incubation and washed again three times. The excitation wavelength for Eu^{3+} is 320–400 nm, produced with xenon flash lamp and an appropriate filter (UG11; Schott, Mainz, Germany). Bandpass filter at 615 nm wavelength and 10 nm bandwith is used for 80% of transmission (Ferroperm, Vedbaek, Denmark). Long lifetime of fluorescence, large Stokes shift, and sharp fluorescent peaks of europium enable the use of time-resolved imaging to distinguish the specific fluorescence from background autofluorescence.[2] After a 300 μs delay a time-resolved fluorescence image is obtained. The TRFI–ICA value is calculated using the mean intensity of islet fluorescence minus background fluorescence and expressed as counts per pixel (cpp; pixel = 18 μm × 18 μm).

TRFI–ICA IN COMPARISON TO CONVENTIONAL ICA

We have now used TRFI–ICA measurement in parallel with measurement of conventional ICA in a large number of ICA-positive and ICA-negative samples. The comparison of these two methods has shown that TRFI has at least the accuracy of the conventional method in determining ICA[3] with over

10 times better signal-to-noise ratio[1] and more stable pattern of titers during the disease process when samples have been collected at 3- to 12-month intervals since birth until the development of T1DM.[3] TRFI–ICA has also been found to be slightly more prevalent in recent-onset T1DM than conventional ICA,[1] and children progressing to T1DM have had higher TRFI–ICA value than the ICA-positive children remaining nondiabetic, even when the children had been matched for the number of positive autoantibodies.[3]

The linear, continuous scale of TRFI–ICA, the disappearance of need for serial dilutions, and the absence of need of reference serum may help determine molecular characteristics, such as avidity,[4] of ICA that have remained obscure so far.

REFERENCES

1. RULLI, M. *et al.* 1997. Time-resolved fluorescence imaging in islet cell autoantibody quantitation. J. Immunol. Methods **208:** 169–179.
2. SEVEUS, L. *et al.* 1992. Time-resolved fluorescence imaging of europium chelate label in immunohistochemistry and in situ hybridization. Cytometry **13:** 329–338.
3. VUORINEN, P. *et al.* 2005. Time-resolved fluorescence imaging of islet cell autoantibodies during progression to type 1 diabetes in the prospective DIPP cohort. Poster presented at the IDS-8. Awaji Island, Japan.
4. RULLI, M. & O. SIMELL. 1999. Avidity of islet cell autoantibodies in non-diabetic children and children with insulin-dependent diabetes. Autoimmunity **31:** 187–193.

MHC Class I Chain-Related Gene-A Is Associated with IA2 and IAA but Not GAD in Swedish Type 1 Diabetes Mellitus

MANU GUPTA,[a] JINKO GRAHAM,[b] BRIAN McNEENY,[b] MARIAN ZARGHAMI,[c] MONA LANDIN-OLSSON,[d] WILLIAM A. HAGOPIAN,[e] JERRY PALMER,[d] ÅKE LERNMARK,[c] AND CARANI B. SANJEEVI[a]

[a]*Department of Molecular Medicine, Karolinska Institutet, S-17176 Stockholm, Sweden*

[b]*Department of Statistics and Actuarial Science, Simon Fraser University, Burnaby V5A 1S6, Canada*

[c]*Department of Medicine, University of Washington, Seattle 98195-7710, Washington*

[d]*Department of Medicine, University of Lund, Lund 98108, Sweden*

[e]*Pacific Northwest Research Institute, Seattle 98195, Washington*

ABSTRACT: In type 1 diabetes mellitus (T1DM), the frequency of antibodies against insulin (IAA), glutamic acid decarboxylase-65 (GAD65), ICA512/IA2 (IA2), and islet cell antigens (ICA) vary with human leukocyte antigen (HLA) composition of the patient. IAA, IA2 autoantibodies, and ICA are increased in DQ8 positives; GAD65 antibodies are increased in DQ2 positives. MHC class I chain-related gene-A (MICA) is another genetic marker that has been proposed to be associated with T1DM. In this article, we looked at microsatellite polymorphism of MICA and its association with autoantibodies (IAA, IA2, and GAD65) in Swedish T1DM patients and if the association explains its importance in early events in autoimmune response. We studied 635 T1DM patients between 0–35 years. Frequency of MICA5/5 was positively associated with the formation of IAA and IA2 antibodies considered individually or in combination (odds ratio [OR], 95% CI, *P*c: [IAA+ versus IAA–] : 4.94, 2.09–11.62, <0.0005; [IA2+ versus IA2–] : 2.65, 1.52–4.59, 0.0015; [IAA and/or IA2+ versus rest]: 9.83, 2.37–40.78, <0.0015; [IAA and IA2+ versus rest]: 3.51, 2.01–6.15, <0.0015). Also, –5.1/5.1 was increased in IAA+ patients compared to IAA– patients (2.82, 1.64–4.83, <0.0005). All patients positive for –5/5 developed at least one of the three antibodies.

Address for correspondence: Dr. C.B. Sanjeevi, Karolinska Institute, Department of Molecular Medicine, Karolinska Hospital Campus, CMM; L5:01, S-17176, Stockholm, Sweden. Voice: +46-8-51776254; fax: +46-8-51776179.
e-mail: sanjeevi.carani@ki.se

Ann. N.Y. Acad. Sci. 1079: 229–239 (2006).
doi: 10.1196/annals.1375.036

Frequency of MICA5.1 was decreased in IAA+ (0.54, 0.36–0.81, 0.017), in IA2A+ (0.63, 0.45–0.88, 0.04), in IAA and/or IA2A+ (0.52, 0.33–0.84, 0.044), and in IAA and IA2A+ (0.55, 0.39–0.78, 0.0055) patients when compared with patients negative for corresponding antibodies. Frequency of MICA9, 5/5.1, and 5.1/9 was decreased in IAA+ compared to IAA– patients (0.51, 0.32–0.79, 0.021; 0.22, 0.11–0.44, <0.005; and 0.39, 0.22–0.69, 0.026, respectively). Frequency of MICA9 and –5.1/9 was also decreased in IAA and/or IA2 antibody-positive patients while MICA5/5.1 decreased in patients positive for IAA and IA2 antibody both together. IAA and IA2 antibodies are believed to appear early during the autoimmune reaction against beta cells. Thus, according to our data, MICA–5/5 and –5.1/5.1 is associated with early autoimmunity in T1DM patients. Our study suggests that MICA gene polymorphism is associated with autoantibody formation and that the polymorphism especially MICA5/5 and –5.1/5.1 are important in early events of autoimmune reaction.

KEYWORDS: **T1DM; MICA; GAD65; IA2; IAA**

INTRODUCTION

Type 1 diabetes (T1DM) is an autoimmune disease marked by infiltration of mononuclear cells into the pancreatic islets.[1] Autoantibodies that develop against islet antigens like insulin (IAA), glutamic acid decarboxylase-65 (GAD65), ICA512/IA2 (IA2), and islet cell antibodies (ICAs) are the markers for the disease.[2,3] ICAs, the traditional marker of T1DM can be detected in around 70–90% of T1DM at and prior to disease onset and between 0% and 5% healthy control subjects. ICAs have multiple and variable target molecules including GAD65 and IA2.[3,4] In majority of the T1DM cases, immune reaction against islet antigens and consequent formation of autoantibodies begins much before the disease is diagnosed clinically.[5–7] Retrospective studies have shown that >90% of T1DM patients are positive for either antibody at diagnosis.[8] For this reason, autoantibody markers have been used as markers for screening programs.[3]

Human leukocyte antigen (HLA) class II molecules-DQ and -DR are known to be the genetic markers of T1DM.[9] DR3-DQA1*0501-DQB1*0201 (DR3-DQ2) and DR4-DQA1*0301-DQB1*0302 (DR4-DQ8) are positively associated with the disease and DR15-DQA1*0102-DQB1*0602 (DR15-DQ6) is negatively associated with the disease in Swedish Caucasians.[10]

It has been reported that frequency of immune markers, such as IAA, GAD65 autoantibodies, IA2 autoantibodies, and ICA varies with age at clinical onset, gender, and HLA composition of the patients.[11–13] In Swedish T1DM, IAA, IA2 autoantibodies, and ICA are increased in DQ8 positives and are inversely related to age-at-onset; GAD65 autoantibodies are increased in DQ2 positives and are positively associated with age-at-onset; GAD65 autoantibodies and ICA are increased in females while IA2 autoantibodies are increased in male patients.[11]

Among many other genes, besides HLA class II, which have been linked with T1DM, one is MHC class I chain-related gene-A (MICA).[14–16] MICA is a member of MIC family that consists of five genes: MICA, -B, -C, -D and -E. Of these, MIC-C, MIC-D, and MIC-E are pseudogenes while MICA and MIC-B are functional genes. MICA gene is located telomeric to the tumor necrosis factor (TNF-α) gene between the B-associated transcript (BAT-1) and the HLA-B genes. MICA gene codes for MHC class I-like molecules with three distinct extracellular domains (α 1, 2, and 3), a transmembrane (TM) segment, and a cytoplasmic tail, each coded by a separate exon. Unlike classical class I molecules, MICA lacks association with β2-microglobulin.[17]

Sequence analysis of exon 5 (which codes the TM region of the protein) of MICA gene has revealed trinucleotide repeat (GCT) polymorphism.[18] So far, 5 alleles of the exon 5 of the MICA gene, which consist of 4, 5, 6, or 9 repetitions of GCT, or 5 repetitions of GCT with an additional insertion of G (GGCT) have been identified.[18] These alleles have accordingly been named A4, A5, A6, A9, and A5.1. Also, MICA carries numerous nonsynonymous polymorphisms in the sequence encoding extracellular region in the α-2 domain.[19,20]

MICA molecules are stress induced and their expression has been recognized on intestinal epithelium and epithelial tumors. MICA molecules act as ligands for an activating receptor NKG2D on NK cells, γδ T-cells, and CD8αβ-T cells.[17,21] MICA molecules can be expressed on cell surface under stress conditions, for example, viral infection.[21] Recently, NK cells have been shown to contribute to beta cell destruction after CBV4 infection in NOD mice with perturbed interferon signaling in beta cells.[22] Though little is known about the role of MICA in autoimmunity, based on the above facts, we speculate that certain environmental factors, for example, viruses can act as inducers of MICA in the islets and that activation of NKG2D receptor bearing NK cells or αβ-T cells through MICA may be one of the mechanism of initiation of T1DM pathogenesis. In this regard, microsatellite polymorphism in MICA gene TM region has been shown to be associated with T1DM in various populations.[14–16,23–26]

If MICA has a role in autoimmune response to β cell antigens, which eventually leads to formation of autoantibodies to insulin, GAD65, IA2, and ICA, we speculate that the polymorphism of MICA gene might be associated with the presence of autoantibodies. In this article, we looked if the microsatellite polymorphism of MICA is associated with autoantibody formation and if the association explains its importance in early events in autoimmune response.

SUBJECTS AND METHODS

The present analysis is based on data from two population-based matched case–control studies described elsewhere.[10] Patients received diagnoses and classifications according to the World Health Organization (WHO) criteria. In the first study, all incident patients with T1DM who were younger than 15 years and received a diagnosis anywhere in Sweden between September 1, 1986 and December 31, 1987 were asked to participate. Matched control subjects were selected as described.[27] The second study comprised incident patients with diabetes who were 15- to 34-years old and received their diagnosis anywhere in Sweden between January 1, 1987 and December 31, 1988; matched control patients were also ascertained.[28] The protocol for patient registration and sampling was the same regardless of age. The two studies administered over overlapping years included a total of 971 incident patients with T1DM and 702 control subjects. Of these, DNA samples from 670 patients (male = 397 and female = 273) and 534 healthy controls (male = 274 and female = 260) were available for MICA typing. The current report is based on data from patients alone. The study was approved by the ethics committee of Karolinska Institute, Stockholm, Sweden and informed consent was obtained from all participating patients and controls.

METHODS

Genetic Markers

MICA Genotyping

MICA alleles were determined using a fluorescence-based automated fragment size analysis. The TM region of the MICA gene (exon 5) was amplified by polymerase chain reaction (PCR) using 5′-CCTTTTTTTCAGGGAAAGTGC-3′ as the forward primer and 5′-CCTTACCATCTCCAGAAACTGC-3′ as the reverse primer.[18] The reverse primer was labeled at the 5′ end with the fluorescent reagent HEX or 6-FAM (Pharmacia Biotech, Bjorkgatan, Sweden). The 12.5-μL PCR containing 20 ng of genomic DNA was carried out in a programmable thermal controller (PTC-100; MJ Research, Inc., Oldendorf, Germany). Following amplification, the numbers of GCT trinucleotide repeat units were determined using Perkin-Elmer ABI 373 DNA sequencer (Perkin-Elmer, Norwalk, CT) and output file was analyzed with Genescan and Genotyper softwares (Perkin-Elmer). MICA genotyping for the exon 5 microsatellite polymorphism was successfully determined for 635 of 670 diabetic patients.

HLA Typing

HLA typing of DQA1 and DQB1 was carried out by PCR amplification of the second exon of the genes followed by dot blot hybridizations using sequence-specific oligo probes and by restriction fragment length polymorphism for DR typing.[29,30] Results for these have already been published.[10,11,29] The number of individuals for whom both MICA and HLA-DR were available were 601 patients.

Immune Markers

Insulin Antibodies

IAA measured by radiobinding assay using acid–charcoal extraction and cold insulin displacement have been described elsewhere.[31,32] IAA measurements were available on 557 patients.

Glutamate Decarboxylase Autoantibodies

For 0–15 years, antibodies to radiolabeled human Mr 65,000 GAD65 were quantified by immunoprecipitation assay using fluorographic densitometry as described earlier.[33,34] For 15- to 35-year olds, GAD65 were radiolabeled by coupled *in vitro* transcription and translation, as described.[35] Positive and negative control sera were included in each assay and the antibody levels were expressed as an index defined as (cpm in unknown sample-negative control) / (positive control–negative control). GAD65 autoantibody index measurements were available on 618 patients.

IA2 or ICA512

Antibodies to ICA512/IA2 were measured by radiobinding immunoassay.[36] The 3′ portion of the ICA512cDNA: residues 602–979 (corresponding to the cytoplasmic portion of the protein) was amplified by RT-PCR from human HTB-14 glioblastoma cells.[37] *In vitro* translation with ^{35}S-methionine yielded a polypeptide of 46 kDa highly precipitable by diabetic sera. Radiobinding assays used scintillation counting of protein A-Sepharose pellets. The levels of IA2 were expressed as index calculated with the same formula as used for GAD65 radioassay. The results for IA2 were available for 615 patients.

Statistical Analysis

The odds ratio (OR) was calculated as described previously.[38,39] Differences in allele or genotype frequencies between the antibody-positive diabetics and the antibody-negative diabetics were tested by the χ^2 method. Yates' correction or the Fisher's exact tests were used when necessary. The P values were corrected (P_c) for the number of comparisons, according to the number of alleles or genotypes observed among diabetic subjects (5 for MICA alleles; 15 for MICA genotypes, and 52 for MICA–HLA haplotypes). A $P_c < 0.05$ was considered significant.

RESULTS

MICA and Single Antibody

IAA

Frequency of MICA –5/5 and –5.1/5.1 were significantly increased in IAA-positive group compared to IAA-negative group (OR, 95% confidence interval [CI], *P*c: 4.94, 2.09–11.62, <0.0005 and 2.82, 1.64–4.83, <0.0005, respectively). Among alleles, frequency of MICA5.1 and MICA9 (OR, 95% CI, *P*c: 0.54, 0.36–0.81, 0.017 and 0.51, 0.32–0.79, 0.021, respectively) and among genotypes frequency of MICA5/5.1 and –5.1/9 were significantly decreased in IAA-positive patients compared to IAA-negative patients (OR, 95% CI, *P*c: 0.22, 0.11–0.44, <0.005 and 0.39, 0.22–0.69, 0.026, respectively) (TABLE 1).

IA2 Autoantibodies

Frequency of MICA5/5 was significantly increased (OR, 95% CI, *P*c: 2.65, 1.52–4.59, 0.0015) and MICA5.1 (OR, 95% CI, *P*c: 0.63, 0.45–0.88, 0.04) was decreased in IA2 autoantibody-positive patients compared to IA2 autoantibody-negative patients (TABLE 1). We did not observe any signifi-

TABLE 1. Frequency of MICA alleles and genotypes in T1DM patients between 0 and 35 years of age positive for IAA and those positive for IA2A versus those negative for corresponding autoantibodies

	IAA+ $n = 408$	%	IAA− $n = 149$	%	IA2+ $n = 372$	%	IA2− $n = 243$	%
MICA5	149	36.52	57	38.26	151	40.59	81	33.33
MICA5.1	**221**	**54.17**	**102**	**68.45**[a]	**201**	**54.03**	**158**	**65.02**[g]
MICA6	63	15.44	37	24.83	59	15.86	51	20.99
MICA9	**62**	**15.20**	**39**	**26.17**[b]	63	16.94	56	23.05
MICA5/5	**70**	**17.16**	**6**	**4.02**[c]	**65**	**17.47**	**18**	**7.40**[h]
MICA5/5.1	**16**	**3.92**	**23**	**15.43**[d]	28	7.53	20	8.23
MICA5.1/5.1	**114**	**27.94**	**18**	**12.08**[e]	84	22.58	49	20.16
MICA5.1/9	**30**	**7.35**	**25**	**16.78**[f]	30	8.06	36	14.81

a = 0.54, 0.36–0.81, 0.017.
b = 0.51, 0.32–0.79, 0.021.
c = 4.94, 2.09–11.62, <0.0005.
d = 0.22, 0.11–0.44, <0.005.
e = 2.82, 1.64–4.83, <0.0005.
f = 0.39, 0.22–0.69, 0.026.
g = 0.63, 0.45–0.88, 0.04.
h = 2.65, 1.52–4.59, 0.0015.

cant differences in frequencies of other MICA alleles or genotypes in IA2 autoantibody-positive compared to -negative patients.

GAD65 Autoantibodies

None of the alleles or genotypes of MICA were associated with the presence or absence of GAD65 autoantibodies (data not shown).

MICA and Two Antibodies

IAA/IA2 Autoantibodies

When patients positive for either IAA or IA2 autoantibodies were compared with those negative for both antibodies, frequency of MICA–5/5 was increased (OR, 95% CI, *P*c: 9.83, 2.37–40.78, <0.0015) while that of MICA –5.1 and –9 as well as –5.1/9 were decreased in those with antibody positivity (OR, 95% CI, *P*c: 0.52, 0.33–0.84, 0.044; 0.48, 0.29–0.80, 0.032 and 0.35, 0.19–0.65, 0.02, respectively) (TABLE 2).

When patients positive for both IAA and IA2 autoantibodies were compared with those negative for either or both the antibodies, frequency of MICA5/5 was increased (OR, 95% CI, *P*c: 3.51, 2.01–6.15, <0.0015) while that of MICA5.1 and –5/5.1 was decreased in those with antibody positivity (OR, 95% CI, *P*c: 0.55, 0.39–0.78, 0.0055 and 0.34, 0.16–0.69, 0.037, respectively) (TABLE 2).

GAD65/IA2 Autoantibodies

When patients positive for either GAD65 autoantibodies or IA2 autoantibodies were compared with those negative for both antibodies or when patients positive for both GAD65 autoantibodies and IA2 autoantibodies were compared with those negative for either or both the antibodies, frequencies of none of the alleles or genotypes of MICA differed significantly in any group (data not shown).

MICA and Three Antibodies

All patients with any of the three antibodies were positive for MICA5/5 and none of the patients with zero antibodies was positive for MICA5/5. MICA6 was decreased in the group carrying any of the three antibodies (OR, 95% CI, *P*c: 0.26, 0.12–0.56, 0.0045) or in group with all three antibodies (OR, 95% CI, *P*c: 0.21, 0.09–0.49, 0.0025) when compared to the group with no antibodies (data not shown).

MICA and HLA Together and Autoantibodies

In all the stratifications done above according to the presence or absence of one or two antibodies, we also analyzed MICA alleles (5, 5.1, 6) together with DR3, with DR4 and with DR3-DR4 (heterozygous). We did not find any difference in frequencies of MICA–HLA combinations when stratified for the presence or absence of autoantibodies.

DISCUSSION

MICA is Associated with Autoantibody Formation

In our study, MICA5/5 was associated with the formation of both IAA and IA2 antibodies considered either individually or together. MICA5.1/5.1 was also associated with the formation of IAA alone. MICA5.1 was negatively associated with the formation of either IAA or IA2 antibodies considered

TABLE 2. Frequency of MICA alleles and genotypes in T1DM patients (0–35 years) positive for IAA or IA2 versus those negative for both autoantibodies (2a); positive for both IAA and IA2 versus those negative for either autoantibody

	IAA or IA2+		IAA or IA2−	
	$N = 439$	%	$N = 99$	%
MICA5	170	38.72	33	33.33
MICA5.1	**240**	**54.67**	**69**	**69.69**[a]
MICA6	71	16.17	24	24.24
MICA9	**70**	**15.95**	**28**	**28.28**[b]
MICA5/5	**74**	**16.86**	**2**	**2.02**[c]
MICA5/5.1	28	6.38	11	11.11
MICA5.1/5.1	110	25.06	16	16.16
MICA5.1/9	**34**	**7.70**	**19**	**19.2**[d]
	IAA & IA2+		IAA & IA2−	
	$N = 279$	%	$N = 259$	%
MICA5	110	39.43	93	35.91
MICA5.1	**141**	**50.54**	**168**	**64.86**[e]
MICA6	38	13.62	57	22.01
MICA9	41	14.70	57	22.01
MICA5/5	**58**	**20.79**	**18**	**6.94**[f]
MICA5/5.1	**11**	**3.94**	**28**	**10.81**[g]
MICA5.1/5.1	76	27.24	50	19.31
MICA5.1/9	18	6.45	35	13.51

$a = 0.52$, 0.33–0.84, 0.044.
$b = 0.48$, 0.29–0.80, 0.032.
$c = 9.83$, 2.37–40.78, <0.0015.
$d = 0.35$, 0.19–0.65, 0.020.
$e = 0.55$, 0.39–0.78, 0.0055.
$f = 3.51$, 2.01–6.15, <0.0015.
$g = 0.34$, 0.16–0.69, 0.037.

individually or in combination. MICA–9 and –5.1/9 were negatively associated with IAA and with IAA and/or IA2 antibody formation while MICA–5/5.1 was negatively associated with IAA formation and with formation of both IAA and IA2 antibodies together. We did not find polymorphism in MICA gene to be associated either with GAD65 antibody formation or ICA formation. The present study, to our knowledge, is the first one to show the association between MICA gene polymorphism and autoantibody formation in T1DM.

MICA is Important in Early Events During Autoimmunity

In majority of cases of T1DM, IAA, and IA2 antibodies are believed to appear first.[40] MICA molecules are a part of innate immune system that interact with and activate NK cells and $\gamma\delta$ T.[17] The role of polymorphic MICA molecules in T1DM pathogenesis is not known. However, we speculate that after an environmental trigger, for example, viral infection, MICA molecules are upregulated, probably, on pancreas or beta cells in specific. These MICA molecules being a part of innate immune system apparently play a role in the initial stages of autoimmune reaction. In this regard, it is a very interesting observation that MICA gene polymorphism especially genotype 5/5 is associated with the formation IAA and IA2 antibodies, which are believed to form early during the autoimmune reaction. Another interesting observation was that all subjects carrying MICA5/5 developed at least one of the three antibodies tested. Thus, the presence of MICA5/5 in addition to IAA or IA2 would be a valuable marker for prediction strategies.

MICA5.1 has been associated with older onset of T1DM.[16] Also, frequency of GAD65 antibodies is positively and IAA and IA2 antibodies is negatively associated with the age-at-onset of the disease.[11] In our analysis, MICA5.1 was negatively associated with the formation of IAA and IA2 antibodies considered individually or in combination. Interestingly, MICA5.1 was associated with the formation of GAD65 antibodies before correction of P value ($P = 0.043$, $Pc =$ NS; data not shown). This hints toward the importance of MICA5.1 in GAD65 antibody formation, which is a marker for the older onset of T1DM.

In conclusion, our study suggests that (*a*) MICA gene polymorphism is associated with autoantibody formation and (*b*) MICA gene polymorphism especially MICA5/5 and –5.1/5.1 are important in early events of autoimmune reaction.

REFERENCES

1. Schranz, D.B. & A. Lernmark. 1998. Immunology in diabetes: an update. Diabetes Metab. Rev. **14:** 3–29.
2. Christie, M.R. *et al.* 1994. Antibodies to islet 37k antigen, but not to glutamate decarboxylase, discriminate rapid progression to IDDM in endocrine autoimmunity. Diabetes **43:** 1254–1259.

3. BONIFACIO, E. & P.J. BINGLEY. 1997. Islet autoantibodies and their use in predicting insulin-dependent diabetes. Acta Diabetol. **34:** 185–193.
4. BORG, H. *et al.* 2000. Islet cell antibody frequency differs from that of glutamic acid decarboxylase antibodies/IA2 antibodies after diagnosis of diabetes. Acta Paediatr. **89:** 46–51.
5. LINDBERG, B. *et al.* 1999. Islet autoantibodies in cord blood from children who developed type I (insulin-dependent) diabetes mellitus before 15 years of age. Diabetologia **42:** 181–187.
6. SEISSLER, J. *et al.* 1996. Combined screening for autoantibodies to IA-2 and antibodies to glutamic acid decarboxylase in first degree relatives of patients with IDDM. The DENIS Study Group. Deutsche Nikotinamid Interventions-Studie. Diabetologia **39:** 1351–1356.
7. TUOMILEHTO, J. & H. YLIHARSILA. 1998. Antibodies as predictors of insulin-dependent diabetes mellitus before the clinical onset. Nutrition **14:** 403–405.
8. DECOCHEZ, K. *et al.* 2000. High frequency of persisting or increasing islet-specific autoantibody levels after diagnosis of type 1 diabetes presenting before 40 years of age. The Belgian Diabetes Registry. Diabetes Care **23:** 838–844.
9. REDONDO, M.J. & G.S. EISENBARTH. 2002. Genetic control of autoimmunity in type I diabetes and associated disorders. Diabetologia **45:** 605–622.
10. GRAHAM, J. *et al.* 1999. Negative association between type 1 diabetes and HLA DQB1*0602- DQA1*0102 is attenuated with age at onset. Swedish Childhood Diabetes Study Group. Eur. J. Immunogenet. **26:** 117–127.
11. GRAHAM, J. *et al.* 2002. Genetic effects on age-dependent onset and islet cell autoantibody markers in type 1 diabetes. Diabetes **51:** 1346–1355.
12. LESLIE, R.D., M.A. ATKINSON & A.L. NOTKINS. 1999. Autoantigens IA-2 and GAD in type I (insulin-dependent) diabetes. Diabetologia **42:** 3–14.
13. VANDEWALLE, C.L. *et al.* 1995. High diagnostic sensitivity of glutamate decarboxylase autoantibodies in insulin-dependent diabetes mellitus with clinical onset between age 20 and 40 years. Belgian Diabetes Registry. J. Clin. Endocrinol. Metab. **80:** 846–851.
14. GUPTA, M. *et al.* 2003. Association between the transmembrane region polymorphism of MHC class I chain related Gene-A and type 1 diabetes mellitus in Sweden. Hum. Immunol. **64:** 553–561.
15. GAMBELUNGHE, G. *et al.* 2000. Association of MHC class I chain-related A (MIC-A) gene polymorphism with type I diabetes. Diabetologia **43:** 507–514.
16. GAMBELUNGHE, G. *et al.* 2001. Two distinct MICA gene markers discriminate major autoimmune diabetes types. J. Clin. Endocrinol. Metab. **86:** 3754–3760.
17. BAHRAM, S. 2000. MIC genes: from genetics to biology. Adv. Immunol. **76:** 1–60.
18. OTA, M. *et al.* 1997. Trinucleotide repeat polymorphism within exon 5 of the MICA gene (MHC class I chain-related gene A): allele frequency data in the nine population groups Japanese, Northern Han, Hui, Uygur, Kazakhstan, Iranian, Saudi Arabian, Greek and Italian. Tissue Antigens **49:** 448–454.
19. GROH, V. *et al.* 1998. Recognition of stress-induced MHC molecules by intestinal epithelial gammadelta T cells. Science **279:** 1737–1740.
20. BRAUD, V.M., D.S. ALLAN & A.J. MCMICHAEL. 1999. Functions of nonclassical MHC and non-MHC-encoded class I molecules. Curr. Opin. Immunol. **11:** 100–108.
21. GROH, V. *et al.* 2001. Costimulation of CD8alphabeta T cells by NKG2D via engagement by MIC induced on virus-infected cells. Nat. Immunol. **2:** 255–260.
22. FLODSTROM, M. *et al.* 2002. Target cell defense prevents the development of diabetes after viral infection. Nat. Immunol. **3:** 373–382.

23. LEE, Y.J. *et al.* 2000. Polymorphism in the transmembrane region of the MICA gene and type 1 diabetes. J. Pediatr. Endocrinol. Metab. **13:** 489–496.
24. ZAKE, L.N. *et al.* 2002. MHC class I chain-related gene alleles 5 and 5.1 are transmitted more frequently to type 1 diabetes offspring in HBDI families. Ann. N. Y. Acad. Sci. **958:** 309–311.
25. PARK, Y. *et al.* 2001. MICA polymorphism is associated with type 1 diabetes in the Korean population. Diabetes Care **24:** 33–38.
26. KAWABATA, Y. *et al.* 2000. Age-related association of MHC class I chain-related gene A (MICA) with type 1 (insulin-dependent) diabetes mellitus. Hum. Immunol. **61:** 624–629.
27. LANDIN-OLSSON, M. *et al.* 1992. Predictive value of islet cell and insulin autoantibodies for type 1 (insulin-dependent) diabetes mellitus in a population-based study of newly-diagnosed diabetic and matched control children. Diabetologia **35:** 1068–1073.
28. LANDIN-OLSSON, M. *et al.* 1992. Islet cell and thyrogastric antibodies in 633 consecutive 15- to 34-yr-old patients in the diabetes incidence study in Sweden. Diabetes **41:** 1022–1027.
29. SANJEEVI, C.B. *et al.* 1995. Polymorphic amino acid variations in HLA-DQ are associated with systematic physical property changes and occurrence of IDDM. Members of the Swedish Childhood Diabetes Study. Diabetes **44:** 125–131.
30. KOCKUM, I. *et al.* 1999. Complex interaction between HLA DR and DQ in conferring risk for childhood type 1 diabetes. Eur. J. Immunogenet. **26:** 361–372.
31. PALMER, J.P. *et al.* 1983. Insulin antibodies in insulin-dependent diabetics before insulin treatment. Science **222:** 1337–1339.
32. HEGEWALD, M.J. *et al.* 1992. Increased specificity and sensitivity of insulin antibody measurements in autoimmune thyroid disease and type I diabetes. J. Immunol. Methods **154:** 61–68.
33. HAGOPIAN, W.A. *et al.* 1993. Quantitative assay using recombinant human islet glutamic acid decarboxylase (GAD65) shows that 64K autoantibody positivity at onset predicts diabetes type. J. Clin. Invest. **91:** 368–374.
34. HAGOPIAN, W.A. *et al.* 1995. Glutamate decarboxylase-, insulin-, and islet cell-antibodies and HLA typing to detect diabetes in a general population-based study of Swedish children. J. Clin. Invest. **95:** 1505–1511.
35. FALORNI, A. *et al.* 1994. Radioimmunoassay detects the frequent occurrence of autoantibodies to the Mr 65,000 isoform of glutamic acid decarboxylase in Japanese insulin-dependent diabetes. Autoimmunity **19:** 113–125.
36. KAWASAKI, E. *et al.* 1996. Autoantibodies to protein tyrosine phosphatase-like proteins in type I diabetes. Overlapping specificities to phogrin and ICA512/IA-2. Diabetes **45:** 1344–1349.
37. LAN, M.S. *et al.* 1994. Molecular cloning and identification of a receptor-type protein tyrosine phosphatase, IA-2, from human insulinoma. DNA Cell Biol. **13:** 505–514.
38. MIETTINEN, O. 1976. Estimability and estimation in case-referent studies. Am. J. Epidemiol. **103:** 226–235.
39. WOOLF, B. 1955. On estimating the relation between blood group and disease. Ann. Hum. Genet. **19:** 251–253.
40. WINTER, W.E., N. HARRIS & D. SCHATZ. 2002. Immunological markers in the diagnosis and prediction of autoimmune type 1a diabetes. Clin. Diabetes **20:** 183–191.

Predominance of the Group A Killer Ig-Like Receptor Haplotypes in Korean Patients With T1D

YONGSOO PARK,[a] HEEJIN CHOI,[a] HYEWON PARK,[a] SUKYUNG PARK,[a] EUN-KYUNG YOO,[b] DUKHEE KIM,[b] AND CARANI B. SANJEEVI[c]

[a]*Department of Internal Medicine, Hanyang University Hospital, Seoul 471-020 South Korea*

[b]*Department of Pediatrics, Yonsei University Severance Hospital, Seoul 471-020 South Korea*

[c]*Department of Molecular Medicine, Karolinska Institute, Stockholm, Sweden*

ABSTRACT: **Type 1 diabetes (T1D) is a T cell-mediated autoimmune disease in which pancreatic β cells are selectively destroyed. Although autoimmune diseases are driven by inappropriate adaptive immunity, innate immunity may play a role in the development of T1D. To study the potential involvement of innate immunity in the pathogenesis of autoimmune disease, we investigated associations of the genes for 14 different killer Ig-like receptors (KIRs), the well-characterized receptors in natural killer cells, with Korean T1D patients. Genetic association analyses revealed that some of the *KIR* genes were associated with T1D. *KIR2DL5* and *2DS2* genes were present at significantly low frequency in Korean T1D patients ($P < 10^{-4}$). We did not detect any influence of ligand distribution on KIR association. With the haplotype assignments, 53% of the KIR haplotypes in the control are of type A. Compared with the control ($P < 10^{-3}$) and autoantibody-negative patients ($P < 10^{-2}$), the group A haplotype predominates in Korean patients with T1D. The *KIR* gene is associated with T1D and distribution differences between T1D and controls were not influenced by the *HLA* genes (*DR-DQ-A-C*). T1D, at least in Koreans, is associated with *KIR* genes, especially in the group A KIR haplotypes. There is a close relationship between innate and adaptive immunity.**

KEYWORDS: **KIR; innate immunity; type 1 diabetes; Korea**

Address for correspondence: Yongsoo Park, M.D., Department of Internal Medicine, Hanyang University Hospital, 249-1 Kyomun-dong, Kuri, Kyunggi-do, 471-020 Seoul, South Korea. Voice: 82-31-560-2239; fax: 82-31-553-7369.

e-mail: parkys@hanyang.ac.kr

Ann. N.Y. Acad. Sci. 1079: 240–250 (2006). © 2006 New York Academy of Sciences.
doi: 10.1196/annals.1375.037

INTRODUCTION

The immune system is adapted to fight infections while maintaining homeostasis and comprises two arms, one recognizing molecular patterns and the other recognizing molecular details, which are called innate and adaptive immune systems, respectively.[1] An immediate immune response is normally generated by the innate immune system in response to invading environmental signals. The less rapid adaptive immune response follows the innate response, as it also did in evolutionary terms. In contrast to the almost infinite adaptivity of the acquired immune system, the innate immune system uses only a few, relatively inflexible, cell populations such as natural killer (NK) cells. The early host defense has an additional role in determining the nature of downstream adaptive immune responses.[1–3]

Type 1 diabetes (T1D) is a T cell-mediated autoimmune disease in which insulin-producing pancreatic β cells are selectively destroyed.[4] A characteristic feature of autoimmune diseases is the selective targeting of a single cell type, organ, or tissue by a certain population of autoreactive T and B cells. Since the adaptive immune system can preferentially recognize self-molecules, autoimmune disease is generally considered to be driven by an inappropriate adaptive immune response.[1,2] Destructive autoimmunity is, however, the final consequence of a complex multistep process and is strongly aggravated by inflammation.[5] Microorganisms can induce or promote inflammatory events and can intervene at any step of the inflammatory response. Each step in the inflammatory process is controlled by a multitude of mechanisms, including those of innate immunity, and either supports or suppresses the development of autoimmunity.[2,5,6]

NK cells, a critical subset of innate effectors, play important roles in immune defense by killing infected cells directly and by producing inflammatory cytokines.[1,2,7] During the progression of autoimmune diseases, NK cells are frequently present in many of the target organs such as the pancreas.[7] NK cells in the target organs, as well as those in peripheral lymphoid tissues, might be involved in the regulation of immune responses to autoantigens.[7] NK cells are critical in the initiation of adaptive T cell responses.[7] NK cell activity is, however, partially controlled through interactions between killer Ig-like receptors (KIRs) and their respective HLA class I ligands.[8] KIRs are members of Ig-superfamily and express molecules with either two or three extracellular Ig-like domains.[8,9] In humans, 16 *KIR* genes are clustered in a 150-kb region of human chromosome 19 called the leukocyte receptor complex (LRC). Plasticity in the *KIR* gene family creates synergistic combinations of allelic polymorphism and variable gene content, which individualize the KIR genotype. In this study of a Korean population, we analyzed the KIR genotype to investigate the role of innate immunity in the development of T1D.

SUBJECTS, MATERIALS, AND METHODS

Study Population

For this investigation, 139 T1D patients were selected randomly from the Korean Seoul Registry (incidence = 0.6/100,000/year).[10] All patients were unrelated and undergoing insulin therapy upon hospital discharge, less than 15 years of age, and residents of Seoul at the time of onset of the disease. The criteria for classification of T1D were as determined by the ADA Commission criteria.[11] Seventy-four were males, 65 were females; their mean current age was 13.4 ± 7.7 years. Their mean age at diagnosis was 7.9 ± 4.4 years with a mean duration of diabetes of 4.5 ± 3.5 years. One hundred thirty-two nondiabetic control subjects, with no family history of diabetes, were selected from the same geographic area.[12] Sixty-eight were males and 64 were females. Their mean current age was 37.3 ± 17.6 years. The epidemiologic procedures developed for selecting T1D patients and nondiabetic control subjects are those employed for the WHO Multinational DiaMond Molecular Epidemiology Study.[13] Of 139 T1D probands, the panel of 442 first-degree family members of 128 T1D patients was also studied for the KIR haplotypic assignment. All the patients or their parents gave their informed consent to the study, as appropriate. The study protocol was approved by the Institutional Review Board of Hanyang University, Seoul, South Korea.

Molecular Typing and Autoantibody Measurement

Peripheral blood lymphocytes from all donors were used for the *KIR* gene typing and molecular typing of the HLAs, A and C. Polymerase chain reaction (PCR)-based sequence-specific primer typing for 14 *KIR* genes was performed with primer sets as described previously[14] (TABLE 1). PCR was performed using 1.25 U of *Taq* DNA polymerase (Takara, Otsu, Japan) in 25 μL reactions at a magnesium concentration of 1.5 mM and 200–300 ng of template DNA. Concentrations for each primer set were optimized in PCR reactions with genomic DNA from several control individuals of known KIR genotype. Primers specific for DQA were included as internal positive controls at a final concentration of 0.8 μM in each mixture. The PCR conditions were initial denaturation for 2 min at 95°C, 10 cycles of 20 s at 94°C, 10 s at 65°C, 90 s at 72°C; and 20 cycles of 20 s at 94°C, 20 s at 61°C, 90 s at 72°C; and final extension of 7 min at 72°C. All reactions were conducted in an oil-free thermal cycler (PE 9600, Applied Biosystems, Foster City, CA), with hotstart procedures. Reaction products were electrophoresed on 0.9% agarose gel (Gibco-BRL, Grand Island, NY) at 100 V for 60 min and visualized by ethidium bromide staining. The presence of each *KIR* gene was determined by a band of the expected size. Individuals were determined negative for a *KIR*

TABLE 1. Sequences of the primers for the PCR-based sequence-specific primer typing of 14 human *killer Ig-like receptor* (*KIR*) genes

Locus	Primer	Sequences
KIR2DL1	Forward	5′-actcactccccctatcagg-3′
	Reverse	5′-ctgcaggacaaggtcacat-3′
KIR2DL2	Forward	5′-acttccttctgcacagagaa-3′
	Reverse	5′-gccctgcagagaacctaca-3′
KIR2DL3	Forward	5′-ccttcatcgctggtgctg-3′
	Reverse	5′-caggagacaactttggatca-3′
KIR2DL4	Forward	5′-aggacaagcccttctgc-3′
	Reverse	5′-ggaaagagccgaagcatc-3′
KIR2DL5	Forward	5′-tgcctcgaggaggacat-3′
	Reverse	5′-ccggctgggctgagagt-3′
KIR3DL1	Forward	5′-ccatyggtcccatgatgct-3′
	Reverse	5′-agagagaaggtttctcatatg-3′
KIR3DL2	Forward	5′-cggtcccttgatgcctgt-3′
	Reverse	5′-gaccacacgcagggcag-3′
KIR3DL3	Forward	5′-ggaacctacagatgttgc-3′
	Reverse	5′-tagttgacctgggaacccg-3′
KIR3DS1	Forward	5′-ggcagaatattccaggagg-3′
	Reverse	5′-aggggtccttagagatcca-3′
KIR2DS1	Forward	5′-tctccatcagtcgcatgar-3′
	Reverse	5′-agggcccagaggaaagtt-3′
KIR2DS2	Forward	5′-tgcacagagaggggaagta-3′
	Reverse	5′-cacgctctctcctgccaa-3′
KIR2DS3	Forward	5′-tcactccccctatcagttt-3′
	Reverse	5′-gcatctgtaggttcctcct-3′
KIR2DS4	Forward	5′-ctggccctcccaggtca-3′
	Reverse	5′-ggaatgttccgttgatgc-3′
KIR2DS5	Forward	5′-agagaggggacgtttaacc-3′
	Reverse	5′-ggaaagagccgaagcatc-3′

gene when a band of the expected size was absent in the presence of a band for the DQA control.

HLA class I high-resolution typing for A and C was carried out using the DYNAL RELI SSO reverse lineblot typing kit (Dynal Biotech Inc., Lafayette Hill, PA) by PCR-SSOP techniques.[15] In brief, genomic DNA was coamplified in a single PCR with biotinylated primers specific for the second and third exons of the relevant locus. The resultant PCR product was then denatured and subsequently hybridized to a set of unlabeled oligonuleotide probes immobilized on a nylon membrane. Membranes were subsequently incubated with streptavidin–horseradish peroxidase enzyme conjugates. Following stringent washing, bound probe was detected by means of a colorimetric detection system using the substrate tetramethylbenzidine. The pattern of probes hybridizing to a given sample indicated the identity of the alleles represented in the PCR product. The strip contained 57 probes for HLA A and 36 probes for HLA C. All had been previously typed for *HLA DR-DQ* and MHC class I chain-related gene A(*MICA*) genes.[10]

Glutamic acid decarboxylase (GAD) and IA-2 antibody measurements were done by radioligand binding assays using *in vitro*-transcribed and -translated antigens. These radioassays were performed using a 96-well plate format as described previously.[16] The positive and negative control sera were included in every assay, and the antibody levels were expressed as an index defined as (cpm in the unknown sample − negative control)/(positive control − negative control). "Positive" was based on the 99th percentile of sera from 132 healthy control subjects. The interassay coefficient of variation (CV) and intra-assay CV were as follows: GAD, 11.7% ($n = 9$) and 10.0% ($n = 10$); IA-2, 11.7% ($n = 9$) and 10.0% ($n = 10$).

Statistical Methods

Differences in the KIR genotype/haplotype distributions and in the proportions of patients positive for islet autoantibodies were determined using the χ^2 test with Yates' correction (two tailed). When the expected frequency was <5, Fisher's exact test was then used. The Bonferroni correction for multiple comparisons was applied. We also calculated the odds ratio (OR) using the Woolf formula[17] to assess the susceptibility effect of the *KIR* genes, with Haldane's formula as appropriate.[18] In the assessment of the KIR haplotypes underlying KIR genotypes, KIR group A haplotypes were defined by the combination of the *KIR2DL1*, *2DL3*, *2DS4*, and *3DL1* genes and the absence of the genes characterizing B haplotypes, *KIR2DS1*, *2DS2*, *2DS3*, *2DS5*, *2DL5*, and *3DS1*. Conversely, KIR group B haplotypes were defined by the presence of one or more of the *KIR2DS1*, *2DS2*, *2DS3*, *2DS5*, *2DL5*, and *3DS1* genes. Assignment of the genotype comprising two B haplotypes was supported by the absence of *2DS4* and *3DL1* genes characteristic of A haplotype.[8] Data from family-based samples allowed unambiguous assignment of each gene to the KIR haplotypes in all families.

RESULTS

Our study aimed to investigate associations of the *KIR* genes in Korean T1D patients and controls. The panel of 139 Korean T1D patients and 132 healthy, unrelated controls were typed for the 14 human *KIR* genes. Some of the *KIR* genes were associated with T1D (TABLE 2). *KIR2DL5* gene was present at significantly lower frequency in T1D patients (OR = 0.1, 95% CI: 0.08–0.3, $P_c < 10^{-5}$). *KIR2DS2* gene was also present at significantly lower frequency in T1D patients (OR = 0.3, 95% CI: 0.2–0.5, $P_c < 10^{-4}$). Nearly, all panel members typed positive for the three framework genes, *2DL4*, *3DL2*, and *3DL3* as well as *2DL1* and *2DL3*.

Although we do not know the ligand information for 2DL5, we stratified all HLA C and A alleles according to the 2DL5 positivity. We could not find any

TABLE 2. *KIR* gene frequencies in T1D patients and control subjects

	Case (%)	Control (%)	OR (99% CI)	P_c value*
2DL1	138 (99.3)	132 (100)	0.35 (0.04–3.76)	NS
2DL2	64 (46.0)	46 (34.8)	1.59 (0.95–2.68)	NS
2DL3	137 (98.6)	130 (98.5)	1.05 (0.15–7.62)	NS
2DL4	136 (97.8)	129 (97.7)	1.05 (0.17–6.67)	NS
2DL5	59 (42.4)	111 (84.1)	0.14 (0.08–0.26)	$<10^{-5}$
3DL1	134 (96.4)	127 (96.2)	1.06 (0.26–4.32)	NS
3DL2	136 (97.8)	130 (98.5)	0.70 (0.12–5.22)	NS
3DL3	134 (96.4)	131 (99.2)	0.20 (0.03–1.83)	NS
3DS1	50 (36.0)	49 (37.1)	0.95 (0.56–1.61)	NS
2DS1	47 (33.8)	58 (43.9)	0.65 (0.39–1.10)	NS
2DS2	28 (20.1)	62 (47.0)	0.28 (0.16–0.50)	$<10^{-4}$
2DS3	14 (10.1)	13 (9.8)	1.03 (0.43–2.43)	NS
2DS4	134 (96.4)	127 (96.2)	1.06 (0.26–4.32)	NS
2DS5	31 (22.3)	44 (33.3)	0.57 (0.32–1.02)	NS

*P_c were determined by multiplying the P value by 14 statistically analyzed *KIR* genes.
NS = not significant.

difference in the distribution of HLA C and HLA A alleles between 2DL5+ and 2DL5− patients (TABLE 3). Only the HLA C*8 allele appeared to increase in T1D patients with 2DL5 ($P = 0.07$, P_c = NS). When we consider the slight increase of C*8 allele in T1D patients versus controls (data not shown), the decrease of 2DL5 in T1D patients was independent of the HLA C. We also could not find any difference in the distribution of HLA C alleles, especially that of the group I HLA C alleles, between 2DS2+ and 2DS2− patients (data not shown).

When we assessed the haplotype underlying KIR genotypes for the individual patients and controls, 29 and 27 different KIR genotypes were found in

TABLE 3. Comparison of the HLA C allele frequencies between T1D patients with and without 2DL5

	2DL5+ ($n = 116$) N	2DL5− ($n = 166$) N	P_c value*
C*01	32 (27.6%)	52 (31.3%)	NS
C*02	0	1 (0.6%)	NS
C*03	29 (25.0%)	33 (19.9%)	NS
C*04	4 (3.4%)	4 (2.4%)	NS
C*05	0	3 (1.8%)	NS
C*06	0	10 (6.0%)	NS
C*07	16 (13.8%)	18 (10.8%)	NS
C*08	20 (17.2%)	16 (9.6%)	NS
C*12	1 (0.9%)	2 (1.2%)	NS
C*14	11 (9.5%)	24 (14.4%)	NS
C*15	3 (2.6%)	3 (1.8%)	NS

*P_c were determined by multiplying the P value by 11 statistically analyzed HLA C alleles.
NS = not significant.

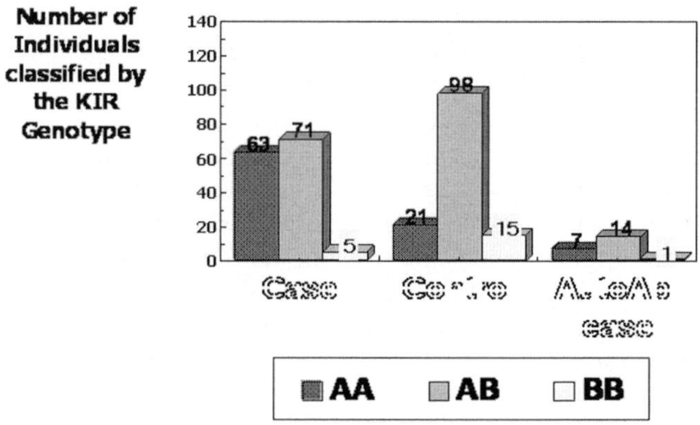

FIGURE 1. Distribution of the genotypes composed of the group A and B KIR haplotypes in T1D patients and controls.

patients and controls, respectively. The most common KIR genotype accounted for 38% of the patients and 23% of the controls, respectively. With these haplotype assignments, 53% of the KIR haplotypes in the control group are of type A and 47% are of type B (Fig. 1). Compared with the control group ($P < 10^{-3}$) and autoantibody-negative patients ($P < 10^{-2}$), the group A haplotype predominates in Korean patients with T1D.

DISCUSSION

Innate immunity has recently been found to be important in determining the fate of autoimmune responses.[6] The function of the innate immune response is to confer prompt self-protection by clearing pathogens or inhibiting their spread.[19,20] In this process, several molecules can be released, such as antigens derived from destroyed pathogens and/or normal components of host cells. These products can trigger the release of inflammatory mediators, including IL-1, IL-6, IL-12, IL-18, TNF, and NO. These molecules can amplify T cells to enhance self-protection against infected cells but, on the other hand, can also affect the development of destructive autoimmunity.[2,5,6] In this study, we demonstrate that some of the *KIR* genes are associated with T1D and the differential distribution of the KIR between T1D and controls was not influenced by the previously known major genetic determinants of T1D (HLA class I, class II, or class III genes) in the Korean population. The deviated *KIR* gene distribution in T1D patients was not influenced by the presence or absence of the islet autoantibodies (GAD or IA-2). As far as we know, this is the first definite report suggesting the association of T1D susceptibility with NK cell receptors (KIR). There has been one report showing that increased numbers of activating *KIR* genes existed in T1D patients, but with marginal significance.[21] They suggested that the activating *KIR* genes might contribute to the pathogenesis of T1D by influencing the immune response when they are present with their ligands, and the genetic imbalance between KIR and their HLA class I ligands may enhance the activation of T cells with a low affinity for pancreatic self-antigens, thereby contributing to the pathogenesis of T1D. In contrast, we found a significant decrease in the activating KIR, especially in the KIR 2DS2 in T1D patients. Even when we subdivided the patients with KIR 2DS2 with and without the group I HLA C ligands, the difference persisted. The discrepancies between the previous study and our study regarding the influences of *KIR* genes on T1D might be explained by the lack of family study to investigate the haplotype assessment and/or marginal significance. The referenced group[21] did not correct for the multiple comparison.

Effector T cell responses can be modulated by competing positive or negative signals transduced by NK cell receptors.[22] Important NK cell function is to regulate by NK receptors that interact with MHC class I molecules on target cells, performing "missing self-recognition."[7] In this sense, the hypothesis that autoreactivity in T1D is associated with increased frequencies of activating KIRs in the absence of regulation by inhibitory KIRs appears to be tempting. Independent segregation of *HLA* and *KIR* genes, along with KIR specificity for particular HLA allotypes, raises the possibility that any given individual may express KIR molecules for which no ligand is present. Subjects with activating *KIR* genes are susceptible to developing psoriatic arthritis, another autoimmune disease, only when HLA ligands for their homologous inhibitory receptors are missing.[23] Absence of ligands for inhibitory KIRs could potentially lower the threshold for NK cell activation mediated through activating receptors. Although information is accumulating on the diversity and promiscuity of the ligands for KIR, the role of activating receptors is less well understood. Both inhibitory KIR 2DL2 and activating KIR 2DS2 share ligands, group I HLA C alleles, with different specificities.[9]

It has been clearly shown that HLA class I molecules are associated with T1D. In our study, HLA C*14, which is usually accompanied by the A*33, was decreased in T1D patients, especially in those without autoantibodies. In addition, C*01 and C*15 were positively and negatively associated with T1D, respectively. MICA-A*6 was negatively associated with T1D. These influences might be dependent on surrounding HLA markers in linkage disequilibrium(LD). Multiple candidate genes in the HLA together with the strong LD in the HLA make it difficult to pinpoint the locus responsible for the true independent T1D susceptibility. The specific HLA class I alleles, A and C, were associated with T1D in Koreans and may, in combination with the differential distribution of KIRs, significantly modify disease risk. Study of KIR diversity in several human populations has led to the description of many different haplotypes and genotypes.[8,9] Two broad groups of human KIR haplotypes are defined. Group A haplotypes contain fewer expressed *KIR* genes and most include *KIR2DS4* and possibly *KIR2DL4* as the only activating receptor genes. Group A haplotypes are extensively diversified by allelic polymorphism. Group B haplotypes contain diverse combinations of activating *KIR* genes and many are characterized by the presence of *KIR2DL5*. The overall trend appears for activating KIR to be more diverse and more rapidly evolving than their inhibitory counterparts. Whereas group A and group B KIR haplotypes segregate at comparable frequencies in Caucasian populations, the more variable B haplotypes are more prevalent in other ethnic groups (Australian aborigines and Asian-Indians). A recent report studying the diversity of KIR genotypes implies that group A KIR haplotypes prevail in the Japanese population[24] like the Korean. It is thus of interest to determine whether populations subjected to strong pressure from infection have higher frequencies of activating NK cell receptors than populations where such pressure was less strong.

The mechanisms by which NK cells modulate adaptive immune responses are not entirely clear.[24] MHC-class-I-specific NK cell receptors comprise two families of molecules, one made of immunoglobulin superfamily domains and the other resembling C-type lectins. Genomic linkage analysis in NOD mice has revealed several idd loci. Genes conferring susceptibility to diabetes in NOD mice have been mapped to a region on chromosome 6 designated the natural killer–gene complex (NKC), which contains a cluster of genes preferentially expressed by NK cells, including NKG2D.[25] Profound dysregulation of NKG2D expressed on most NK cells and certain T cell subsets, and its MIC ligands, might cause autoreactive T cell stimulation, promoting autoimmune diseases.[22] We studied KIR located in LRC rather than receptors in NKC. Since NK cell activity is also controlled through interactions involving NKG2D and others and their respective ligands, besides the KIR, these genes may be associated with T1D susceptibility. Thus, we conclude that the *KIR* genes were associated with and might play a role in the development of T1D, and the differential distribution between T1D and controls was not influenced by HLA class I or *MICA* genes in the Korean population. From these, we might suggest that there is a close relationship between innate and adaptive immunities. Innate immunity may prime or promote an aggressive adaptive immune response.

ACKNOWLEDGMENT

This work was supported by the grants from Korea Science and Engineering Foundation (R01-2005-10075).

REFERENCES

1. Parham, P. 2000. The Immune System. Garland Publishing. New York.
2. Beyan, H., L.R. Buckley, N. Yousaf, *et al.* 2003. A role for innate immunity in type 1 diabetes? Diabetes Metab. Res. Rev. **19:** 89–100.

3. FRANTZ, S., R.A. KELLY & T. BOURRCIER. 2001. Role of TLR-2 in the activation of nuclear factor B by oxidative stress in cardiac myocytes. J. Biol. Chem. **276:** 5197–5203.
4. PARK, Y. & G.S. EISENBARTH. 2000. Natural history of type 1 diabetes. *In* Diabetes Mellitus: a fundamental and Clinical Text, 2nd ed. S. Taylor, D. LeRoith & J. Olefsky, Eds.: 347–362. Lippincott Williams & Wilkins. Philadelphia, PA.
5. JANEWAY, C.A. 2001. How the immune system works to protect the host from infection: a personal view. Proc. Natl. Acad. Sci. USA **98:** 7461–7468.
6. BACH, J.F. 2003. Autoimmune diseases as the loss of active "self-control." Ann. N. Y. Acad. Sci. **998:** 161–177.
7. MACKAY, I. & F.S. ROSEN. 2000. Innate immunity. N. Engl. J. Med. **343:** 338–343.
8. MCQUEEN, K.L. & P. PARHAM. 2002. Variable receptors controlling activation and inhibition of NK cells. Curr. Opin. Immunol. **14:** 615–621.
9. CARRINGTON, M. & P. NORMAN. 2003. The KIR Gene Cluster. NCBI. Bethesda.
10. PARK, Y. & G.S. EISENBARTH. 2001. Genetic susceptibility factors of type 1 diabetes in Asians and their functional evaluation. Diabetes Metab. Res. Rev. **17:** 2–11.
11. REPORT OF THE EXPERT. 2000. Committee on the diagnosis and classification of diabetes mellitus. Diabetes Care **23**(Suppl 1): S4–S19.
12. PARK Y, H. LEE., C.R. SANJEEVI. & G.S. EISENBARTH. 2002. MIC-A Polymorphism is associated with type 1 diabetes in the Korean population. Diabetes Care **24:** 33–38.
13. PARK, Y., K. KO, S. YANG & THE WHO DIAMOND MOLECULAR EPIDEMIOLOGY SUB-PROJECT GROUP. 1996. Molecular epidemiology of insulin-dependent diabetes mellitus (IDDM) in Korea. Diabetes Res. Clin. Pract. **34**(S)**:** S55–S59.
14. GOMEZ-LOZANO, V. 2002. Genotyping of killer-cell immunoglobulin like receptors (KIR) by the polymerase chain reaction: an update. Tissue Antigens **59:** 184–193.
15. BUGAWAN, T.L., W. KLITZ, M. ALEJANDRINO, *et al.* 2002. The association of specific HLA class I and II alleles with type 1 diabetes among Filipinos. Tissue Antigens **59:** 452–469.
16. PARK, Y., K. KO, S. YANG, *et al.* 2001. Evaluation of the efficacy of multiple autoantibody screening in Korean patients with IDDM. Acta Diabetol. **37:** 213–217.
17. WOOLF, B. 1955. On estimating the relation between blood group and diseases. Ann. Eugen. **19:** 251–253.
18. HALDANE, S. 1956. The estimation and significance of the logarithm of a ratio of frequencies. Ann. Hum. Genet. **20:** 309–311.
19. ZHAO, Z.S., F. GRANUCCI, L. YEH, *et al.* 1998. Molecular mimicry by herpes simplex virus-type 1: autoimmune disease after viral infection. Science **279:** 1344–1347.
20. SHI, F.D., H.B. WONG, H. LI, *et al.* 2000. Natural killer cells determine the outcome of B cell-mediated autoimmunity. Nat. Immunol. **1:** 245–251.
21. VAN DER SLIK, A.R., B.P.C. KOELEMAN, W. VERDUIJN, *et al.* 2003. KIR in type 1 diabetes. Disparate distribution of activating and inhibitory natural killer cell receptors in patients versus HLA-matched control subjects. Diabetes **52:** 2639–2642.
22. GROH, V., A. BRUHL, H. EL-GABALAWY, *et al.* 2003. Stimulation of T cell autoreactivity by anomalous expression of NKG2D and its MIC ligands in rheumatoid arthritis. Proc. Natl. Acad. Sci. USA **100:** 9452–9457.
23. MARTIN, M.P., G. NELSON, J.H. LEE, *et al.* 2002. Cutting edge: susceptibility to psoriatic arthritis: influence of activating killer Ig-like receptor genes in the absence of specific HLA-C alleles. J. Immunol. **169:** 2818–2822.

24. YAWATA, M., N. YAWATA, K.L. MCQUEEN, *et al.* 2002. Predominance of group A KIR haplotypes in Japanese associated with diverse NK cell repertoires of KIR expression. Immunogenetics **54:** 543–550.
25. GHOSH, S., S.M. PALMER, N.R. RODRIGUES, *et al.* 1993. Polygenic control of autoimmune diabetes in nonobese diabetic mice. Nat. Genet. **4:** 404–409.

Frequency of CTLA-4 Gene CT60 Polymorphism May Not Be Affected by Vitamin D Receptor Gene Bsm I Polymorphism or HLA DR9 in Autoimmune-Related Type 1 Diabetes in the Japanese

YASUHIKO KANAZAWA,[a] YOSHIKO MOTOHASHI,[b] SATORU YAMADA,[c] YOICHI OIKAWA,[a] TOSHIKATSU SHIGIHARA,[a] YOSHIAKI OKUBO,[a] TARO MARUYAMA,[d] AND AKIRA SHIMADA[a]

[a]*Department of Internal Medicine, Keio University School of Medicine, Tokyo 160-8582, Japan*

[b]*Department of Internal Medicine, Tokyo Metropolitan Otsuka Hospital, Tokyo 170-8476, Japan*

[c]*Department of Internal Medicine, Kitasato Institute Hospital, Tokyo 108-8642, Japan*

[d]*Department of Internal Medicine, Saitama Social Insurance Hospital, Saitama-city, Saitama 336-0002, Japan*

ABSTRACT: One of the CTLA-4 SNPs, +6230G>A (CT60), has recently been reported to be related to susceptibility to type 1 diabetes and autoimmune thyroid disease. We have previously reported an association between acute-onset type 1 diabetes in Japanese and the Vitamin D receptor (VDR) gene Bsm I large B polymorphism, which is related to the Th1-type response. Moreover, we found a significant correlation between autoimmune-related type 1 diabetes with HLA DR9 and detection of GAD-reactive Th1 (T helper 1)-type cells. In the present article, we tried to clarify whether the frequency of one of the CTLA-4 SNPs, +6230G>A (CT60), is affected by the VDR gene Bsm I polymorphism or by HLA DR9 in Japanese type 1 diabetics. The frequency of the CT60 GG genotype did not appear to be affected by either the VDR gene Bsm I large B polymorphism or HLA DR9.

KEYWORDS: CTLA-4; Vitamin D receptor; HLA; type 1 diabetes

Address for correspondence: Akira Shimada, M.D., Ph.D., Department of Internal Medicine, Keio University School of Medicine, 35 Shinanomachi, Shinjuku-ku, Tokyo 160-8582, Japan. Voice: +81-3-3353-1211; ext: 62383; fax: +81-3-5269-3219.
e-mail: asmd@sc.itc.keio.ac.jp

Ann. N.Y. Acad. Sci. 1079: 251–256 (2006).
doi: 10.1196/annals.1375.038

INTRODUCTION

Most of the type 1 diabetes mellitus is thought to be caused by autoimmunity to the islets of Langerhans in the pancreas. Various molecules are thought to be involved in the pathogenesis of some autoimmune diseases. CTLA-4 is a costimulatory molecule that is capable of regulating effector cells by competing with CD28. It has been reported that single nucleotide polymorphisms (SNPs) of this molecule are associated with certain autoimmune diseases, such as type 1 diabetes and autoimmune thyroid disease. Recently, Ueda and colleagues reported that one of the SNPs of this molecule, +6230G>A (CT60), might be related to susceptibility of type 1 diabetes and Graves' disease.[1] On the other hand, 1,25-dihydroxyvitamin D3 [1,25$(OH)_2$D3] is considered to have the capacity of modulating T helper1 (Th1)/Th2 balance and cytokine expression,[2] and its specific nuclear receptor is known to be present on monocytes and activated T lymphocytes.[3] We have previously reported that a higher frequency of the large B allele in the Vitamin D receptor (VDR) gene Bsm I polymorphism is observed in acute-onset type 1 diabetic patients as compared to controls.[4] In regard to HLA DR9, which is considered to be a susceptible HLA type in Japanese type 1 diabetic patients, we have also reported that the number of GAD-specific interferon-γ (IFN-γ)-producing T cells is increased in Japanese autoimmune-related type 1 diabetic patients with HLA DR9.[5] So in the present article, we tried to clarify whether the frequency of the CTLA-4 gene +6230G>A (CT60) polymorphism in Japanese autoimmune-related type 1 diabetic patients is affected by either the VDR Bsm large B allele or HLA DR9.

METHODS

Patients

Blood samples were obtained from 72 "autoimmune-related" type 1 diabetic patients ("autoimmune DM": 31 male and 41 female, mean onset age 35.4 ± 1.8 years) who were proven to possess at least one of the islet-associated autoantibodies (anti-GAD65 antibody, IA-2 antibody, or insulin autoantibody), and from 39 healthy controls who had normal glucose tolerance, no autoimmune disease, no autoantibodies, and no family history of diabetes mellitus. Type 1 diabetic patients were recruited from Keio University Hospital or Saitama Social Insurance Hospital. Informed consent was obtained from all the subjects, and institutional review board approval was obtained.

Autoantibody Measurement

Screening for anti-GAD65 antibody (GADA) was performed using a recombinant human GAD65 kit (RSR Ltd., Cardiff, UK), and "positive" was defined as a value above mean +3 SD of that in healthy subjects (an index > 1.3 U/mL). Screening for IA-2 antibody (an index > 0.010) and insulin autoantibody (IAA) (>50 nU/mL) was performed as previously described.[6,7] When at least one of GADA, IA-2 antibody, or IAA was positive, those patients were defined as "islet-associated autoantibody positive."

Analysis of CTLA-4 Gene +6230G>A (CT60) Polymorphism and VDR Gene Bsm I Polymorphism

After obtaining informed consent from recruited subjects, we extracted DNA from peripheral blood, which was then analyzed for these two gene polymorphisms, the CT60 and the VDR Bsm I, by PCR–RFLP method. First, in regard to the CTLA-4 gene +6230G>A (CT60) polymorphism, referring to the CTLA-4 gene sequence (accession no. AF 225900), PCR amplification of the region containing the polymorphism was performed using the forward primer in the 3′ UTR region (5′-CTTTGCACCAGCCATTACCT-3′) and the reverse primer in the 3′ UTR region (5′-AGGGGAGGTGAAGAACCTGT-3′). The PCR conditions used in the present study were as follows: 94°C for 5 min, and 35 cycles using the following temperature profile; 94°C for 30 s, 58°C for 30 s, 72°C for 30 s, and final elongation for 5 min. The PCR products were 163-bp long and were digested with Nla III at 37°C for 2 hours, and then subjected to electrophoresis in 2% agarose gel containing ethidium bromide. There were two types of lengths of restriction fragments; 134 bp and 29 bp (G allele), and 91 bp, 43 bp, and 29 bp (A allele). The genotype was determined from the length of fragments; that is, AA, AG, GG.[1]

In regard to the VDR gene Bsm I polymorphism, referring to the VDR gene sequence (accession no. I33554), PCR amplification of the region containing the polymorphism was performed using the forward primer in exon 7 (5′-CAACCAAGACTACAAGTACCGCGTCAGTGA-3′) and the reverse primer in intron 8 (5′-AACCAGCGGAAGAGGTCAAGGG-3′). The PCR conditions used in the present study were as follows; 95°C for 5 min, and 30 cycles using the following temperature profile: 95°C for 1 min, 56°C for 1 min, 72°C for 1 min, and final elongation for 10 min. The PCR products were 825-bp long (B allele) and were digested with Bsm I at 65°C for 1 h, and then subjected to electrophoresis in 2% agarose gel containing ethidium bromide. The lengths of the restriction fragments were 649 and 176 bp (b allele).[4]

HLA Typing

HLA class II antigen (HLA DR alleles) of the subjects was examined by sequence-based typing of serum.

TABLE 1. Frequency of CTLA-4 gene CT60 polymorphism

CT60 genotype	AA	AG	GG
"Autoimmune DM"	11.2% (8/71)	31.0% (22/71)	57.7% (41/71)
Control	2.6% (1/39)	43.6% (17/39)	53.8% (21/39)

P value: N.S. (AA+AG versus GG) by χ^2 test.

Statistical Analysis

Comparisons of genotype frequency and allele frequency between groups were performed using χ^2 test, or Fisher's exact test (if needed).

RESULTS

Frequency of CTLA-4 CT60 GG Genotype in Japanese Autoimmune Diabetic Patients

First, we examined the frequency of the CT60 GG genotype in Japanese autoimmune-related type 1 diabetic patients and control subjects. There was no significant difference in the frequency of the CT60 GG genotype between the groups ("autoimmune diabetics" 57.7% versus controls 53.8%, TABLE 1). This indicates that the CT60 GG genotype may not affect susceptibility to autoimmune-related type 1 diabetes mellitus in Japanese.

CTLA-4 CT60 GG Genotype may not be Affected by VDR Gene Bsm I Polymorphism in Japanese Autoimmune Diabetic Patients

We then evaluated the correlation between the frequency of the CT60 GG genotype and possession of the VDR Bsm I large B allele in "autoimmune diabetic" patients. As shown in TABLE 2, the frequency of the CT60 GG genotype did not differ regardless of the possession of the VDR large B allele. This indicates that the CT60 GG genotype seems not to be affected by possession of the VDR large B allele in Japanese autoimmune-related diabetic patients.

TABLE 2. Frequency of CTLA-4 gene CT60 polymorphism in "autoimmune DM" patients in relation to VDR gene polymorphism

CT60 genotype	AA	AG	GG
Large B allele (+)	10.5% (2/19)	42.1% (8/19)	47.4% (9/19)
Large B allele (−)	11.1% (3/27)	22.2% (6/27)	66.7% (18/27)

P value: N.S. (AA+AG versus GG) by χ^2 test.

TABLE 3. Frequency of CTLA-4 gene CT60 polymorphism in "autoimmune DM" patients with or without HLA DR9

CT60 genotype	AA	AG	GG
HLA DR9 (+)	12.0% (3/25)	24.0% (6/25)	64.0% (16/25)
HLA DR9 (−)	11.1% (3/27)	26.0% (7/27)	63.0% (17/27)

P value: N.S. (AA+AG versus GG) by χ^2 test.

HLA DR9 may not Affect Frequency of CT60 GG Genotype in Japanese Autoimmune Diabetic Patients

To clarify the relationship between the CT60 GG genotype frequency and the possession of HLA DR9 in Japanese autoimmune-related patients, we investigated the difference in the frequency of the CT60 GG genotype between "autoimmune diabetic" subjects with or without HLA DR9. There was no significant difference between the groups (TABLE 3). This indicates that possession of HLA DR9, which is related to autoimmune type 1 diabetes in Japanese, did not affect the frequency of the CTLA-4 gene CT60 polymorphism in autoimmune-related type 1 diabetic patients.

DISCUSSION

Type 1 diabetes is caused by insulin deficiency, associated with T cell-mediated autoimmunity to β cells of the pancreas. Most autoimmune diseases are considered to result from a failure in the mechanisms of the immune systems that establish and maintain tolerance to self. It has been reported that common allelic variation in the expression levels of alternative spliced forms of a key negative regulator of T cell immune response, CTLA-4, may be a primary determinant of susceptibility to autoimmune diseases.[1] However, contrary to the previous report, we did not find a significant difference in the frequency of the CT60-susceptible GG genotype between Japanese autoimmune diabetic patients and healthy controls.

Recently, some VDR gene polymorphisms were shown to be associated with autoimmune diseases. We previously reported that a higher frequency of the VDR Bsm I large B allele is observed in acute-onset type 1 diabetics than in controls.[4] As CTLA-4 is considered to be the regulatory molecule of T lymphocyte response, and vitamin D is capable of modulating Th1 response, we suspected that both susceptible alleles may affect each other. However, no significant relationship was found in the present study group. Our previous report indicated that a higher frequency of the large B allele is found in overall or acute-onset type 1 diabetic patients, but not in slow-onset type 1 diabetics.[4] Because the number of subjects in the present study was relatively small, we only evaluated the frequency of both alleles in the overall “autoimmune diabetes” group, which was not divided by onset-pattern categories. Therefore, further analysis may be needed to reach a conclusion.

In Japanese, HLA DR4 and DR9 are considered to be the major susceptible genes for type 1 diabetes.[8] We have reported that a higher number of IFN-γ-producing GAD-reactive T cells are detected in Japanese autoimmune-related diabetic patients with HLA DR9.[5] So, we focused on HLA DR9 in relation to the CTLA-4 gene CT60 polymorphism. In the present study, however, regardless of the possession of DR9, the frequency of the CT60 GG genotype was not statistically significantly different.

In the present study, we could not find any evidence of involvement of the CT60 GG genotype in autoimmune diabetes in Japanese, even concentrating on patients possessing the VDR Bsm I large B allele or HLA DR9. Further evaluation is needed to conclude whether the CT60 GG genotype is really involved in susceptibility to type 1 diabetes.

REFERENCES

1. Ueda, H., J.M.M. Howson, J.A. Todd, *et al.* 2003. Association of the T-cell regulatory gene CTLA4 with susceptibility to autoimmune disease. Nature **423:** 508–511.
2. Rigby, W.F., S. Denome & M.W. Fanger. 1987. Regulation of lymphokine production and human T lymphocyte activation by 1,25-dihydroxyvitamin D3. Specific inhibition at the level of messenger RNA. J. Clin. Invest. **79:** 1659–1664.
3. Provvedini, D.M. & S.C. Manolagas. 1989. 1Alpha, 25-dihydroxyvitamin D3 receptor distribution and effects in subpopulations of normal human T lymphocytes. J. Clin. Endocrinol. Metab. **68:** 774–779.
4. Motohashi, Y., S. Yamada, T. Yanagawa, *et al.* 2003. Vitamin D receptor gene polymorphism affects onset pattern of type 1 diabetes. J. Clin. Endocrinol. Metab. **88:** 3137–3140.
5. Itoh, A., A. Shimada, *et al.* 2004. GAD-reactive T cells were mainly detected in autoimmune-related type 1 diabetic patients with HLA, DR9. Ann. N. Y. Acad. Sci. **1037:** 33–40.
6. Kasuga, A., Y. Ozawa, T. Maruyama, *et al.* 1997. Autoantibody against ICA 512 did not improve test sensitivity for slowly progressive IDDM in adults. Diabetes Care **20:** 679–680.
7. Maruyama, T., A. Kasuga, Y. Ozawa, *et al.* 1997. Glutamic acid decarboxylase 65 (GAD 65) antibodies and insulin autoantibodies in Japanese patients with non-insulin dependent diabetes mellitus. Endocr. J. **44:** 43–51.
8. Maruyama, T., A. Shimada, A. Kasuga, *et al.* 1994. Analysis of MHC class II antigens in Japanese, IDDM by a novel HLA-typing method, hybridization protection assay. Diabetes Res. Clin. Pract. **23:** 77–84.

Genetic and Functional Evidence Supporting *SUMO4* as a Type 1 Diabetes Susceptibility Gene

CONG-YI WANG, ROBERT PODOLSKY, AND JIN-XIONG SHE

Center for Biotechnology and Genomic Medicine, Medical College of Georgia, Augusta, Georgia 30912, USA

ABSTRACT: Genomewide linkage analyses since the early 1990s suggested over 20 genomic intervals that may contain susceptibility genes for type 1 diabetes. However, the identification of the specific genes in these intervals presents a formidable challenge due to a number of difficulties associated with genetic mapping and cloning of genes implicated in complex diseases. One of the difficulties is due to the presence of many weak and different susceptibility genes in different patients and populations, a phenomenon known as genetic heterogeneity. In 2004, we reported the cloning of a novel small ubiquitin-like modifier (*SUMO*) gene, *SUMO4*, in the *IDDM5* interval on chromosome 6q25, and presented strong genetic and functional evidence suggesting that *SUMO4* is a susceptibility gene for type 1 diabetes mellitus (T1DM). In this article, we will summarize genetic association data suggesting that *SUMO4* is consistently associated with T1DM in the Asian populations while the association is more heterogeneous in the Caucasian populations. We will also discuss the possible molecular pathways through which sumoylation may regulate T1DM and autoimmunity.

KEYWORDS: susceptibility; genetic heterogeneity; linkage; association; pathogenesis; risk assessment; odds ratio (OR); autoimmunity; sumoylation; NF-κB; IκBα; oxidative stress; antioxidant enzyme

INTRODUCTION

Type 1 diabetes mellitus (T1DM) is an autoimmune disease characterized by specific destruction of the insulin-secreting beta cells of the pancreatic islets.[1–3] It is believed that susceptibility to T1DM is determined by interactions of multiple genes with unknown environmental factors.[4] Because the autoimmune process begins many years before the onset of clinical diabetes, it is difficult

Address for correspondence: Dr. Cong-Yi Wang, Center for Biotechnology and Genomic Medicine, Medical College of Georgia, 1120 15th Street, CA4098, Augusta, GA 30912. Voice: 706-721-3508; fax: 706-721-3688.
e-mail: cwang@mcg.edu

Ann. N.Y. Acad. Sci. 1079: 257–267 (2006).
doi: 10.1196/annals.1375.039

to ascertain the nature of environmental triggers. Therefore, a great deal of research has been focused on identifying T1DM susceptibility genes in the past two decades. Despite the success in identifying over 20 different genomic intervals showing suggestive or significant linkage, the susceptibility genes encoded in these regions remain largely elusive. One major difficulty is that a large number of genes probably influence T1DM susceptibility, with each gene only having a weak effect that is difficult to be detected by linkage analysis. To further complicate matters, different patients, families, ethnic groups, or races may have a different subset of genes, which, in combination, are responsible for their disease onset (known as genetic heterogeneity). Furthermore, gene–gene interaction and gene–environment interaction add additional complications that contribute to the difficulty in identifying T1DM susceptibility genes.

In 2004, we reported small ubiquitin-like modifier 4 (*SUMO4; IDDM5*) as the first T1DM susceptibility gene identified by the positional cloning approach. We discovered the M55V substitution within the *SUMO4* gene and showed that the mutation is associated with increased risk for T1DM in multiple ethnic groups.[5] Our functional study revealed that the M55V substitution results in a significant reduced sumoylation function for SUMO4, indicating its possible role in T1DM pathogenesis. Subsequent studies from other research groups have confirmed *SUMO4* association for T1DM susceptibility in the Asian populations.[6,7] However, association with *SUMO4* is not consistently observed in the European Caucasians, raising doubt about the validity of our initial report. Here, we will review the genetic and functional evidence supporting an important role of *SUMO4* in T1DM pathogenesis.

LINKAGE EVIDENCE FOR *IDDM5* ON CHROMOSOME 6q25

The *IDDM5* locus was initially localized to chromosome 6q25 by a genome scan,[8] which provided suggestive evidence for linkage at the *ESR* marker (n = 96; maximum lod score [MLS] = 1.82, $P = 0.003$; $\lambda s = 1.66$). Linkage was also obtained in the U.S. families ($n = 84$; MLS = 1.18, $P = 0.017$; $\lambda s = 1.18$), but not in an independent UK data set ($n = 102$).[8] A subsequent genome scan using 105 Caucasian families by our research group provided linkage evidence for *D6S446* (MLS = 2.8) and for *D6S264* (MLS = 2.0) on 6q25 and 6q27, respectively, suggesting that the 6q25-q27 interval may contain two distinct T1DM susceptibility genes, that is, *IDDM5* and *IDDM8*.[9] A follow-up study by Davies and co-workers using 334 sib-pair families further confirmed the existence of *IDDM5* and *IDDM8* within the genomic interval on 6q25-q27.[10]

Using 30 microsatellite markers flanking the 6q25-q27 region and an expanded data set, we obtained strong linkage evidence that confirmed three *IDDM* susceptibility intervals including *IDDM5*.[11] This fine mapping study narrowed the *IDDM5* locus to a 5-cM region of genomic DNA between markers *D6S476* and *D6S473*. The strongest linkage evidence for *IDDM5* was obtained at *ESR*, giving an MLS of 4.5, which met the standard for a significant linkage (MLS = 4.5). Our results were later confirmed by an independent study.[12] Interestingly, there was no linkage evidence for *IDDM5* in the UK data set. Indeed, the percentage of gene sharing for *IDDM5* in the UK data set (47%) is lower than the randomly expected 50% and significantly lower than what was observed in the U.S. data set ($P = 0.006$).[11]

FINE MAPPING OF THE *IDDM5* LOCUS

To further narrow the disease interval, we performed fine mapping using single nucleotide polymorphisms (SNPs) densely spaced in the *IDDM5* region by linkage disequilibrium (LD) analysis. The initial phase used a case–control association study design that includes patients and ethnically and geographically matched controls from multiple countries.[5] Markers with suggestive association evidence were further confirmed using family-based association studies with 944 families. One of the SNPs (*001Msp*) showed very strong association with T1DM in the U.S. Caucasian data set ($P = 9.7 \times 10^{-5}$) and French/Spanish data set ($P = 0.03$). Similar trend of transmission was also observed in the Mexican American, Italian, Chinese/Korean data sets although statistical significance in individual data set was not reached due to small sample size. Overall, the association between *001Msp* and T1DM was highly significant in the combined data set ($P < 3 \times 10^{-7}$). Interestingly, we did not observe any evidence for association in the UK data set, which showed significant difference from the remaining data set ($P < 0.004$). These results suggest a significant genetic heterogeneity.

To identify the susceptibility gene in the interval, 13 additional polymorphic SNPs flanking *001Msp* and encompassing a 320-kb genomic region were analyzed in all diabetic families. These data mapped the *IDDM5* locus to a genomic region of 197-kb between *493Ras* and *454Msp* ($P = 0.05$). This region contains only one previously known gene, *TAB2*, which plays a very important role in the interleukin-1 (IL-1) signaling pathway.[13–16] A novel candidate gene named *SUMO4* was identified within the interval. *SUMO4* belongs to the *SUMO* gene family, which is required for viability of most eukaryotic cells, including yeast, nematodes, fruit flies, and vertebrate cells in culture.[17] A 163A>G mutation within the CUE domain of *SUMO4* was identified. The mutation results in the amino acid met55 to val substitution (M55V). Met55 encoded by the A allele is evolutionarily conserved among diverse species and the substituted G allele (val55), is strongly associated with increased risk for T1DM.[5] However, the percentage of transmission for the G allele (val55) in the British families is significantly lower (44%) than the randomly expected 50% ($P = 0.0003$), an observation consistent with the heterogeneity observed in our previous linkage studies.

GENETIC HETEROGENEITY IN THE EUROPEAN CAUCASIANS

Association between the M55V SNP and T1DM was independently reported by another group.[18] This study analyzed a total of 478 families, of which 222 were originated from UK. In contrast to our finding in the non-UK data set but consistent with our finding in the UK data set, the A allele (met55) of *SUMO4* is transmitted more frequently from parents to affected children (57.1%, $P < 0.0004$). Subsequently, association between M55V of *SUMO4* and T1DM was not replicated in two studies of European Caucasians.[19,20] These results raised some doubt about the validity of the reported association.

A number of possibilities could be responsible for the discrepant association with *SUMO4*, including genotyping mistakes, random variation due to small sample size, spurious association, genetic heterogeneity, or population differences in gene–gene and gene–environment interactions. We ruled out genotyping mistakes by regenotyping of a subset of the samples. Spurious association is unlikely responsible for the observed association because of the family-based association study design. Our sample size was also sufficiently large, and the possibility for association caused by random variation was very low.

VALIDATION OF *SUMO4* AS A T1DM SUSCEPTIBILITY GENE

In our initial report, we observed significant association between *SUMO4* and T1DM in two Asian populations (Chinese and Korean, TABLE 1). The association was independently confirmed in a Korean case–control cohort consisting of 386 individuals with T1DM and 553 normal controls.[6] Consistent with the initial report, the GG and AG genotypes had a higher frequency in affected individuals (62.0%) than that in matched controls (52.1%), with a relative risk (RR) of 1.5 ($P < 0.003$) (TABLE 1). More recently, Noso and co-workers provided additional evidence supporting a significant association between T1DM and *SUMO4* in Asians (TABLE 1).[7] This study includes a large cohort of 1113 Japanese (472 cases and 641 controls) and 171 Korean subjects (69 cases and 102 controls). Once again, the G allele (val55) is significantly more common in Japanese diabetic patients than in controls (odds ratio [OR] = 1.43, $P < 0.005$). A similar trend was also observed in Korean subjects (OR = 1.75). In combined data from Japanese and Korean subjects, the G allele was significantly associated with T1DM (OR = 1.46, $P = 0.00083$).[7] A meta-analysis of nonoverlapping case–control data sets from Asia showed highly significant association (OR = 1.5, $P = 1.5 \times 10^{-6}$) (TABLE 2). No heterogeneity was detected among Asian populations (TABLE 2).

Given the results from the Asian populations, there is little doubt that *SUMO4* is a T1DM susceptibility gene. However, the issue is less settled in

TABLE 1. Summary of published case–control association results for M55V of *SUMO4*

Data sets		GG (%)	AG (%)	AA (%)	GG + AG (%)
Guo *et al.*[5]					
Florida data set	T1DM: 244	83 (34.0)	114 (46.7)	47 (19.3)	197 (80.7)
	Control: 274	58 (21.2)	134 (48.9)	82 (29.9)	192 (70.1)
	P-value	0.001	NS	0.005	0.005
Spanish data set	T1DM: 170	47 (27.6)	93 (54.7)	30 (17.7)	140 (82.3)
	Control: 151	39 (25.8)	81 (53.6)	31 (20.6)	120 (79.4)
	P-value	NS	NS	NS	NS
Taiwan, China	T1DM: 96	5 (5.2)	51 (53.2)	40 (41.6)	56 (58.4)
	Control: 191	18 (9.4)	78 (40.8)	95 (49.8)	96 (50.2)
	P-value	NS	0.048	NS	NS
Mainland China	T1DM: 96	18 (18.8)	38 (40.0)	40 (41.2)	63 (58.8)
	Control: 188	15 (7.9)	86 (45.7)	87 (46.4)	101 (53.6)
	P-value	0.007	NS	NS	NS
Korean data set	T1DM: 97	19 (19.6)	47 (48.5)	31 (31.9)	66 (68.1)
	Control: 112	12 (10.7)	48 (42.9)	52 (46.4)	60 (53.6)
	P-value	NS	NS	0.03	0.03
Wang *et al.*[21]					
Florida data set	T1DM: 197	66 (33.5)	90 (45.7)	41 (20.8)	156 (79.2)
	Control: 1,060	268 (25.3)	534 (50.4)	258 (24.3)	802 (75.7)
	P-value	0.01	NS	NS	NS
Park *et al.*[6]					
Korean data set	T1DM: 386	52 (13.5)	187 (48.5)	147 (38.0)	239 (62.0)
	Control: 553	58 (10.5)	230 (41.6)	265 (47.9)	288 (52.1)
	P-value	NS	<0.04	<0.003	<0.003
Noso *et al.*[7]					
Japanese data set	T1DM: 472	43 (9.1)	234 (49.6)	195 (41.3)	277 (58.7)
	Control: 641	64 (9.9)	256 (40.0)	321 (50.1)	320 (50.1)
	P-value	NS	0.001	<0.004	<0.004
Korean data set	T1DM: 69	9 (13)	31 (45.0)	29 (42)	40 (58)
	Control: 102	11 (10.8)	34 (33.3)	57 (44.1)	57 (55.9)
	P-value	NS	NS	NS	NS
Smyth *et al.*[19]					
UK data set	T1DM: 3,442	898 (26.2)	1,769 (51.7)	775 (22.1)	2667 (77.9)
	Control: 3,788	1007 (26.6)	1856 (49.0)	925 (24.4)	2863 (75.6)
	P-value	NS	0.04	0.056	0.056
Combined Florida data set	T1DM: 441	149 (33.8)	204 (46.3)	88 (19.9)	353 (80.1)
	Control: 1,334	326 (24.4)	668 (50.1)	340 (25.5)	994 (74.5)
	P-value	0.0001	NS	0.02	0.02

the Caucasian populations. Similar trend of association between *SUMO4* and T1DM was observed in several populations studied in our initial report. The strongest evidence was from the North-Central Florida data set (TABLE 1). In addition to the initial data set, we also analyzed a new Florida cohort consisting of 196 individuals with T1DM and 1060 matched controls. A significant association for the G allele (val55) of *SUMO4* was obtained (OR = 1.5, $P = 0.01$).[21] When we combined this new cohort with the initial Florida case–control data

TABLE 2. Meta-analysis of published results

Race	Models	OR	Confidence interval	P (association)	P (heterogeneity)
Case–control studies					
Asian	Fixed effects	1.46	1.25–1.70	1.6×10^{-6}	0.97
Caucasian	Fixed effects	1.15	1.04–1.28	0.005	0.17
Combined	Fixed effects	1.24	1.14–1.35	5.6×10^{-7}	0.17
Family-based studies					
Asian	Fixed effects	1.67	0.99–2.82	0.06	0.17
Caucasian	Random effects	1.00	0.93–1.06	0.93	0.0006
Combined	Random effects	1.00	0.94–1.07	0.93	0.0005

set (244 cases and 274 controls), the evidence is further enhanced (OR = 1.6, $P = 0.0001$, TABLE 1).[21] In the large UK case–control data set studied by Smyth and co-workers, there is also marginally significant association consistent with the initial finding[19] (TABLE 1). Given prior observation of significant association, this data set indeed provides additional support for association between SUMO4 and T1DM in Caucasians. Association between *SUMO4* and T1DM was also confirmed using transmission disequilibrium test in diabetic families in our initial studies. However, the association has not been confirmed in additional family-based data sets. The reason for the discrepant observations between case–control and family-based studies are still unknown at this time. It is possible that the observed associations in case–control studies are due to spurious association. This is unlikely as strong associations are observed in the Asian populations and consistent association was observed in three different Caucasian populations studied so far (TABLE 1). The most likely possibility is that the family-based studies did not have sufficient sample size to detect weak association. It is, therefore, important to analyze additional Caucasian case–control cohorts to determine whether *SUMO4* is only associated with T1DM in some Caucasian populations. Given the small OR expected, the sample size will have to be very large to confirm the association.

Genetic heterogeneity has often been blamed for the inconsistent observations on disease association across different populations or ethnic groups. Although heterogeneity was not observed in the case-control studies in either Asians or Caucasians (TABLE 2), significant heterogeneity was observed in the Caucasian family data sets (TABLE 2). However, the cause for the heterogeneity remains to be determined. One possible explanation for the heterogeneity is that the *IDDM5* interval may contain multiple T1DM susceptibility genes, which may contain both susceptible and protective alleles that are in different linkage disequilibrium patterns in different populations. This phenomenon has already been observed for the *DRB1* and *DQA1/DQB1* genes in the HLA region.[22] Further studies should be performed to determine whether similar phenomenon also occurs in the *IDDM5* region.

FUNCTIONAL DIFFERENCE FOR THE SUMO4 M55V SNP

SUMO proteins are a highly conserved protein family found in all eukaryotes.[17] SUMO and ubiquitin are distantly related in amino acid sequence but share the same structural folding. Both ubiquitin and SUMO are covalently conjugated to substrates by an isopeptide bond through their carboxyl termini. However, unlike ubiquitin, which usually leads to protein degradation, SUMO addition to a target protein mediates posttranslational modification, that is, sumoylation.[17] Extensive studies in the past few years indicated that sumoylation is a remarkably versatile regulatory mechanism of protein function involved in the regulation of immune response and cellular apoptosis with implication in signal transduction, protein targeting, DNA repair, and RNA processing.[17,23]

SUMO4 is the fourth *SUMO* member identified in the human genome.[5] Phylogenetic analyses revealed that *SUMO4* is more similar to *SUMO1* in terms of amino acid sequence and functional properties. Unlike other *SUMO* members, *SUMO4* expression is more restricted to immune tissues and pancreatic islets,[17] suggesting that it may be a potent regulator for immune response.[5,17] We demonstrated that SUMO4 conjugates to IκBα and stabilizes IκBα from signal-induced degradation. As a result, SUMO4 negatively regulates NF-κB, a pivotal transcription factor involved in immune response.[17]

The M55 residue, located in the CUE domain of SUMO4, has been found to be evolutionarily conserved among diverse species.[5,17] The M55V substitution changes a PKC phosphorylation site (at position 54–56), which appears to be important for the molecular conformation and functional activity of SUMO4. Indeed, we found a significant reduction in sumoylation function for the high risk SUMO4 V55 variant.[5] HEK293 cells transfected with the SUMO4*V55 isoform showed 5.5-fold higher NF-κB-dependent transcriptional activity than that of cells transfected with the SUMO4*M55 isoform upon IL-1β stimulation. Furthermore, the M55V substitution resulted in more than threefold higher *IL12-p40*, an NF-κB-dependent gene expression *in vivo.*[5] Consistent with our observations, Bohren and co-workers demonstrated a decreased enhancing capability for heat shock transcription factors for the SUMO4*V55 variant.[24] These results provided additional support for a role of SUMO4 in T1DM pathogenesis.

MOLECULAR PATHWAYS FOR SUMO4 IN T1DM PATHOGENESIS

The molecular mechanisms by which SUMO4 contributes to T1DM pathogenesis are still elusive. Our recent studies suggested a negative feedback network for SUMO4 in the NF-κB signaling pathway. Upon signal-induced activation, NF-κB upregulates the expression of a number of immune reactive genes in response to stimulation (e.g., inflammatory cytokines and costimulatory molecules); moreover, it also activates the transcription of inhibitors to tightly control the immune responsive potency. We now have evidence suggesting that SUMO4 may be involved in this critical process as NF-κB can activate the transcription of *SUMO4*, a negative regulator for NF-κB activity.[17,23] In addition to regulating NF-κB activity, SUMO4 may also play an important role in regulating the activities of several other key transcription factors, such as AP-1 and STAT proteins as well as heat shock proteins. These pathways are known to be implicated in autoimmune diseases.

There is also compelling evidence that autoimmune-mediated cellular stress is implicated in the pathogenesis of islet destruction during the development of T1DM.[25,26] Recently, we used HEK293 cell as a model to characterize SUMO4 substrate proteins in cells undergoing serum starvation-induced cellular stress.[23] This systematic analysis further suggested a possible role for SUMO4 in the regulation of oxidative stress during the destruction of pancreatic islets. SUMO4-associated substrates were analyzed by two-dimensional ployacrylamide gel electrophoresis (2D PAGE) and subsequent MALDI-TOF/TOF analyses. By this approach, we identified 90 SUMO4-associated substrate proteins. Of note, a major group of SUMO4-associated substrates comprise the anti-stress proteins, including antioxidant enzymes (e.g., Cu/ZnSOD, catalase, and peroxiredoxins), chaperones (e.g., HSP70 and Grp58) and stress defense proteins (e.g., valosin-containing protein and TXNDC4, ER). Our study also identified many SUMO4-associated substrates involved in the regulation of DNA repair and synthesis, RNA processing, and protein degradation.[23] By Western blot analysis, we further demonstrated that SUMO4 sumoylates several crucial transcription factors involved in the regulation of cellular stress, such as AP-1, AP-2α, STAT1 and 3, and glucocorticoid receptor (GR).

We performed functional studies to demonstrate the effect of sumoylation on the stress-associated transcription factors. Luciferase reporter and electrophoretic mobility shift assays (EMSA) suggested that SUMO4 sumoylation represses the transcriptional activity for AP-1 and AP-2α, while it enhances DNA-binding capacity for GR.[23] GR is an endogenous antagonist for NF-κB and AP-1.[17] It has been demonstrated that oxidative events regulate AP-1 and NF-κB transactivation, which in turn activate the expression of numerous cytokines,[27,28] a major source of autoimmune-mediated beta cell stress during the development of T1DM.[25] Therefore, SUMO4 sumoylation of these transcription factors could be a mechanism for the regulation of intracellular stress.[17,29,30] For example, AP-2α is a repressor for MnSOD expression,[31] a primary antioxidant enzyme that is critical for maintaining normal cell function and survival. SUMO4 sumoylation could enhance MnSOD expression by repressing AP-2α transcriptional activity. However, the effects of SUMO4 sumoylation on antioxidant enzymes, such as Cu/ZnSOD, are yet to be established. On the basis of the known effects of sumoylation, SUMO4 sumoylation of these antistress proteins could be a protective mechanism against intracellular stress by: (*a*) competing with ubiquitylation and thus stabilizing key antistress proteins by protecting them against degradation; and (*b*) targeting these proteins to specific subcellular organelles for detoxification of reactive oxygen species (ROS) produced as a result of the cellular stress.[23] These observations suggest a potential role for SUMO4 in the regulation of cellular stress, which could have a significant implication in autoimmune-mediated beta cell death during the development of T1DM.

CONCLUSIONS AND FUTURE PERSPECTIVES

Despite the discrepant associations observed for *SUMO4* to T1DM susceptibility in the Caucasian populations, *SUMO4* has been found to be consistently associated with T1DM in the Asian populations. Further studies are required to determine whether genetic heterogeneity or different linkage disequilibrium patterns are responsible for the discrepancies observed in Caucasians. The essential roles for sumoylation in several biological processes have been well established.[32–35] There is increasing evidence that perturbation of the sumoylation function may play an important role in T1DM and other autoimmune diseases. Elucidation of the roles of sumoylation in T1DM should provide novel insights into the pathogenesis of the disease and possibly new intervention strategies.

ACKNOWLEDGMENTS

Research activities by the authors described in the present review were supported by the CIGP program (RI00329) of the Medical College of Georgia, MCG Research Funding (HI00105G), the American Diabetes Association (1-05-JF-47), the Juvenile Diabetes Research Foundation International (1-2004-235) to CYW, and the National Institute of Child Health and Development (HD37800) to JXS. The authors declare that they have no competing financial interest.

REFERENCES

1. LOVISELLI, A., V.M. SOLINAS, E.G. MAMELI, *et al.* 1999. Genetic markers and insulin-dependent diabetes mellitus (IDDM) in Sardinia. Anthropol. Anz. **57:** 25–32.
2. ILONEN, J., O. SIMELL, M. KNIP & H.K. AKERBLOM. 1998. Screening for genetic IDDM risk and prevention trials in infancy. Diabetes Metab. Rev. **14:** 188.
3. LOHMANN, T., J. SESSLER, H.J. VERLOHREN, *et al.* 1997. Distinct genetic and immunological features in patients with onset of IDDM before and after age 40. Diabetes Care **20:** 524–529.

4. KITAGAWA, T., H. FUJITA, S. TSUKASA, *et al.* 1987. Early phase of juvenile IDDM–environmental and genetic intervention. Acta Paediatr. Jpn. **29:** 47–53.
5. GUO, D., M. LI, Y. ZHANG, *et al.* 2004. A functional variant of SUMO4, a new IkappaBalpha modifier, is associated with type 1 diabetes. Nat. Genet. **36:** 837–841.
6. PARK, Y., S. PARK, J. KANG, *et al.* 2005. Assessing the validity of the association between the SUMO4 M55V variant and risk of type 1 diabetes. Nat. Genet. **37:** 112–113.
7. NOSO, S., H. IKEGAMI, T. FUJISAWA, *et al.* 2005. Genetic heterogeneity of SUMO4 M55V variant with susceptibility to type 1 diabetes. Diabetes **54:** 3582–3586.
8. DAVIES, J.L., Y. KAWAGUCHI, S.T. BENNETT, *et al.* 1994. A genome-wide search for human type 1 diabetes susceptibility genes. Nature **371:** 130–136.
9. LUO, D.F., M.M. BUI, A. MUIR, *et al.* 1995. Affected-sib-pair mapping of a novel susceptibility gene to insulin-dependent diabetes mellitus (IDDM8) on chromosome 6q25-q27. Am. J. Hum. Genet. **57:** 911–919.
10. DAVIES, J.L., F. CUCCA, J.V. GOY, *et al.* 1996. Saturation multipoint linkage mapping of chromosome 6q in type 1 diabetes. Hum. Mol. Genet. **5:** 1071–1074.
11. LUO, D.F., R. BUZZETTI, J.I. ROTTER, *et al.* 1996. Confirmation of three susceptibility genes to insulin-dependent diabetes mellitus: IDDM4, IDDM5 and IDDM8. Hum. Mol. Genet. **5:** 693–698.
12. DELEPINE, M., F. POCIOT, C. HABITA, *et al.* 1997. Evidence of a non-MHC susceptibility locus in type I diabetes linked to HLA on chromosome 6. Am. J. Hum. Genet. **60:** 174–187.
13. JIANG, Z., J. NINOMIYA-TSUJI, Y. QIAN, *et al.* 2002. Interleukin-1 (IL-1) receptor-associated kinase-dependent IL-1-induced signaling complexes phosphorylate TAK1 and TAB2 at the plasma membrane and activate TAK1 in the cytosol. Mol. Cell Biol. **22:** 7158–7167.
14. QIAN, Y., M. COMMANE, J. NINOMIYA-TSUJI, *et al.* 2001. IRAK-mediated translocation of TRAF6 and TAB2 in the interleukin-1-induced activation of NFkappa B. J. Biol. Chem. **276:** 41661–41667.
15. TAKAESU, G., J. NINOMIYA-TSUJI, S. KISHIDA, *et al.* 2001. Interleukin-1 (IL-1) receptor-associated kinase leads to activation of TAK1 by inducing TAB2 translocation in the IL-1 signaling pathway. Mol. Cell Biol. **21:** 2475–2484.
16. TAKAESU, G., S. KISHIDA, A. HIYAMA, *et al.* 2000. TAB2, a novel adaptor protein, mediates activation of TAK1 MAPKKK by linking TAK1 to TRAF6 in the IL-1 signal transduction pathway. Mol. Cell **5:** 649–658.
17. LI, M., D. GUO, C.M. ISALES, *et al.* 2005. SUMO wrestling with type 1 diabetes. J. Mol. Med. **83:** 504–513.
18. OWERBACH, D., L. PINA & K.H. GABBAY. 2004. A 212-kb region on chromosome 6q25 containing the TAB2 gene is associated with susceptibility to type 1 diabetes. Diabetes **53:** 1890–1893.
19. SMYTH, D.J., J.M. HOWSON, C.E. LOWE, *et al.* 2005. Assessing the validity of the association between the SUMO4 M55V variant and risk of type 1 diabetes. Nat. Genet. **37:** 110–111.
20. QU, H., B. BHARAJ, X.Q. LIU, *et al.* 2005. Assessing the validity of the association between the SUMO4 M55V variant and risk of type 1 diabetes. Nat. Genet. **37:** 111–112.
21. WANG, C.Y., P. YANG & J.X. SHE. 2005. Assessing the validity of the association between the SUMO4 M55V variant and risk of type 1 diabetes. Nat. Genet. **37:** 112–113.

22. SHE, J.X. 1996. Susceptibility to type I diabetes: HLA-DQ and DR revisited. Immunol. Today **17:** 323–329.
23. GUO, D., J. HAN, B.L. ADAM, *et al.* 2005. Proteomic analysis of SUMO4 substrates in HEK293 cells under serum starvation-induced stress. Biochem. Biophys. Res. Commun. **337:** 1308–1318.
24. BOHREN, K.M., V. NADKARNI, J.H. SONG, *et al.* 2004. A M55V polymorphism in a novel SUMO gene (SUMO-4) differentially activates heat shock transcription factors and is associated with susceptibility to type I diabetes mellitus. J. Biol. Chem. **279:** 27233–27238.
25. EIZIRIK, D.L. & T. MANDRUP-POULSEN. 2001. A choice of death–the signal-transduction of immune-mediated beta-cell apoptosis. Diabetologia **44:** 2115–2133.
26. EIZIRIK, D.L., B. KUTLU, J. RASSCHAERT, *et al.* 2003. Use of microarray analysis to unveil transcription factor and gene networks contributing to Beta cell dysfunction and apoptosis. Ann. N. Y. Acad. Sci. **1005:** 55–74.
27. WANG, S.Y., R. FENG, Y. LU, *et al.* 2005. Inhibitory effect on activator protein-1, nuclear factor-kappaB, and cell transformation by extracts of strawberries (Fragaria x ananassa Duch). J. Agric. Food Chem. **53:** 4187–4193.
28. KRIEHUBER, E., W. BAUER, A.S. CHARBONNIER, *et al.* 2005. Balance between NF-kappaB and JNK/AP-1 activity controls dendritic cell life and death. Blood **106:** 175–183.
29. SHAO, R., E. RUNG, B. WEIJDEGARD & H. BILLIG. 2006. Induction of apoptosis increases SUMO-1 protein expression and conjugation in mouse periovulatory granulosa cells in vitro. Mol. Reprod. Dev. **73:** 50–60.
30. LEE, Y.S., M.S. JANG, J.S. LEE, *et al.* 2005. SUMO-1 represses apoptosis signal-regulating kinase 1 activation through physical interaction and not through covalent modification. EMBO Rep. **6:** 949–955.
31. ZHU, C.H., Y. HUANG, L.W. OBERLEY & F.E. DOMANN. 2001. A family of AP-2 proteins down-regulate manganese superoxide dismutase expression. J. Biol. Chem. **276:** 14407–14413.
32. NEVE, R.L. 2003. A new wrestler in the battle between alpha- and beta-secretases for cleavage of APP. Trends Neurosci. **26:** 461–463.
33. LI, Y., H. WANG, S. WANG, *et al.* 2003. Positive and negative regulation of APP amyloidogenesis by sumoylation. Proc. Natl. Acad. Sci. USA **100:** 259–264.
34. STEFFAN, J.S., N. AGRAWAL, J. PALLOS, *et al.* 2004. SUMO modification of Huntingtin and Huntington's disease pathology. Science **304:** 100–104.
35. UEDA, H., J. GOTO, H. HASHIDA, *et al.* 2002. Enhanced SUMOylation in polyglutamine diseases. Biochem. Biophys. Res. Commun. **293:** 307–313.

No Association of *TLR2* and *TLR4* Polymorphisms with Type I Diabetes Mellitus in the Basque Population

IZORTZE SANTIN,[a] JOSE RAMON BILBAO,[a,b] GUIOMAR PÉREZ DE NANCLARES,[a] BEGOÑA CALVO,[a] AND LUIS CASTAÑO[a,c]

[a]*Endocrinology and Diabetes Research Group,* [b]*Department of Nursing, and* [c]*Department of Pediatrics, Hospital de Cruces, Barakaldo, University of the Basque Country, Bilbao, E48903 Bizkaia, Spain*

ABSTRACT: The destruction of pancreatic β cells that occurs in type 1 diabetes mellitus (T1DM) is mediated by the immune system, and evidence has accumulated supporting the implication of innate immune mediators. Toll-like receptors (TLRs) participate in the first line of immune defense through antigen recognition, and their ligands are mostly exogenous but can be host-derived as well. To test the possible role of TLRs in the development of T1DM, we studied different SNPs of *TLR2* (N199N, S450S, R677W, and R753Q) and *TLR4* (D299G, T399I, and S400N) in Basque families with T1DM. Several positions analyzed were not polymorphic in the Basque population. Genetic association analysis failed to demonstrate any association of these polymorphisms of *TLR2* and *TLR4* with T1DM in our population. The differences in *TLR4* haplotype transmission to affected and unaffected offspring are indicative of a possible implication of *TLR4* in disease risk but differences did not reach statistical significance.

KEYWORDS: *TLR2*; *TLR4*; type 1 diabetes; SNP; Basque

INTRODUCTION

Type I diabetes mellitus (T1DM) is an organ-specific autoimmune disorder that involves both genetic and environmental factors. The destruction of pancreatic β cells is mediated by immune response and, although the role of the adaptive immune system in autoimmune diseases has been clearly established, there is growing evidence to implicate the innate arm of the immune response in these disorders.[1] Toll-like receptors (TLRs) are members of a family of receptors encoded by different TLR genes (*TLR1–13*) that are expressed in many

Address for correspondence: Luis Castaño, M.D., Ph.D., Endocrinology and Diabetes Research Group, Hospital de Cruces, Barakaldo E48903 Bizkaia, Spain. Voice: +34-94-600-6099; fax: +34-94-600-6076.
e-mail: lcastano@hcru.osakidetza.net

**Ann. N.Y. Acad. Sci. 1079: 268–272 (2006). © 2006 New York Academy of Sciences.
doi: 10.1196/annals.1375.040**

tissues and cell types and participate in antigen recognition. TLRs are type I transmembrane receptors, which are characterized by an extracellular leucine-rich (LRR) domain and an intracellular toll/IL-1 receptor (TIR) domain. LRRs are involved in antigen recognition and signal transduction, whereas, TIR is a conserved protein–protein interaction module. TLR ligands are quite diverse in structure and origin, and are mostly exogenous molecules, but certain endogenous molecules can act as ligands for TLRs. *TLR2*, encoded at *4q32*, has been shown to be involved in the recognition of a broad range of microbial proteins, but it is able to recognize MIP-2 and SPA molecules, which are host derived. *TLR4*, encoded at *9q32-33* and expressed predominantly in the cells of immune system, including macrophages and dendritic cells, interacts with many ligands, such as bacterial lipopolysaccharide but also with endogenous molecules (HSP60, HSP70, and fibrinogen, among others). In this article, we studied different polymorphisms of *TLR2* and *TLR4* in order to test the possible association of the disease with TLR genes in the Basques.

MATERIALS AND METHODS

Subjects

Our study population consisted of 70 Basque families (81 T1DM patients and 239 first-degree relatives) with at least one member with T1DM (42 male and 39 female [age at onset 14.5 ± 9.9 years]).

TLR2 *and* TLR4 *Genotyping*

Four positions in *TLR2* (Asn199Asn, Ser450Ser, Arg677Trp, and Arg753Gln) and three positions in *TLR4* (Asp299Gly, Thr399Ile, and Ser400Asn) were genotyped by specific PCR amplification and direct sequencing using ABI3100-Avant sequencing apparatus (Applied Biosystems, Foster City, CA). The primers used for amplification and sequencing were designed by *Fast PCR V3.6* program (www.biocenter.helsinki.fi/bi/bare-1_html/oligos.htm) and are available upon request.

Association Studies

Allele frequency for each locus was calculated and its contribution to the disease was determined by affected family-based controls (AFBAC) or Transmission Disequilibrium Test (TDT) approach depending on the heterozygosity degree of the parents. Haplotypes for *TLR2* and *TLR4* were built using the program *"Haplotype Estimation,"* which is available at www.bioinf.mdc-berlin.de/projects/hap. The distribution of allele and haplotype frequencies

TABLE 1. Wild-type allele frequencies (%) in T1DM and AFBAC, showing no differences between groups

Gene	Position	Nucleotide change	T1DM ($n = 81$)	AFBAC ($n = 239$)
TLR2	*Asn199Asn*	597 T>C	54	53
	Ser450Ser	1350 T>C	100	100
	Arg677Trp	2029 C>T	100	100
	Arg753Gln	2258 G > A	100	99,5
TLR4	*Asp299Gly*	896 A>G	86,9	87,3
	Thr399Ile	1196 C>T	86,6	87,9
	Ser400Asn	1199 G>A	100	100

in T1DM patients and AFBAC were compared in contingency tables using Fisher's exact test.

RESULTS

In our population, there were three positions in *TLR2* (pos. 450, pos. 667, and pos. 753) and one position in *TLR4* (pos. 400) that were not polymorphic. The remaining SNPs were polymorphic but allele distribution in T1DM patients and AFBAC did not show significant differences (TABLE 1). Four different haplotypes were observed for each gene (TABLE 2) and no significant differences in distribution were observed between disease and AFBAC groups. TDT test was performed to test the transmission of the three less frequent *TLR2* haplotypes and the two most discordant *TLR4* haplotypes, but transmission to T1DM offspring and healthy children, although different, did not reach statistical significance.

DISCUSSION

TLR1–13 encode receptors predominantly expressed in tissues involved in immune function, as well as those exposed to the external environment.

TABLE 2. Haplotype distribution in T1DM and AFBAC groups and TDT analysis

		Frequencies		TDT Analysis		
Gene	Haplotype	*DM*	*AFBAC*	Transmitted	Nontransmitted	*P*
TLR2	*Asn-Ser (TT)*	68	54	—	—	—
	Asn-Ser (CT)	39	51	9	10	n.s.
	Asn-Ser (TC)	2	1	2	1	n.s.
	Asn-Ser (CC)	10	10	32	48	n.s.
TLR4	*Asp-Thr-Ser*	90	89	—	—	—
	Gly-Ile Ser	11	7	8	4	n.s.
	Asp-Ile-Ser	2	5	1	5	n.s.
	Gly-Thr-Ser	4	3	—	—	n.s.

Studies on TLRs indicate that they are essential elements in host defense against antigens (exogenous as well as host derived) by activating the innate immune system, a prerequisite for the induction of adaptive immunity.[2] Innate immunity has recently been found to be important in determining the fate of autoimmune responses and thus, TLRs could be involved in the development of autoimmune diseases, like T1DM.[3] In order to test the possible association of TLRs with T1DM, we analyzed different polymorphisms in *TLR2* and *TLR4* genes in Basque families with T1DM but no evidence of association was found.

The first evidences of TLR genes involvement in autoimmunity come from extensive studies in different autoimmune diseases. A recent study has associated polymorphisms of *TLR2* with T1DM in Korean population.[4] Other studies have associated *TLR4* polymorphisms with several autoimmune diseases, such as Crohn's disease or ulcerative colitis in Caucasian populations.[5,6] Nevertheless, other studies have revealed that those polymorphisms of *TLR2* and *TLR4* have no association with other autoimmune diseases: in Austrians, no association of *TLR4* polymorphisms with multiple sclerosis[7] and in Spanish population, no evidence of association of *TLR2* and *TLR4* polymorphisms with rheumatoid arthritis nor systemic lupus erythematosus has been observed.[8] There are several possible reasons for these differences between groups. First, *TLR2* and *TLR4* polymorphisms analyzed may well not be the etiologic mutation. Second, linkage disequilibrium patterns between these *TLR2* and *TLR4* variants and the actual etiologic mutation somewhere else in this region may be different in the Basque population compared to those populations where positive associations have been observed. Third, it is possible that penetrance of these *TLR2* and *TLR4* polymorphisms could be reduced by other interacting genes or environmental factors, specific of the Basque population. Finally, in view of the similar allele distribution between T1DM and AFBAC groups in our population, a larger sample size may be needed to find association, which is probably not very strong, compared to the effect of the major susceptibility loci. Nevertheless, despite our negative results, TLR genes remain possible candidate genes for autoimmune diseases, including T1DM.

ACKNOWLEDGMENTS

This work was funded by grants RGDM-G03/212 and RCMN-C03/08 from the Instituto de Salud Carlos III of the Spanish Ministry of Health. IS is supported by a predoctoral fellowship from the University of the Basque Country. JRB, BC, and GPN are FIS researchers supported by the Spanish Ministry of Health Fellowships no. 99/3076, 03/0062, and 03/0064, respectively.

REFERENCES

1. Wen, L. *et al.* 2004. The effect of innate immunity on autoimmune diabetes and the expression of Toll-like receptors on pancreatic islets. J. Immunol. **172:** 3173–3180.

2. SINGH, B.P. *et al.* 2003. Toll-like receptors and their role in innate immunity. Curr. Sci. **85:** 1156–1164.
3. BEYAN, H. *et al.* 2003. A role for innate immunity in type 1 diabetes? Diabetes Metab. Res. Rev. **19:** 89–100.
4. PARK, Y. *et al.* 2004. Association of the polymorphism for toll-like receptor 2 with type 1 diabetes susceptibility. Ann. N. Y. Acad. Sci. **1037:** 170–174.
5. FRANCHIMONT, D. *et al.* 2004. Deficient host-bacteria interactions in inflammatory bowel disease? The toll-like receptor (TLR)-4 Asp299gly polymorphism is associated with Crohn's disease and ulcerative colitis. Gut **53:** 987–992.
6. TÖRÖK, H.P. *et al.* 2004. Polymorphisms of the lipopolysaccharide-signaling complex in inflammatory bowel disease: association of a mutation in the toll-like receptor 4 gene with ulcerative colitis. Clin. Immunol. **112:** 85–91.
7. REINDI, M. *et al.* 2003. Mutations in the gene for toll-like receptor 4 and multiple sclerosis. Tissue Antigens **61:** 85–88.
8. SÁNCHEZ, E. *et al.* 2004. Polymorphisms of toll-like receptor 2 and 4 genes in rheumatoid arthritis and systemic lupus erythematosus. Tissue Antigens **63:** 54–57.

Association of SUMO4 M55V Polymorphism with Autoimmune Diabetes in Latvian Patients

SAIKIRAN K. SEDIMBI,[a] ARUN SHASTRY,[a] YONGSOO PARK,[b] INGRIDA RUMBA,[c] AND CARANI B. SANJEEVI[a]

[a]*Department of Molecular Medicine and Surgery, Karolinska Institute, Stockholm S-171 76, Sweden*

[b]*Department of Internal Medicine, Hanyang University Hospital, Kuri, Kyunggi-do, Korea 471-020*

[c]*Faculty of Medicine, University of Latvia, Riga LV-1001, Latvia*

Abstract: Small ubiquitin-related modifier (SUMO4), located in IDDM5, has been identified as a potential susceptibility gene for type 1 diabetes mellitus (T1DM). The novel polymorphism M55V, causing an amino acid change in the evolutionarily conserved met55 residue has been shown to activate the nuclear factor κB (NF-κB), hence the suspected role of SUMO4 in the pathogenicity of T1DM. The M55V polymorphism has been shown to be associated with susceptibility to T1DM in Asians, but not in Caucasians. Latent autoimmune diabetes in adults (LADA) is a slowly progressive form of T1DM and SUMO4 M55V has not been studied in LADA to date. The current study aims to test whether Latvians are similar to Caucasians in susceptibility to autoimmune diabetes (T1DM and LADA), with respect to SUMO4 M55V. We studied, age- and sex-matched, Latvian T1DM patients ($n = 100$) and healthy controls ($n = 90$) and LADA patients ($n = 45$) and healthy controls ($n = 95$). SUMO4 M55V polymorphism was analyzed using polymerase chain reaction (PCR)–restriction fragment length polymorphism (RFLP). The allelic frequencies of the A and G alleles were compared with HLA DR3–DR4-positive and HLA DR3-DR4-negative patients to identify any potential relation between HLA DR3–DR4 and SUMO4 M55V. We found no significant association between SUMO4 M55V and T1DM susceptibility in Latvians, the results being in concurrence with the previous studies in Caucasians of British and Canadian origin. Comparison of the A and G alleles with HLA DR3–DR4 did not result in any significant *P* values. No significant association was found between SUMO4 M55V and LADA. SUMO4 M55V is not associated with susceptibility to T1DM and

Address for correspondence: Dr. C.B. Sanjeevi, M.D., Ph.D., Karolinska Institute, Department of Molecular Medicine, Karolinska Hospital Campus, CMM L5:01, S-17176, Stockholm, Sweden. Voice: +46-8-51776254; fax: +46-8-51776179.
e-mail: sanjeevi.carani@ki.se

**Ann. N.Y. Acad. Sci. 1079: 273–277 (2006). © 2006 New York Academy of Sciences.
doi: 10.1196/annals.1375.041**

LADA in Latvians, and Latvians exhibit similarity to other Caucasians with respect to association of SUMO4 M55V with autoimmune diabetes.

KEYWORDS: **SUMO4; M55V; autoimmune diabetes; LADA**

INTRODUCTION

Diabetes mellitus is a group of metabolic disorders resulting from defects in insulin secretion, action, or both. It has been broadly classified as type 1 diabetes mellitus (T1DM) and type 2 diabetes mellitus (T2DM)[1] based on the etiology of the disease. T1DM is characterized by T cell-mediated (autoimmune) destruction of insulin secreting β cells. β cell autoantigens presented to the $CD4^+$ T cells, activate them causing the release of interleukin-2 (IL-2). IL-2 activates β cell antigen-specific $CD8^+$ cytotoxic T cells, which are involved in destruction of the β cells.[1] T1DM has been shown to be a polygenic trait, associated with several loci, with the major locus at major histocompatibility complex.[2]

T2DM patients who test positive for autoantibodies are referred to as slowly progressive IDDM (SPIDDM), type 1.5 diabetes, and latent autoimmune diabetes in adults (LADA); the latter is the most commonly used term. Despite the presence of autoantibodies, the progression of the β cell destruction is slow. LADA was found to occur in approximately 10% of the T2DM patients aged above 35 years and 25% of the patients aged below 35 years. Vatay *et al.*,[3] indicated differences in the genetic backgrounds of T1DM and LADA. They suggested that the low presence of the TNF2 allele in LADA patients might be a reason for the slow progression of the disease. Sanjeevi *et al.*,[4] showed the difference in association of MIC-A alleles (5 in T1DM and 5.1 in LADA) and HLA (DR3–DQ2 in LADA and DR4–DQ8 in T1DM).

Recent studies in the IDDM5 interval have revealed the association of a novel gene, small ubiquitin-related modifier 4 (SUMO4), to TIDM. Fifteen single nucleotide polymorphisms (SNPs) were analyzed and a 163A→G SNP was found to cause a M55V amino acid substitution in an evolutionarily conserved residue met55 of SUMO4, with susceptibility to T1DM, but with contradicting susceptibility alleles.[5,6] Subjects with Asian origin showed that the possession of the G allele was significantly associated with increased risk of T1DM,[7,8] whereas Caucasian subjects with European descent showed no association or even an association of the A allele with the disease.[6,9]

SUMO4 is an intron-less gene situated within the intron 6 of the MAP3K7IP2 gene. It encodes a 95 amino acid protein that negatively regulates the transcriptional activity of nuclear factor κB (NF-κB). Bohren *et al.*[6] postulated that the higher levels of activated heat shock protein transcription factors, by met55 variant, might have a protective effect over the val55 variant. They also demonstrated that the met55 variant suppresses NF-κB compared to val55 variant.

Guo *et al.*,[5] suggested that the M55V substitution might result in an increased cellular response to stimulation, resulting in higher levels of NF-κB activity, which causes the transcription of the genes involved in β cell destruction. Hence a direct implication of SUMO4 M55V in pathogenesis of T1DM is very much possible; though the functional details need to be worked out.

Latvians are Caucasians by origin. Killer cell immunoglobulin-like receptor genes (KIR) have been worked out in a Latvian cohort with T1DM by Sanjeevi *et al.*[4] The current study aims to test the hypothesis that Latvians are similar to Europeans (Caucasians) with respect to the susceptibility of SUMO4 M55V to T1DM and whether this susceptibility extends to LADA. This is because the association of the M55V of SUMO4 with LADA has not been studied till date.

Subjects

For SUMO4 M55V SNP analysis, we used 100 T1DM patients and 90 healthy, age- and sex-matched individuals from Latvia. The age at disease onset was from a few months to 18 years. Disease duration was less than 5 years. Study material previously has been typed for HLA-DQ and DR genes, MICA, tumor necrosis factor (TNF)-microsatellite polymorphisms, and KIR genes. For M55V analysis in LADA, 46 patients and 95 healthy, age- and sex-matched individuals were studied. Autoantibodies (GAD65 and IA2) were detected using radioligand-binding assay using protein A Sepharose (RIA) and HLA-DQA1, DQB1, and DRB1 were typed previously.[10]

Methods

SUMO4 M55V was amplified by PCR-SSP, following the protocol of Park *et al.*[7] The PCR product was run on a 2% agarose gel, with a 100-bp DNA marker to verify the amplification. Restriction fragment length polymorphism (RFLP) was performed using Taq 1 restriction enzyme (Invitrogen, Carlsbad, CA). RFLP products were run on a 2.5% agarose gel and documented using a gel documentation system. The AA, AG, and GG bands were distinguished based on their size. Allele frequencies were analyzed using χ^2 test and P values less than or equal to 0.05 were considered significant.

RESULTS AND DISCUSSION

The results of the M55V polymorphism in LADA patients are shown in TABLE 1 and that of T1DM patients are shown in TABLE 2. We found no significant difference in the presence of alleles in patients and healthy controls in both study groups. Studies by Guo *et al.*[5] showed that the G allele was associated with susceptibility to T1DM. But, results obtained by Smyth *et al.*,[9]

TABLE 1. Association of M55V of SUMO4 in Latvian LADA patients

		Patients	Controls	Odds ratio	*P* value
	N (%)	46	95		
Genotype	AA	8 (17.39)	26 (27.36)	0.56 (0.23–1.35)	0.19
	AG	21 (45.65)	47 (49.47)	0.86 (0.42–1.74)	0.67
	GG	17 (36.95)	22 (23.15)	1.95 (0.91–4.16)	0.08
Allele	A	37 (40.21) (*n*=92)	99 (52.10) (*n*=190)	0.62 (0.37–1.02)	0.06
	G	55 (59.78) (*n*=92)	91 (47.89) (*n*=190)	1.62 (0.98–2.67)	0.06
Phenotype	G	38 (82.61)	69 (72.63)	1.30 (0.54–3.12)	0.55

in a larger population (including patients from UK, United States, Northern Ireland, Finland, Romania, and Norway) showed no evidence of M55V association with T1DM. The possession of the G allele was shown to be related to susceptibility to T1DM in Asians. In a meta-analysis, Noso *et al.*,[8] pointed out that the inclusion of Caucasian data leads to a weak association of the G allele with T1DM. The current study supports the findings of Smyth *et al.*,[9] in that, there is no significant association between SUMO4 M55V polymorphism and T1DM. Though T1DM and LADA are thought to have different genetic backgrounds, the aspect of SUMO4 M55V variant appears to be the same, that is, no significant association.

We also compared the HLA high-risk alleles HLA-DR3 and -DR4 with SUMO4 M55V polymorphism. Comparison between HLA-DR3 or -DR4-positive patients with HLA-DR3 or -DR4-negative patients with SUMO4 M55V did not show any significant association. When the presence or absence of HLA-DR3 and HLA-DR4 alleles was compared individually with M55V polymorphism no significant *P* values were observed. A combination of HLA-DR3 and -DR4 (both present) versus the rest with M55V was tested, no association was found. When HLA-DR4-positive and -negative patients were studied taking the presence of autoantibodies into consideration, with M55V,

TABLE 2. Association of M55V of SUMO4 in Latvian T1DM patients

		Patients	Controls	Odds ratio	*P* value
	N (%)	95	77		
Genotype	AA	21 (22.10)	26 (33.76)	0.56 (0.28–1.09)	0.08
	AG	47 (49.47)	34 (44.15)	1.24 (0.68–2.26)	0.48
	GG	27 (28.42)	17 (22.07)	1.40 (0.70–2.82)	0.34
Allele	A	89 (46.84) (*n* = 190)	86 (55.84) (*n* = 154)	0.70 (0.45–1.07)	0.09
	G	101 (53.15) (*n* = 190)	68 (44.15) (*n* = 154)	1.44 (0.94–2.20)	0.09
Phenotype	G	74 (77.89)	51 (66.23)	1.80 (0.92–3.52)	0.08

no association was found. Heterogeneity seems to play a role in disease susceptibility. Another possibility might be the environmental conditions, which can trigger the SUMO4-related pathway of pathogenesis in T1DM, but in all cases functional evidence can only be accepted as direct proof.

ACKNOWLEDGMENTS

We acknowledge the Swedish Institute for supporting Saikiran and Arun Shastry with a stipendium. We thank Prof. R. Banerjee (IIT Kharagpur, India). The study was supported by grants from Swedish Medical Research Council to CBS, Swedish Diabetes Association, Swedish Child Diabetes Fund, and Karolinska Institute.

REFERENCES

1. YOON, J.W., *et al.* 2005. Autoimmune destruction of pancreatic beta cells. Am. J. Ther. **12:** 580–591.
2. DAVIES, J.L., *et al.* 1994. A genome-wide search for human type 1 diabetes susceptibility genes. Nature **371:** 130–136.
3. VATAY, A., *et al.* 2002. Differences in the genetic background of latent autoimmune diabetes in adults (LADA) and type 1 diabetes mellitus. Immunol. Lett. **84:** 109–115.
4. SANJEEVI, C.B., *et al.* 2002. Genetics of latent autoimmune diabetes in adults. Ann. N. Y. Acad. Sci. **958:** 107–111.
5. GUO, D., *et al.* 2004. A functional variant of SUMO4, a new IkBα modifier, is associated with type 1 diabetes. Nat. Genet. **36:** 837–841.
6. BOHREN, K.M., *et al.* 2004. A M55V polymorphism in a novel SUMO gene (SUMO4) differentially activates heat shock transcription factors and is associated with susceptibility to type 1 diabetes mellitus. J. Biol. Chem. **279:** 27233–27238.
7. PARK, Y., S. PARK, S. YANG & D. KIM. 2005. Assessing the validity of the association between the SUMO4 M55V variant and risk of type 1 diabetes. Nat. Genet. **37:** 112.
8. NOSO, S., *et al.* 2005. Genetic heterogeneity in association of the SUMO4 M55V variant with susceptibility to type 1 diabetes. Diabetes **54:** 3582–3586.
9. SMYTH, D.J., *et al.* 2005. Assessing the validity of the association between the SUMO4 M55V variant and risk of type 1 diabetes. Nat. Genet. **37:** 110–111.
10. SANJEEVI, C.B., *et al.* 1999. Association of HLA class II alleles with different subgroups of diabetes mellitus in eastern India identify different associations with IDDM and malnutrition-related diabetes. Tissue Antigens **54:** 83–87.

A Second Component of HLA-Linked Susceptibility to Type 1 Diabetes Maps to Class I Region

YUMIKO KAWABATA,[a,b] HIROSHI IKEGAMI,[a,b] TOMOMI FUJISAWA,[a] SHINSUKE NOSO,[a] KATSUAKI ASANO,[a] YOSHIHISA HIROMINE,[a] AND TOSHIO OGIHARA[a]

[a]*Department of Geriatric Medicine, Osaka University Graduate School of Medicine, Osaka 565-0871, Japan*

[b]*Department of Endocrinology, Metabolism and Diabetes, Kinki University School of Medicine, Osaka-Sayama, Osaka 589-8511, Japan*

ABSTRACT: Type 1 diabetes is a polygenic disease with a major susceptibility locus, *IDDM1*, located in the human leukocyte antigen (HLA) region. Although class II loci, *DR* and *DQ* genes in particular, are major components of *IDDM1*, accumulating lines of evidence indicated that *IDDM1* consists of multiple components and that non-class II genes in addition to class II genes contribute to susceptibility to and/or age-at-onset of type 1 diabetes. To identify a second component of *IDDM1*, we investigated the association of a panel of polymorphisms in 2.2 Mb region of the HLA encompassing from class II to class I regions with type 1 diabetes. Polymorphisms types were: *DRB1* and *DQB1* in class II; two microsatellite markers, *BAT2-GT* and *TNFa* in class III; and, five microsatellite markers, *STR-MICA, MIB, C1-3-1, C2-4-4,* and *C3-2-10* in class I region. A total of >200 Japanese patients and healthy control subjects were studied. Class II *DRB1* 0405* and *DQB1* 0401* were significantly associated with susceptibility to, but not with age-at-onset of, type 1 diabetes. *C1-3-1,* located near C locus, was significantly associated with not only susceptibility to, but also age-at-onset of type 1 diabetes. These data suggest that a second component of *IDDM1* maps to the HLA class I region, contributing to susceptibility to as well as age-at-onset of type 1 diabetes.

KEYWORDS: type 1 diabetes mellitus; genetics; human leukocyte antigen; class I; susceptibility

Address for correspondence: Dr. Hiroshi Ikegami, Department of Endocrinology, Metabolism and Diabetes, Kinki University School of Medicine, 377-2 Ohno-higashi, Osaka-Sayama, Osaka 589-8511, Japan. Voice: +81-72-366-0221; ext.: 3123
e-mail: ikegami@med.kindai.ac.jp

Ann. N.Y. Acad. Sci. 1079: 278–284 (2006).
doi: 10.1196/annals.1375.042

INTRODUCTION

Type 1 diabetes mellitus is a multifactorial disease, which is caused by autoimmune destruction of insulin-producing β cells of the pancreas. Both in animal models and humans, type 1 diabetes is a polygenic trait, with a major locus encoded by the major histocompatibility complex (MHC) on chromosome 6p21 and several other loci throughout the genome contributing to disease susceptibility. However, a number of evidence indicated that the penetrance of these loci is influenced by environmental factors. The incidence of type 1 diabetes varied markedly among different countries, ranging from 0.1/100,000 per year (in China and Venezuela) to over 35/100,000 per year (in Finland and Sardinia), and the incidence has been rising worldwide and particularly increasing in younger age groups. These epidemiological data also support the view that susceptibility to type 1 diabetes is determined by a combination of genetic and environmental factors.

Although class II loci, *DR* and *DQ* genes in particular, are the major components of *IDDM1*, accumulating lines of evidence indicated that *IDDM1* consists of multiple components and that non-class II genes in addition to class II genes contribute to susceptibility to and/or age-at-onset of type 1 diabetes. In present article, to identify the second component of *IDDM*, we investigated the association of a panel of polymorphisms in 2.2 Mb region of the human leukocyte antigen (HLA) encompassing from class II to class I regions with type 1 diabetes.

SUBJECTS AND METHODS

Subjects ($n > 200$) consisted of Japanese patients with type 1 diabetes and healthy control subjects. HLA-*DRB1* and *DQB1* alleles were determined by PCR-RFLP methods.[1,2] Seven microsatellite markers within the HLA region, *BAT2-GT*, *TNFa*, *STR-MICA*, *MIB*, *C1-3-1*, *C2-4-4* and *C3-2-10*, were genotyped using a fluorescence-based method. *BAT2-GT* and *TNFa* allele belong to class III region. Other five markers belong to class I region. Allele frequencies were compared between patients and control subjects. Mean age-at-onset was compared between patients with and without each allele.

RESULTS

Class II *DQB1∗0401* and *DRB1*0405* were significantly associated with susceptibility to type 1 diabetes. *C1-3-1* was also significantly associated with susceptibility to type 1 diabetes (TABLE 1). When the subjects were divided into two groups according to the presence or absence of disease susceptible HLA-class II DR haplotypes at *IDDM1*, the degree of association of the

TABLE 1. Odds ratio for susceptible alleles of polymorphic markers genotyped

	DQB1	*DRB1*	*BAT2-GT*	*TNFa*	*STR- MICA*	*MIB*	*C1-3-1*	*C2-4-4*	*C3-2-10*
OR	2.6*	3.1*	2.4*	1.8	1.7	1.9	2.7*	2.0	1.8

*Significant association (corrected $P < 0.05$). OR = odds ratio.

C1-3-1 with type 1 diabetes was almost similar, irrespective of class II susceptible haplotypes. The mean age-at-onset in patients with *C1-3-1* was significantly younger than those without. *DQB1* and *DRB1* were not associated with age-at-onset of type 1 diabetes.

DISCUSSION

Type 1 diabetes is a polygenic disease with a major susceptibility gene, *IDDM1,* located in the HLA region. Strong association of class II DR4 (*DRB1**0405-DQB1*0401*) and DR9 (*DRB1*0901-DQB1*0303*) haplotypes to susceptibility to type 1 diabetes in the present study is consistent with this.

The contribution of HLA to susceptibility to type 1 diabetes was first indicated by the association with HLA-B8 and -B15, and then with the HLA-DR3 and -DR4 antigens encoded at the *DRB1* locus. Subsequently, the *DQB1* and *DQA1* genes were shown to be more strongly associated with type 1 diabetes, and the DQ molecule was favored as the primary susceptibility factor. Recently, several genome scans for linkage to type 1 diabetes have been performed and these studies indicated that a gene or genes in the HLA region (*IDDM1*) at 6p21 have the strongest impact on the disease risk. Cox *et al*. reported a LOD score of 65.8.[3] The strong linkage disequilibrium, however, within the HLA region makes it difficult to identify a gene (or genes) responsible for susceptibility to type 1 diabetes.

Studies in both humans and animal models have shown that particular alleles of the class II MHC loci, *HLA -DQA1*, *-DQB1,* and *-DRB1* in humans and *A* and *E* in mice, are closely associated with susceptibility to type 1 diabetes. In humans, particular combinations of class II HLA haplotypes have been shown to confer very strong susceptibility to type 1 diabetes, that is, heterozygotes for DR3 (*DRB1*0301-DQB1-0201*) and DR4 (*DRB1*0401-DQB1*0302*) in Caucasians and homozygotes for DR9 (*DRB1*0901-DQB1*0303*) in Asians.[2] In contrast, a particular DQ6 molecule, encoded by *DQA1*0102-DQB1*0602*, confer dominant protection against type 1 diabetes in both Caucasian and Asian populations.[2]

As for *HLA-DR* genes, the frequencies of only certain *HLA-DR4*-associated *DRB1* alleles are increased among type1 diabetic patients. The effect of *DR4* subtypes appear to range from most to least predisposing.[4] Cucca *et al.*[5]demonstrated that the different risk categories are determined by the predicted structure and action of the peptide-binding pockets, P1 and P4, of the

DRB1 molecule. The observation that several different class II HLA alleles and combinations of alleles may be associated with the disease allowed researchers to search a common factor to these alleles which is responsible to susceptibility. Certain amino acids of the *HLA-DQB1* and *-DRB1* chains correlate well with disease susceptibility to and protection against type 1 diabetes. In particular, residue 57, which is located in pocket 9, of the DQβ chain has been reported to correlate with susceptibility to and protection from type 1 diabetes: aspartic acid at this position (Asp57) with neutral to protective effect, alanine with very strong susceptibility, valine with susceptibility, and serine with weak susceptibility. Kwok *et al.* found that the residue 57 has a pronounced role in the function of class II molecules with respect to peptide binding.[6] Asp57 of DQβ chain, however, is not associated with type 1 diabetes in Japanese because two haplotypes, *DRB1*0405-DQB1*0401* and *DRB1*0901-DQB1*0303,* strongly associated with type 1 diabetes in the present study do not have Asp57. *DQB1*0401*, however, possesses a substituted amino acid at residue 56, which is also in pocket 9 and may therefore influence the function of this pocket, from other *DQB1* allele with Asp 57.

In addition to class II loci, the present study suggested the contribution of class I region to susceptibility to and age-at-onset of type 1 diabetes. Previous studies in both humans and animal models have also suggested that loci other than class II MHC may also contribute to susceptibility to and heterogeneity in type 1 diabetes. Studies in nonobese diabetic (NOD) mice congenic for a recombinant MHC with the same class II as the NOD, but different class I and class III regions from the NOD mouse, have clearly shown that strong susceptibility linked to the MHC is due to the combined effect of *Idd1* in the class II region and another gene or genes outside the class II region.[7] The second component of MHC-linked susceptibility, designated *Idd16*, was mapped to the less than 10.5 cM region adjacent to, but distinct from the class II MHC region containing class I genes.[7] Subsequent studies suggested that allelic variation of the class I K gene may be responsible for *Idd16*.[8] A second component of the MHC-linked susceptibility to type 1 diabetes was also indicated by other groups using different congenic lines, either in class I K[9] or D[10] regions.

Several lines of evidence in humans also indicated that *IDDM1* consists of multiple components and that non-class II genes in addition to class II genes associated with type 1 diabetes (FIG. 1). A role of HLA genes other than class II genes was first suggested by Thomsen *et al.*[11] and several studies have subsequently supported a role of class I and class III in predisposition to type 1 diabetes, but the number of samples was small in these studies. Stronger evidence has been provided by subsequent studies with systematic typing of microsatellite markers. Moghaddam *et al.*[12] analyzed 11 markers in the *IDDM1* region in 120 patients with type 1 diabetes and 83 control subjects who were fully matched for the high-risk *HLA-DQA1*, and *-DQB1* genotypes. Their study provided strong evidence that two regions, class II region and region around *D6S273,* ~200 kb centromeric of *TNF* in class III region, contribute

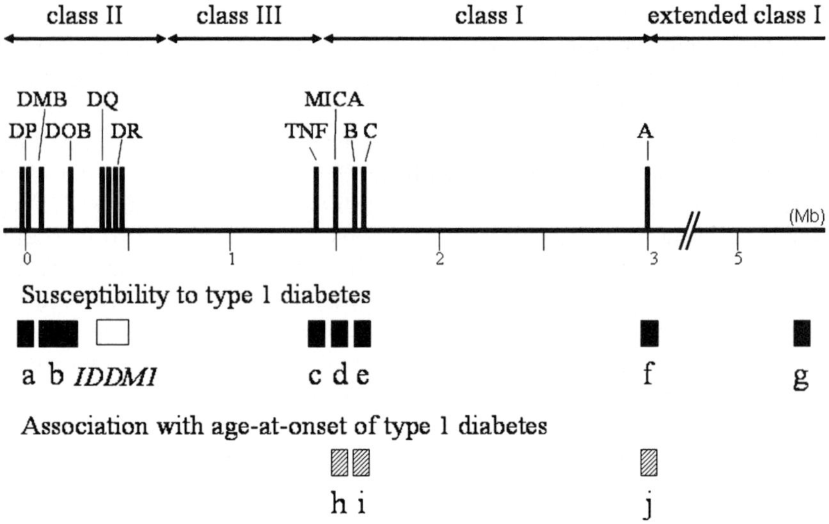

FIGURE 1. Reported susceptibility loci for type 1 diabetes other than *DQ* and *DR* (*IDDM1*) in HLA region. (*a*) Noble, J.A. *et al.* Diabetes 49: 121, 2000; Cucca, F., *et al.* Diabetes 50: 1200, 2001; Cruz, T.D., *et al.* Diabetes 53: 2158, 2004. (*b*) Zavattari, P., *et al.* Hum. Mol. Genet. 10: 881, 2001; Johansson, S., *et al.* Genes Immun. 4: 46, 2003. (*c*) Moghaddam, P.H., *et al. Diabetes* 47: 263, 1998; Lie, B.A., *et al.* Am. J. Hum. Genet. 64: 793, 1999; Zavattari, P., *et al.* Hum. Mol. Genet. 10: 881, 2001; Johansson, S., *et al.* Genes Immun. 4: 46, 2003. (*d*) Gambelunghe, G., *et al.* Diabetologia 43: 507, 2000; Nejentsev. S., *et al.* Diabetes 49: 2217, 2000; Park. Y., *et al.* Diabetes Care. 24:33, 2001; Johansson, S., *et al.* Genes Immun. 4: 46, 2003. (*e*) Nejentsev, S., *et al.* Diabetes 49: 2217, 2000; Gambelunghe, G., *et al.* Diabetologia. 43: 507, 2000; Johansson, S., *et al.* Genes Immun. 4: 46, 2003; Pitkaniemi, J., *et al.* Hum. Hered. 57: 69, 2004, Valdes, A.M. *et al.* Hum Immunol. 66: 301, 2005. (*f*) Noble, J.A. *et al.* Hum. Immunol. 63: 657, 2002. (*g*) Johansson, S., *et al.* Genes Immun. 4: 46, 2003; Lie, B.A. *et al.* Am. J. Hum. Genet. 64: 793, 1999. (*h*) Kawabata, Y., *et al.* Hum. Immunol. 61: 624, 2000; Gambelunghe, G., *et al.* Diabetologia 43: 507, 2000. (*i*) Fujisawa, T., *et al.* Diabetologia 38: 1493, 1995; Pitkaniemi, J., *et al.* Hum. Hered. 57: 69, 2004; Valdes, A.M., *et al.* Hum. Immunol. 66: 301, 2005; Kawabata, Y., *et al.*, 2005. (*j*) Valdes, A.M., *et al.* Diabetes 48: 1658, 1999; Pitkaniemi, J. *et al.* Hum. Hered. 57: 69, 2004.)

to type 1 diabetes susceptibility or protection. Lie *et al.*[13] have scanned 12 Mb of the MHC and flanking chromosomal regions with microsatellite polymorphisms and analyzed the transmission of these marker alleles to diabetic probands from parents who were homozygous for the alleles of the *HLA-DRB1*, *HLA-DQA1*, and *HLA-DQB1* genes, suggesting the presence of an additional type 1 diabetes gene (or genes). Zavattari *et al.*[14] investigated the contribution of non-*DQ/DR* polymorphic makers within a 9.452 Mb region encompassing the whole HLA complex to the disease risk in the founder population of Sardinia, after taking into account linkage disequilibrium with the disease loci

HLA-DQB1, *-DQA1,* and *-DRB1*. Three regions, including *DMB*, *DOB,* and *TNFc*, were identified as risk modifiers using the conditional association test. The individual contributions of these risk modifiers were relatively modest but their combined impact was highly significant.

In the present study, a marker in the class I C region was associated not only with susceptibility, but also with age-at-onset of type 1 diabetes. We previously reported the contribution of class I HLA to age-at-onset of type 1 diabetes,[15] and the observation was confirmed by the present study with a larger number of subjects and more dense markers in the HLA region. Several reports in different ethnic groups suggested that heterogeneity in age-at-onset of type 1 diabetes was determined by gene (or genes) in class I region.[15–18] Contribution of class I and class II genes in different stages in the development of diabetes was also reported in that class II genes are associated with initiation of β cells autoimmunity as measured by the appearance of islet autoantibodies, whereas class I genes are associated with the progression from autoimmunity to clinical disease.[19] Contribution of class I region, B and C loci in particular, to susceptibility to as well as heterogeneity in type 1 diabetes was further supported by recent large-scale studies in Caucasian populations with fixed class II genotypes.[20–22] Altogether, these data suggest that a second component of HLA-linked susceptibility maps to the HLA class I region, contributing to susceptibility to as well as age-at-onset of type 1 diabetes.

ACKNOWLEDGMENT

This work was supported by a Grant-in-Aid for Scientific Research from the Ministry of Education, Science, Sports, Culture, and Technology, Japan.

REFERENCES

1. Ikegami, H., Y. Kawaguchi, E. Yamato, *et al.* 1992. Analysis by the polymerase chain reaction of histocompatibility leukocyte antigen-DR9-linked susceptibility to insulin-dependent diabetes mellitus. J. Clin. Endocrinol. Metab. **75:** 1381–1385.
2. Kawabata, Y., H. Ikegami, Y. Kawaguchi, *et al.* 2002. Asian-specific HLA haplotypes reveal heterogeneity of the contribution of HLA-DR and -DQ haplotypes to susceptibility to type 1 diabetes. Diabetes **51:** 545–551.
3. Cox, N.J., B. Wapelhorst, V.A. Morrison, *et al.* 2001. Seven regions of the genome show evidence of linkage to type 1 diabetes in a consensus analysis of 767 multiplex families. Am. J. Hum. Genet. **69:** 820–830.
4. She, J-X. 1996. Susceptibility to type I diabetes: HLA-DQ and DR revisited. Immunol. Today **17:** 323–329.
5. Cucca, F., R. Lampis, M. Congia, *et al.* 2001. A correlation between the relative predisposition of MHC class II alleles to type 1 diabetes and the structure of their protein. Hum. Mol. Genet. **10:** 2025–2037.
6. Kwok, W.W., M.E. Domeier, M.L. Johnson, *et al.* 1996. HLA-DQB1 codon 57 is critical for peptide binding and recognition. J. Exp. Med. **183:** 1253–1258.

7. IKEGAMI, H., S. MAKINO, E. YAMATO *et al.* 1996. Identification of a new susceptibility locus for insulin-dependent diabetes mellitus by ancestral haplotype congenic mapping. J. Clin. Invest. **96:** 1936–1942.
8. INOUE, K., H. IKEGAMI, T. FUJISAWA, *et al.* 2004. Allelic variation in class I K gene as candidate for second component of MHC-linked susceptibility to type 1 diabetes in NOD mouse. Diabetologia **47:** 739–747.
9. HATTORI, M., E. YAMAMOTO, N. ITOH, *et al.* 1999. Homologous recombination of the MHC class I K region defines new MHC-linked diabetogenic susceptibility gene(s) in nonobese diabetic mice. J. Immunol. **163:** 1721–1724.
10. POMERLEAU, D.P., R.J. BAGLEY, D.V. SERREZE, *et al.* 2005. Major histocompatibility complex-linked diabetes susceptibility in NOD/Lt mice: subcongenic analysis localizes a component of *Idd16* at the *H2-D* end of the diabetogenic $H2^{g7}$ complex. Diabetes **54:** 1603–1606.
11. THOMSEN, M., J. MOLVIG, A. ZERBIB, *et al.* 1988. The susceptibility to insulin-dependent diabetes mellitus is associated with C4 allotypes independently of the association with HLA-DQ alleles in HLA-DR3, 4 heterozygotes. Immunogenetics **28:** 320–327.
12. MOGHADDAM, P.H., P. DE KNIFF, B.O. ROEP, *et al.* 1998. Genetic structure of IDDM1. Two separate regions in the major histocompatibility complex contribute to susceptibility or protection. Diabetes **47:** 263–269.
13. LIE, B.A., J.A. TODD, F. POCIOT, *et al.* 1999. The predisposition to type 1 diabetes linked to the human leukocyte antigen complex includes at least one non-class II gene. Am. J. Hum. Genet. **64:** 793–800.
14. ZAVATTARI, P., R. LAMPIS, C. MOTZO, *et al.* 2001. Conditional linkage disequilibrium analysis of a complex disease superlocus, *IDDM1* in the HLA region, reveals the presence of independent modifying gene effects influencing the type 1 diabetes risk encoded by the major *HLA-DQB1*, *-DRB1* disease loci. Hum. Mol. Genet. **10:** 881–889.
15. FUJISAWA, T., H. IKEGAMI, Y. KAWAGUCHI, *et al.* 1995. Class I HLA is associated with age-at-onset of IDDM, while class II HLA confers susceptibility to IDDM. Diabetologia **38:** 1493–1495.
16. VALDES, A.M., G. THOMSON, H.A. ERLICH, *et al.* 1999. Association between type 1 diabetes age of onset and HLA among sibling pairs. Diabetes **48:** 1658–1661.
17. KAWABATA, Y., H. IKEGAMI, Y. KAWAGUCHI, *et al.* 2000. Age-related association of MHC class I chain-related gene A (MICA) with type 1 (insulin-dependent) diabetes mellitus. Hum. Immunol. **61:** 624–629.
18. GAMBELUNGHE, G., M. GHADERI, A. COSENTINO, *et al.* 2000. Association of MHC Class I chain-related A (MIC-A) gene polymorphism with type 1 diabetes. Diabetologia **43:** 507–514.
19. TAIT, B.D., P.G. COLMAN, G. MORAHAN, *et al.* 2003. HLA genes associated with autoimmunity and progression to disease in type 1 diabetes. Tissue Antigens **61:** 146–153.
20. NEJENTSEV, S., Z. GOMBOS, A.-P. LAINE, *et al.* 2000. Non-class II HLA gene associated with type 1 diabetes maps to the 240-kb region near HLA-B. Diabetes **49:** 2217–2221.
21. PITKANIEMI, J., T. HAKULINEN, J. NASANEN, *et al.* 2004. Class I and II HLA genes are associated with susceptibility and age at onset in Finnish families with type 1 diabetes. Hum. Hered. **57:** 69–79.
22. VALDES, A.M., H.A. ERLICH, J.A. NOBLE, *et al.* 2005. Human leukocyte antigen class I B and C loci contribute type 1 diabetes (T1D) susceptibility and age at T1D onset. Hum. Immunol. **66:** 301–313.

Molecular Scanning of the Gene for Programmed Cell Death-1 (PDCD-1) as a Candidate for Type 1 Diabetes Susceptibility

YOSHIHISA HIROMINE,[a] HIROSHI IKEGAMI,[a,b] TOMOMI FUJISAWA,[a] YUMIKO KAWABATA,[a,b] SHINSUKE NOSO,[a] KAORI YAMAJI,[a] KATSUAKI ASANO,[a] AND TOSHIO OGIHARA[a]

[a]*Department of Geriatric Medicine, Osaka University Graduate School of Medicine, Suita, Osaka 565-0871, Japan*

[b]*Department of Endocrinology, Metabolism and Diabetes, Kinki University School of Medicine, 377-2 Ohno-higashi, Osaka-Sayama, Osaka 589-8511, Japan*

ABSTRACT: Multiple genes are involved in the susceptibility to autoimmune type 1 diabetes. The immunoreceptor programmed cell death-1 (PDCD-1), an inhibitory costimulatory molecule regulating peripheral tolerance, was reported to play a role in the development of type 1 diabetes, making the human PDCD-1 gene, *PDCD1*, as a candidate for disease susceptibility. In this article, we sequenced all 5 exons and exon–intron junctions of *PDCD1* in Japanese subjects, and found 10 sequence variants. Preliminary data suggested no association of these polymorphisms with type 1 diabetes. These sequence variants are valuable for further studies to clarify contribution of *PDCD1* to susceptibility to type 1 diabetes.

KEYWORDS: programmed cell death-1 (PDCD-1); autoimmune disease; type 1 diabetes; genetic susceptibility; autoimmunity

INTRODUCTION

Type 1 diabetes mellitus is caused by autoimmune destruction of insulin-producing beta cells of the pancreas. While the development of type1 diabetes is influenced by both environmental and genetic factors, genetic susceptibility

Address for correspondence: Dr. Hiroshi Ikegami, Department of Endocrinology, Metabolism and Diabetes, Kinki University School of Medicine, 377-2 Ohno-higashi, Osaka-Sayama, Osaka 589-8511, Japan.
e-mail: ikegami@med.kindai.ac.jp

Ann. N.Y. Acad. Sci. 1079: 285–288 (2006). © 2006 New York Academy of Sciences.
doi: 10.1196/annals.1375.043

to type 1 diabetes is determined by multiple genes.[1] While the strongest component conferring susceptibility is linked to human leukocyte antigen (HLA) region,[2] termed as *IDDM1*, number of studies so far demonstrated that other susceptible genes that are not linked to HLA are also important for the development of the disease. Most of these non-HLA genes have not yet been clarified, except for a few genes, such as insulin and cytotoxic T lymphocyte antigen 4 (CTLA4) genes. Elucidation of susceptibility genes is not only useful to identify individuals at high risk for type 1 diabetes, but also would facilitate our understanding of the disease pathogenesis, leading to development of novel strategies for more effective methods for prevention and cure of the disease.

Programmed cell death-1 (PDCD-1) is involved in immune responses as an inhibitory regulator and plays a role in the regulation of peripheral tolerance. *In vivo*, blockade of interaction between PDCD-1 and its ligand, PD-L1, has recently been reported to accelerate type 1 diabetes of the non-obese diabetic (NOD) mice,[3] indicating a role for PDCD-1 in the development of type 1 diabetes. PDCD-1 is one of the costimulatory receptor members, which belongs to the B7-CD28 superfamily. CTLA4 is also another member of this family with some sequence homology to PDCD-1. Recently, Ueda *et al*. demonstrated that a polymorphism of *CTLA4* is involved in susceptibility to type1 diabetes and is responsible for *IDDM12*.[4] Given a similarity between CTLA4 and PDCD-1 in molecular structures as well as function with an immunoinhibitory role, *PDCD1* is considered as a candidate gene for susceptibility to the disease.

In this article, to clarify the contribution of *PDCD1* to genetic susceptibility to type 1 diabetes, we screened sequence variations of *PDCD1* in Japanese subjects with or without type 1 diabetes, and some of the sequence variations identified were subjected to association study for type 1 diabetes.

METHODS

For the screening of sequence variants, we studied more than 10 subjects with type 1 diabetes as well as more than 10 subjects without the disease. Genomic DNA was extracted from peripheral blood leukocytes. Primers were designed to cover all 5 exons and exon–intron junctions in the published human *PDCD1* sequence (Ensemble Human Geneview). Polymerase chain reaction (PCR) amplification was performed in TAKARA Ex Taq™ TAKARA LA Taq™ or TAKARA PrimeSTAR™ HS system (TAKARA BIO INC), in a TaKaRa PCR Thermal Cycler. Sequencing was performed using ABI PRISM® BigDye™ Terminators v3.1 Cycle Sequencing Kit (Applied Biosystems, Tokyo, Japan) and an ABI PRISM® 3730 Genetic Analyzer (Applied Biosystems).

Some of the sequence variations identified were genotyped in larger samples (>200) with and without type 1 diabetes by PCR–restriction-fragment length polymorphism (RFLP) methods.

RESULTS

A total of approximate 4000 base pairs, which included all 5 exons, were sequenced. In total, we identified 10 sequence variants, of which 4 variants turned out to be novel. Among the 10 variants, 3 were found in exons, and the C7625T polymorphism was accompanied with an amino acid substitution. PD1.3A polymorphism that was previously reported to be associated with type 1 diabetes in Caucasian,[5] however, was not found to be polymorphic in the Japanese subjects investigated. Preliminary data suggested that none of the polymorphisms were associated with type 1 diabetes.

DISCUSSION

There have been a number of reports studying genetic susceptibility to type 1 diabetes, and more than 20 *IDDM* loci in total have been reported to be linked to or associated with type 1 diabetes. *PDCD1* is on chromosome 2q37.3, where none of the *IDDM* loci have been mapped in the previous genome scans. It does not necessarily mean, however, that *PDCD1* is excluded as a candidate for a susceptibility gene. Recently, several groups demonstrated that genetic predisposition to type 1 diabetes is conferred by *PTPN22,* a human gene encoding lymphoid tyrosine phosphatase (LYP), whose chromosomal location is not overlapped with any of *IDDM* loci mapped to date.[6,7] Therefore, it is still possible that *PDCD1* is involved in genetic susceptibility to type 1 diabetes. Sequence variations identified in the present study will be valuable for further studies to clarify the contribution of *PDCD1* to susceptibility to type 1 diabetes as well as to other autoimmune diseases.

ACKNOWLEDGMENTS

We thank M. Moritani and Y. Tsukamoto for their skillful technical assistance. This work was supported by a Grant-in-Aid for Scientific Research from the Ministry of Education, Science, Sports, Culture, and Technology, Japan.

REFERENCES

1. IKEGAMI, H. & T. OGIHARA. 1996. Genetics of insulin-dependent diabetes mellitus. Endocr. J. **43:** 605–613.
2. YUMIKO KAWABATA, Y., H. IKEGAMI, *et al.* 2002. Asian-specific HLA haplotypes reveal heterogeneity of the contribution of HLA-DR and -DQ haplotypes to susceptibility to type 1 diabetes. Diabetes **51:** 545–551.
3. ANSARI, M.J. *et al.* 2003. The programmed death-1 (PD-1) pathway regulates autoimmune diabetes in nonobese diabetic (NOD) mice. J. Exp. Med. **198:** 63–69.

4. UEDA, H. *et al.* 2003. Association of the T-cell regulatory gene CTLA4 with susceptibility to autoimmune disease. Nature **423:** 505–511.
5. NIELSEN, C. *et al.* 2003. Association of a putative regulatory polymorphism in the PD-1 gene with susceptibility to type 1 diabetes. Tissue Antigens **62:** 492–497.
6. SIMONOVITCH, K.A. 2004. PTPN22 and autoimmune disease. Nat. Genet. **36:** 1248–1249.
7. KAWASAKI, E.,T. AWATA, H. IKEGAMI, *et al.* 2005. Systematic search for single nucleotide polymorphisms in a lymphoid tyrosine phosphatase (PTPN22) gene: association between promoter polymorphism and type 1 diabetes in Asian populations. Am. J. Med. Genet. **140:** 586–593.

Genetic Determinants of Type 1 Diabetes Across Populations

MOHAMED M. JAHROMI[a,b] AND GEORGE S. EISENBARTH[a]

[a]*Barbara Davis Center for Childhood Diabetes, University of Colorado, Health sciences Center, Aurora, Colorado 80010, USA*

[b]*Salmaniya Medical Complex, Ministry of Health, Manama, Kingdom of Bahrain*

ABSTRACT: T1D results from autoimmune-mediated destruction of the pancreatic β cells, a process that is conditioned by multiple genes and environmental factors. The main genetic determinants map to the major histocompatibility complex (MHC), and in particular DR and DQ, although, genes outside the MHC contribute, including the insulin gene, *PTPN22*, and *CTLA-4*. There are remarkable differences in genetic susceptibility to T1D between populations. We believe this variation reflects differing frequencies of diabetes causative and protective alleles and haplotypes, and thus remains a major genetic influence linked to the MHC region not accounted for by DR and DQ alleles. In this article, we discuss global variations in genetic susceptibility to T1D in view of current genetic understanding.

KEYWORDS: type 1A diabetes; insulin; PTPN 22; CTLA- 4

INTRODUCTION

Type 1A diabetes (T1D) is an autoimmune disorder characterized by chronic T-cell-mediated destruction of the insulin-secreting β cells of the pancreatic islet of Langerhans.

T1D is heterogeneous in terms of age at diabetes development with as many adults developing the disorder as children.[1] Genetic susceptibility is dependent on the degree of genetic identity with the proband, and the risk of diabetes in families has a nonlinear correlation with the number of alleles shared with the proband. The highest risk is naturally observed in monozygotic twins (100% sharing) followed by first, second, and third degree relatives (50%, 25%, and 12.5% sharing, respectively).[2]

Address for correspondence: George S. Eisenbarth, MD, PhD, Barbara Davis Center for Childhood Diabetes, University of Colorado Health Sciences Center, Mail Stop B140, PO Box 6511, Aurora, COl 80010. Voice: 303-724-6847; fax: 303-724-6839.
e-mail: George.Eisenbarth@UCHSC.edu

Ann. N.Y. Acad. Sci. 1079: 289–299 (2006).
doi: 10.1196/annals.1375.044

GEOGRAPHIC VARIATION OF T1D

The incidence of T1D is rapidly increasing in multiple regions of the world with a trend toward earlier onset. T1D incidence is highly variable among different populations. The overall ratio of incidence of T1D varies from 0.1/100,000 per year in China to more than 36/100,000 per year in Sardinia and in Finland. This represents a more than 350-fold variation among populations analyzed.[3] The polar equatorial gradient (i.e., north–south gradient) described for disease incidence is not as strong as previously thought (e.g., Sardinia with extremely high incidence). Most populations with very high incidence rates are Europid. High incidence rates have also been noted in Kuwait,[4,5] Oman,[4] and Puerto Rico.[6] In fact, a relatively high-gradient risk has been reported among some non-Europid ethnicities (i.e., admixed partly African [1/100,000 per year in Mauritius versus 15/100,000 per year in Chicago] and Arab [5/100,000 per year in Sudan versus 18/100,000 per year in Kuwait]).[6]

GENETIC OF T1D

There are rare variants of immune-mediated diabetes with single gene mutations including the APS-I syndrome (*AIRE* autoimmune regulator gene) and the IPEX syndrome (*FoxP3* mutation).[7] Multiple genetic factors influence both susceptibility and resistance to the common forms of T1D.[8] Although a significant proportion of patients with T1D lack a family history of the disease, there is significant familial clustering with an average prevalence of 6% in siblings compared to 0.4% in the U.S. Caucasian population. Of note, there is a 3.8% risk of type 1 diabetes in Japanese siblings of patients with T1D compared to 0.01∼0.02% prevalence in the general Japanese population.[9] The sibling ratio (λs) can be calculated as the ratio of the risk to siblings over the disease prevalence in the general population, and thus $\lambda s = 6/0.4 = 15$ and $3.8/0.01 \sim 0.02 = > 100$ for the United States and Japan, respectively.[9]

Both association studies and linkage analysis using various analytical methods have been used to identify susceptibility loci. Using the candidate gene approach, association studies provided evidence for the first two susceptibility loci, the human leukocyte antigen (HLA) region (*IDDM1*) and the insulin gene (*INS*) locus (*IDDM2*). These two loci only contribute a portion of the familial clustering (50% for *IDDM1* and 10% for *INS*), suggesting the existence of additional loci.[10] The next most potent locus for T1D of man was also discovered using a candidate gene approach, namely the LYP (*PTPN22*) gene with an odds ratio of approximately 1.7 for a "missense" mutation that contributes to multiple different autoimmune disorders.[11–13] Recently, however, Cytotoxic T lymphocyte antigen-4 (*CTLA-4*) gene (*IDDM12*) and *SUMO-4* with weak association were described following genome analysis. Both the latter associations appear heterogeneous and dependent on the population (e.g., stronger association of Sumo-4 in Asian populations and lack of association in multiple European populations),[3] and nature of the disease (e.g., *CTLA-4* associated with diabetes with thyroid autoimmunity).[14] Undoubtedly, future genome-wide association studies will reveal more loci, each providing a piece to the genetic puzzle of T1D, but with difficulty of distinguishing false positive from true signals with very weak associations.

THE MAJOR HISTOCOMPATIBILITY COMPLEX, *IDDM1*

The major loci for susceptibility to T1D are located within the HLA region on the short arm of chromosome 6[15] and provide up to 40–50% of the inheritable diabetes risk.[16] The HLA complex was first linked to diabetes when associations with several HLA class I antigens (e.g., HLA-B8, -B18, and -B15) were discovered by serological typing and affected sib-pair analysis showed evidence of linkage.[17–19] With the development of typing reagents, HLA class II alleles (DQ, DR, and DP; in that order of risk) were shown to be even more strongly associated with the disease.[19–21] However, other loci within or near the HLA complex appear to modulate diabetes risk, and add further complexity to the analysis of *IDDM1*-encoded susceptibility.

The great majority of Caucasian patients have HLA-DR3(withDRB1*0301 with DQA1*0501,DQB1*0201,DQ2) or DR4(with DRB1*04 with DQA1*0301,DQB1*0302,DQ8) class II haplotypes and approximately 30–50% of patients are DR3/DR4 heterozygotes.[22] The DR3/DR4 (DQ2, DQ8) genotype confers the highest diabetes risk with a synergistic mode of action.[23] However, DR4/DR9 has been reported to be a highly susceptible haplotype in Japanese. The absence of DR3 haplotypes in the Japanese population may contribute to lower frequency of the disease in Japan.[9,24] On the other hand, in the Chinese population, the DR3/DR9 genotype is highly susceptible.[24] DQ–DR linkage disequilibrium patterns of HLA haplotypes in different populations may explain part of the worldwide differences in the frequency of incidence of T1D[24] (e.g., DRB1*0405-DQB1*0302 is a high-risk haplotype while DRB1*0403-DQB1*0302 is neutral or protective) with different DRB1 alleles modulating high risk provided by high-risk DQ alleles.[25]

Furthermore, DRB1*1501-DQB1*0602 is protective in all populations which have been studied to date.[5,26–33] Analysis of rare "recombinant" haplotype suggests that DQB1*0602 provides protection and not DRB1*1501. FIGURE 1 summarizes odds ratios for DQB1*0602 in multiple populations. A recent report of Swedish patients where 8 individuals with DQB1*0602 and T1D were ascertained (of 971 patients) and haplotypes with the allele 15 of microsatellite D6S265 with DQB1*0602 haplotype had an odds ratio of 0.2 compared to other DQB1*0602 haplotypes with odds ratios of 0.02.[34] We believe it is very likely that in all populations DQB1*0602 is

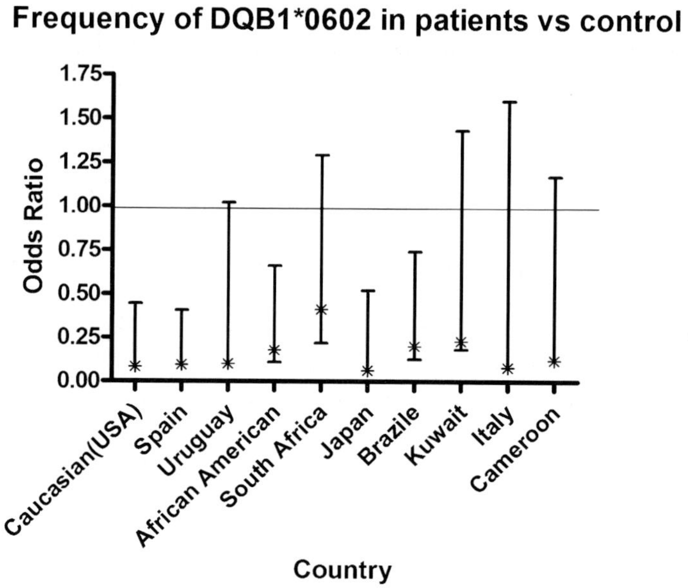

FIGURE 1. Odd ratio below 0.25 in all populations except South Africa. Arrow bars symbolize 95% confidence intervals.[5,26–33]

protective from T1D, and the search for exceptions is important, as it might shed light on the mechanism of potent protection. DQB1*0602 protects from the expression of anti-islet autoantibodies and may further influence progression to diabetes, but for the latter too few individuals expressing multiple autoantibodies have been studied to date.[35,36]

We have recently reported in oral presentation that combined typing of high-risk HLA alleles with analysis of HLA haplotype sharing can identify siblings with an extraordinary genetic risk of T1D (M Rewers Kelly West Lecture, American Diabetes Association 2005). This strongly implicates major genes in addition to DR and DQ alleles. The current ability to determine multiple polymorphisms (thousands) throughout the MHC and multiple studies of conserved haplotypes (e.g., A1-B8-DR3-DQ2 common extended haplotype[37] and Basque A30-B18-DR3-DQ2 haplotype, with the latter conferring increased risk) should enhance the search for these additional MHC linked determinants.

INSULIN GENE (*IDDM2*)

The 4.1 kb region containing the *INS* and its flanking regions contain several polymorphisms in linkage disequilibrium[38] that have been associated with diabetes risk. All the polymorphisms identified within this region lie outside coding sequences. Extensive studies involving polymorphisms in the neighboring HUMTHO1 (tyrosine hydroxylase) and *IGF2* genes provided strong evidence that INS is the main susceptibility determinant in this region.[39–42] Shortly after its discovery,[43] the insulin variable number of tandem repeats (VNTR) was found to be associated with T1D.[44] Susceptibility in the INS region, or the *IDDM2* locus, was initially associated to a VNTR located ~0.5 kb upstream of *INS*.[43,45,46] Homozygosity for the short-class VNTR I alleles is found in ~75–85% of the patients compared to a frequency of 50–60% in the general population, suggesting that it predisposes to T1D. In contrast, homozygosity for the longer class III VNTR alleles is rarely seen in patients and the class III VNTR is believed to confer a dominant protective effect.[44,47,48] The relative risk ratio of the I/I genotype versus I/III or III/III has been reported to be moderate relative to MHC influence (in the 3–5 range) and it accounts for about 10% of the familial clustering of T1D.[49] However, analyses suggest that it is not possible to discriminate effects of the VNTR from other polymorphisms in this region[50,51] and that at least two other polymorphisms (−23HphI and +1140A/C) may be important.[52] Moreover, by measuring the HphI polymorphism (in tight linkage disequilibrium with the VNTR),[38] Metcalfe *et al.*[53] showed that homozygosity for the predisposing INS genotype increases the likelihood that identical twins will be concordant for T1D.

IDDM2-associated susceptibility and resistance may derive from quantitative differences in *INS* transcription in the specialized antigen presenting cells found in thymus and peripheral lymphoid tissues, where production of self-antigens such as proinsulin may be crucial for the shaping and maintaining of a self-tolerant T cell repertoire.[54–56] Such mechanisms may influence the probability of developing autoimmune responses to insulin, a key autoantigen in T1D.[57,58]

LYP GENE: *PTPN22*

LYP (encoded by *PTPN22* gene) belongs to a family of protein tyrosine phosphatases (PTPs) that are involved in modulating T cell activation with recent evidence indicating that the diabetes associated allele (LYP-Trp 620) may result in a "gain of function"[59]and thereby contribute to T cell activation. Bottini and co-workers evaluated a functional polymorphism in LYP (no relation to the lymphopenia gene of the BB rat) in two series of patients with T1D, one from Denver and another from Sardinia.[59] The odds ratio was approximately 1.7, making this polymorphism the most potent after *IDDM1* and *IDDM2*. The polymorphism appears to be a missense mutation that changes an arginine at position 620 to a tryptophan and thereby abrogates the ability of the molecule to bind to the signaling molecule Csk.[59,60] Consistent with a general effect on immune function is the finding that the minor tryptophan encoded allele is associated with a series of autoimmune disorders including T1D, rheumatoid arthritis,[60] and lupus erythematosus.[61] Multiple recent studies have confirmed the association of this missense mutation with T1D including a large study from Great Britain.[62] It is possible that polymorphisms in linkage disequilibrium with R620W determine increased risk of autoimmunity rather than the 620 polymorphism, but this seems unlikely given the rapid confirmation of this polymorphism's association with multiple forms of autoimmune disease in multiple populations and its functional significance. It is well documented that *PTPN22* is a susceptibility gene for T1D in Caucasian populations, but the diabetes-associated polymorphism is not found in the Japanese population.[63]

CYTOTOXIC T LYMPHOCYTE ANTIGEN-4 (*IDDM12*)

CTLA-4 gene is located on chromosome 2q33, is one of the confirmed T1D susceptibility loci. This 300-kb region is known to contain at least three genes: *CD28*, *CTLA-4*, and the inducible costimulatory molecule gene.[3] Genetic and physical mapping has suggested that *CTLA-4* or a gene in close proximity to it may be involved in susceptibility to T1D.[64] *CTLA-4* antigen, which is expressed on activated T cells, is an important factor in T cell regulation.[3,64] Kavvoura and Ioannidis have a meta-analysis on three of them and concluded that the A(49)G gene polymorphism in exon 1 is associated with T1D.[3] They have also reported a significant ethnic variation in that polymorphism. On the other hand, the A(CT60)G gene polymorphism have been studied in parallel with A(49)G in different in Caucasian as well as Asian population.

CONCLUDING REMARKS

A large body of evidence indicates that genetic factors influence both susceptibility to and resistance to T1D. Several chromosomal regions have been linked with the disease, suggesting that this is a polygenic disorder in most families. A few rare families have dramatic Mendelian mutations leading to immune-mediated diabetes.

Although DR and DQ alleles and their linkage disequilibrium pattern can explain a major portion of disease risk, there is evidence for additional genes linked or within the MHC-influencing risk. We believe it is likely that a combination of genes linked to the MHC have a major effect on risk of T1D in addition to the known potent effects of HLA-DR and -DQ alleles. In addition, other genes such as *INS*, *PTPN22,* and *CTLA-4* contribute to pathogenesis and additional genes not linked to the MHC with small but significant effects remain to be defined. Differences in disease risk between populations is likely due in part to the distribution within populations of DR and DQ haplotypes and we hypothesize that major genetic factors, probably linked to the MHC remain to be defined that will contribute to the remarkable population differences in type 1A incidence. Recent technological advances in large scale single nucleotide polymorphism (SNP) typing and the formation of cooperative global genetic study groups should enhance the speed at which true gene(s) for T1D will be uncovered.

ACKNOWLEDGMENTS

This work was supported by the National Institutes of Health (DK32083, DK32493, DK057538), Autoimmunity Prevention Center (AI50964), Diabetes Endocrine Research Center (P30 DK57516), Clinical Research Centers (MO1 RR00069, MO1 RR00051), the Immune Tolerance Network (AI15416), the American Diabetes Association, the Juvenile Diabetes Research Foundation, and the Children's Diabetes Foundation. MMJ has a Fulbright Fellowship.

REFERENCES

1. BARNETT, A.H., C. EFF, R.D. LESLIE, *et al.* 1981. Diabetes in identical twins: a study of 200 pairs. Diabetologia **20:** 87–93.
2. MILLWARD, B.A., L. ALVIGGI, P.J. HOSKINS, *et al.* 1986. Immune changes associated with insulin dependent diabetes may remit without causing the disease: a study in identical twins. Br. Med. J. **292:** 793–796.
3. KAVVOURA, F.K. & J.P. IOANNIDIS. 2005. CTLA-4 gene polymorphisms and susceptibility to T1D mellitus: a HuGE Review and meta-analysis. Am. J. Epidemiol. **162:** 3–16.
4. ABDULLAH, M.A. 2005. Epidemiology of type I diabetes mellitus among Arab children Saudi. Med. J. **26:** 911–917.
5. HAIDER, M.Z., A. SHALTOUT, K. ALSAEID, *et al.* 1999. Prevalence of human leukocyte antigen DQA1 and DQB1 alleles in Kuwaiti Arab children with T1D mellitus. Clin. Genet. **56:** 450–456.
6. KARVONEN, M., M. VIIK-KAJANDER, E. MOLTCHANOVA, *et al.* 2000. Incidence of childhood T1D worldwide. Diabetes Mondiale (DiaMond) Project Group. Diabetes Care **23:** 1516–1526.
7. WILDIN, R.S. & A. FREITAS. 2005. IPEX and FOXP3: clinical and research perspectives. J. Autoimmun. **25**(Suppl): 56–62.
8. ERLICH, H.A., R.L. GRIFFITH, T.L. BUGAWAN, *et al.* 1991. Implication of specific DQB1 alleles in genetic susceptibility and resistance by identification of IDDM siblings with novel HLA-DQB1 allele and unusual DR2 and DR1 haplotypes. Diabetes **40:** 478–481.
9. IKEGAMI, H., Y. KAWAGUCHI, E. YAMATO, *et al.* 1992. Analysis by the polymerase chain reaction of histocompatibility leucocyte antigen-DR9-linked susceptibility to insulin-dependent diabetes mellitus. J. Clin. Endocrinol. Metab. **75:** 1381–1385.
10. FAIN, P. & G.S. EISENBARTH. 2002. Genetics of type 1 diabetes mellitus. *In* Genetics in Endocrinology. J. Baxter, S. Melmed, M. New & L. Martini, Eds.: 37–72. Lippincott Williams & Williams. Philadelphia.
11. SHEEHY, M.J., S.J. SCHARF, J.R. ROWE, *et al.* 1989. A diabetes-susceptible HLA haplotype is best defined by a combination of HLA-DR and -DQ alleles. J. Clin. Invest.**83:** 830–835.

12. MOREL, P.A., J.S. DORMAN, J.A. TODD, *et al.* 1988. Aspartic acid at position 57 of the HLA-DQ beta chain protects against type I diabetes: a family study. Proc. Natl. Acad. Sci. USA **85:** 8111–8115.
13. KHALIL, I., L. D'AURIOL, M. GOBET, *et al.* 1990. A combination of HLA-DQβ Asp57-negative and HLA DQα Arg52 confers susceptibility to insulin-dependent diabetes mellitus. J. Clin. Invest. **85:** 1315–1319.
14. MOCHIZUKI, M., S. AMEMIYA, K. KOBAYASHI, *et al.* 2003. Association of the CTLA-4 gene 49 A/G polymorphism with type 1 diabetes and autoimmune thyroid disease in Japanese children. Diabetes Care **26:** 843–847.
15. SANJEEVI, C.B., C. DEWEESE, M. LANDIN-OLSSON, *et al.* 1997. Analysis of critical residues of HLA-DQ6 molecules in insulin-dependent diabetes mellitus. Tissue Antigens **50:** 61–65.
16. HOOVER, M.L. & R.T. MARTA. 1997. Molecular modelling of HLA-DQ suggests a mechanism of resistance in type I diabetes. Scand. J. Immunol. **45:** 193–202.
17. AWATA, T., T. KUZUYA, A. MATSUDA, *et al.* 1990. High frequency of aspartic acid at position 57 of HLA-DQ B-chain in Japanese IDDM patients and nondiabetic subjects. Diabetes **39:** 266–269.
18. RONNINGEN, K.S., T. IWE, T.S. HALSTENSEN, *et al.* 1989. The amino acid at position 57 of the HLA-DQ beta chain and susceptibility to develop insulin-dependent diabetes mellitus. Hum. Immunol. **26:** 215–225.
19. TODD, J.A., C. MIJOVIC, J. FLETCHER, *et al.* 1989. Identification of susceptibility loci for insulin-dependent diabetes mellitus by trans-racial gene mapping. Nature **338:** 587–589.
20. MIJOVIC, C.H., A.H. BARNETT & J.A. TODD. 1991. Genetics of diabetes. Trans-racial gene mapping studies [review]. Baillieres Clin. Endocrinol. Metab. **5:** 321–340.
21. JENKINS, D., C. MIJOVIC, J. FLETCHER, *et al.* 1990. Identification of susceptibility loci for type I (insulin-dependent) diabetes by trans-racial gene mapping. Diabetologia **33:** 387–395.
22. MIJOVIC, C.H., D. JENKINS, K.H. JACOBS, *et al.* 1991. HLA-DQA1 and -DQB1 alleles associated with genetic susceptibility to IDDM in a black population. Diabetes **40:** 748–753.
23. RONNINGEN, K.S., A. SPURKLAND, B.D. TAIT, *et al.* 1992. HLA class II associations in insulin-dependent diabetes mellitus among Blacks, Caucasiods, and Japanese. *In* HLA 1991 Proceedings of the Eleventh International Histocompatibility Workshop and Conference. K. Tsuji, M. Aizawa & T. Sasazuki, Eds.: 713–722. Oxford University Press. Oxford.
24. SHE, J-X. 1996. Susceptibility to type I diabetes: HLA-DQ and DR revisited. Immunol. Today **17:** 323–329.
25. PARK, Y., J.-X. SHE, S. BABU, *et al.* 2001. Transracial evidence for the influence of the homologous HLA DR-DQ haplotype on transmission of HLA DR4 haplotypes to diabetic children. Tissue Antigens **57:** 185–191.
26. CAILLAT-ZUCMAN, S., I. DJILALI-SAIAH, J. TIMSIT, *et al.* 1997. Insulin dependent diabetes mellitus (IDDM) joint report. 12th International Histocompatibility Workshop Study. *In* Genetic Diversity of HLA. Functional and Medical Implications. D. Charron, Ed.: 389–398. EDK. Paris.
27. ESCRIBANO-DE-DIEGO, J., P. SANCHEZ-VELASCO, C. LUZURIAGA, *et al.* 1999. HLA class II immunogenetics and incidence of insulin-dependent diabetes mellitus in the population of Cantabria (Northern Spain). Hum. Immunol. **60:** 990–1000.

28. MIMBACAS, A., F. PEREZ-BRAVO, P.C. HIDALGO, *et al.* 2003. Association between diabetes type 1 and DQB1 alleles in a case-control study conducted in Montevideo, Uruguay. Genet. Mol. Res. **2:** 29–35.
29. PIRIE, F.J., M.G. HAMMOND, A.A. MOTALA & M.A. OMAR. 2001. HLA class II antigens in South African Blacks with type I diabetes. Tissue Antigens **57:** 348–352.
30. KAWASAKI, E. & K. EGUCHI. 2004. Is Type 1 diabetes in the Japanese population the same as among Caucasians? Ann. N. Y. Acad. Sci. **1037:** 96–103.
31. MBANYA, J.C., E. SOBNGWI & D.N. MBANYA. 2001. HLA-DRB1, -DQA1, -DQB1 and DPB1 susceptibility alleles in Cameroonian type 1 diabetes patients and controls. Eur. J. Immunogenet. **28:** 459–462.
32. PETRONE, A., T.L. BUGAWAN, C.A. MESTURINO, *et al.* 2001. The distribution of HLA class II susceptible/protective haplotypes could partially explain the low incidence of type 1 diabetes in continental Italy (Lazio region). Tissue Antigens **58:** 385–394.
33. HAUACHE, O.M., A.F. REIS, C.S. OLIVEIRA, *et al.* 2005. Estimation of diabetes risk in Brazilian population by typing for polymorphisms in HLA-DR-DQ, INS and CTLA-4 genes. Dis. Markers **21:** 139–145.
34. VALDES, A.M., G. THOMSON, J. GRAHAM, *et al.* 2005. D6S265*15 marks a DRB1*15, DQB1*0602 haplotype associated with attenuated protection from type 1 diabetes mellitus. Diabetologia **48:** 2540–2543.
35. GREENBAUM, C.J., D. CUTHBERTSON, G.S. EISENBARTH, *et al.* 2000. Islet cell antibody positive relatives with HLA-DQA1*0102, DQB1*0602: identification by the Diabetes Prevention Trial-1. J. Clin. Endocrinol. Metab. **85:** 1255–1260.
36. GREENBAUM, C.J., G.S. EISENBARTH, M. ATKINSON, *et al.* 2005. High frequency of abnormal glucose tolerance in DQA1*0102/DQB1*0602 relatives identified as part of the Diabetes Prevention Trial—Type 1 Diabetes. Diabetologia **48:** 68–74.
37. ALPER, C.A., Z. AWDEH & E.J. YUNIS. 1992. Conserved, extended MHC haplotypes. Exp. Clin. Immunogenet. **9:** 58–71.
38. OWERBACH, D. & K.H. GABBAY. 1996. The search for IDDM susceptibility genes: the next generation [review]. Diabetes **45:** 544–551.
39. STEAD, J.D., J. BUARD, J.A. TODD & A.J. JEFFREYS. 2000. Influence of allele lineage on the role of the insulin minisatellite in susceptibility to type 1 diabetes. Hum. Mol. Genet. **9:** 2929–2935.
40. VAFIADIS, P., S.T. BENNETT, E. COLLE, *et al.* 1996. Imprinted and genotype-specific expression of genes at the *IDDM2* locus in pancreas and leukocytes. J. Autoimmun. **9:** 397–403.
41. PALMER, J.P., C.M. ASPLIN, P. CLEMONS, *et al.* 1983. Insulin antibodies in insulin-dependent diabetics before insulin treatment. Science **222:** 1337–1339.
42. VARDI, P., A.G. ZIEGLER, J.H. MATTHEWS, *et al.* 1988. Concentration of insulin autoantibodies at onset of type I diabetes Inverse log-linear correlation with age. Diabetes Care **11:** 736–739.
43. VARDI, P., S.A. DIB, M. TUTTLEMAN, *et al.* 1987. Competitive insulin autoantibody assay. Prospective evaluation of subjects at high risk for development of type I diabetes mellitus. Diabetes **36:** 1286–1291.
44. HASKINS, K. & D. WEGMANN. 1996. Diabetogenic T-cell clones. Diabetes **45:** 1299–1305.
45. YU, L., D.T. ROBLES, N. ABIRU, *et al.* 2000. Early expression of antiinsulin autoantibodies of humans and the NOD mouse: evidence for early determination of subsequent diabetes. Proc. Natl. Acad. Sci. USA **97:** 1701–1706.

46. NASERKE, H.E. & A.-G. ZIEGLER. 2001. Humoral and cellular immune response to insulin. Diabetes Nutr. Metab. **9:** 208–214.
47. PUGLIESE, A., D. BROWN, D. GARZA, *et al.* 2001. Self-antigen presenting cells expressing islet cell molecules in human thymus and peripheral lymphoid organs: phenotypic characterization and implications for immunological tolerance and type 1 diabetes. J. Clin. Invest. **107:** 555–564.
48. SOSPEDRA, M., X. FERRER-FRANCESCH, O. DOMINGUEZ, *et al.* 1998. Transcription of a broad range of self-antigens in human thymus suggests a role for central mechanisms in tolerance toward peripheral antigens. J. Immunol. **161:** 5918–5929.
49. WERDELIN, O., U. CORDES & T. JENSEN. 1998. Aberrant expression of tissue-specific proteins in the thymus: a hypothesis for the development of central tolerance. Scand. J. Immunol. **47:** 95–100.
50. WONG, F.S., J. KARTTUNEN, C. DUMONT, *et al.* 1999. Identification of an MHC class I-restricted autoantigen in type 1 diabetes by screening an organ-specific cDNA library. Nat. Med. **5:** 1026–1031.
51. JOLICOEUR, C., D. HANAHAN & K.M. SMITH. 1994. T-cell tolerance toward a transgenic β-cell antigen and transcription of endogenous pancreatic genes in thymus. Proc. Natl. Acad. Sci. USA **91:** 6707–6711.
52. HEATH, V.L., N.C. MOORE, S.M. PARNELL & D.W. MASON. 1998. Intrathymic expression of genes involved in organ specific autoimmune disease. J. Autoimmun. **11:** 309–318.
53. METCALFE, K.A., G.A. HITMAN, R.E. ROWE, *et al.* 2001. Concordance for type 1 diabetes in identical twins is affected by insulin genotype. Diabetes Care **24:** 838–842.
54. GEENEN, V., I. ACHOUR, F. ROBERT, *et al.* 1993. Evidence that insulin-like growth factor 2 (IGF2) is the dominant thymic peptide of the insulin superfamily. Thymus **21:** 115–127.
55. HOLMES, D.I., N.A. WAHAB & R.M. MASON. 1999. Cloning and characterization of ZNF236, a glucose-regulated Kruppel-like zinc-finger gene mapping to human chromosome 18q22-q23. Genomics **60:** 105–109.
56. COPEMAN, J.B., F. CUCCA, C.M. HEARNE, *et al.* 1995. Linkage disequilibrium mapping of type 1 diabetes susceptibility gene *(IDDM7)* to chromosome 2q31-q33. Nat. Genet. **9:** 80–85.
57. NAKAYAMA, M., N. ABIRU, H. MORIYAMA, *et al.* 2005. Prime role for an insulin epitope in the development of type 1 diabetes in NOD mice. Nature **435:** 220–223.
58. KENT, S.C., Y. CHEN, L. BREGOLI, *et al.* 2005. Expanded T cells from pancreatic lymph nodes of type 1 diabetic subjects recognize an insulin epitope. Nature **435:** 224–228.
59. BOTTINI, N., L. MUSCUMECI, A. ALONSO, *et al.* 2004. A functional variant of lymphoid tyrosine phosphatase is associated with type I diabetes. Nat. Genet. **36:** 337–338.
60. BEGOVICH, A.B., V.E. CARLTON, L.A. HONIGBERG, *et al.* 2004. A missense single-nucleotide polymorphism in a gene encoding a protein tyrosine phosphatase (PTPN22) is associated with rheumatoid arthritis. Am. J. Hum Genet. **75:** 330–337.
61. KYOGOKU, C., C.D. LANGEFELD, W.A. ORTMANN, *et al.* 2004. Genetic association of the R620W polymorphism of protein tyrosine phosphatase PTPN22 with human SLE. Am. J. Hum. Genet. **75:** 504–507.

62. Smyth, D., J.D. Cooper, J.E. Collins, *et al.* 2004. Replication of an association between the lymphoid tyrosine phosphatase locus (LYP/PTPN22) with type 1 diabetes, and evidence for its role as a general autoimmunity locus. Diabetes **53:** 3020–3023.
63. Mori, M., R. Yamada, K. Kobayashi, *et al.* 2005. Ethnic differences in allele frequency of autoimmune-disease-associated SNPs. J. Hum. Genet. **50:** 264–266.
64. Marron, M.P., A. Zeidler, L.J. Raffel, *et al.* 2000. Genetic and physical mapping of a type 1 diabetes susceptibility gene (IDDM12) to a 100-kb phagemid artificial chromosome clone containing D2S72-CTLA4-D2S105 on chromosome 2q33. Diabetes **49:** 492–499.

TNFa-e Microsatellite, HLA-DRB1 and -DQB1 Alleles and Haplotypes in Brazilian Patients Presenting Recently Diagnosed Type 1 Diabetes Mellitus

DIANE M. RASSI,[a] ISABELA J. WASTOWSKI,[a] RENATA T. SIMÕES,[b] SANDRA RODRIGUES,[c] NEIFE N.H.S. DEGHAIDE,[c] CELSO T. MENDES-JUNIOR,[c] AGUINALDO L. SIMÕES,[d] C.P. SOARES,[e] GERALDO A.S. PASSOS,[c,d] AND EDUARDO A. DONADI[a,c]

[a]*Program of Basic and Applied Immunology,* [b]*Department of Pathology,* [c]*Department of Medicine ,* [d]*Department of Genetics, Faculty of Medicine of Ribeirão Preto, University of São Paulo (USP), 14049-900, Ribeirão Preto, São Paulo, Brazil*

[e]*Department of Clinical Analysis, School of Pharmaceutical Sciences, University of São Paulo State (UNESP), 14-801-902, Araraquara, São Paulo, Brazil*

ABSTRACT: TNF microsatellite and HLA class II polymorphisms were studied in 28 recently diagnosed Brazilian patients presenting type 1 diabetes mellitus (T1DM) and in 120 healthy controls. TNFa-e and HLA-DRB1/DQB1 alleles were identified using sets of sequence-specific primers. Compared to controls, the DRB1*03 and DQB1*02 allele groups, TNFa1 allele, and the TNFa4-b5-c1-d4-e3 and TNFa10-b5-c1-d4-e3 haplotypes were overrepresented in patients. TNF microsatellite together with HLA polymorphisms is associated with type 1 diabetes in Brazilian patients, corroborating the participation of the MHC genes in disease susceptibility.

KEYWORDS: type 1 diabetes mellitus; polymorphism; TNF microsatellite; HLA

INTRODUCTION

Few studies have evaluated the human leukocyte antigen (HLA) class III gene polymorphism, particularly the tumar necrosis factor (TNF) region, in type 1 diabetes mellitus (T1DM). TNF region has 12 kb in length and contains

Address for correspondence: Eduardo Antonio Donadi, Division of Clinical Immunology, School of Medicine of Ribeirão Preto, University of São Paulo. Av. Bandeirantes, 3900, 14049-900. Ribeirão Preto, SP, Brazil. Voice: + 55-16-602-3373.
e-mail: eadonadi@fmrp.usp.br

Ann. N.Y. Acad. Sci. 1079: 300–304 (2006). © 2006 New York Academy of Sciences.
doi: 10.1196/annals.1375.045

several polymorphic sites, some of them have been associated with TNF production. *TNFa-f* microsatellites span around the TNF and lymphotoxin loci, exhibiting 14, 7, 2, 7, 4, and 10 alleles, respectively.[1,2] Since many of the TNF cluster polymorphisms have been found to be in linkage disequilibrium with HLA class I and II alleles, in this article we evaluated *TNFa-e* microsatellite and HLA-DR/DQ alleles and haplotypes in Brazilian patients presenting with recently diagnosed T1DM patients.

PATIENTS AND METHODS

Subjects

Twenty-eight Brazilian patients with T1DM aged 4 to 16 years, and 120 healthy children paired to patients for sex and age were studied. The protocol (7945/99) of the study was approved by the local Ethics Committee.

HLA and TNF Microsatellite Typing

HLA-DRB1/DQB1 allele group typing was performed using commercial kits (One-Lambda, Canoga Park, CA,). *TNFa-e* microsatellite primer sequences and DNA amplification conditions are described elsewhere.[1]

Statistical Analysis

The GENEPOP and ARLEQUIN softwares, and the Fisher's exact test were used. The relative risk (RR), and the etiologic (EF) or preventive (PF) fractions were also calculated. The expectation algorithm (EM)[3] was used to infer phase at linked loci from genotypes using the haplotype trend regression (HTR) software.

RESULTS

The frequency of TNF microsatellite alleles in T1DM patients and controls is shown in TABLE 1. The TNFa1 allele frequency ($P = 0.0138$; RR = 3.1; EF = 0.10) was significantly increased in DM-1 patients when compared with controls. The HLA-DR3 allele group ($P = 0.0012$; RR = 2.5; EF = 10.22) and HLA-DQ2 ($P < 0.0001$; RR = 2.5; EF = 0.34) frequencies were significantly increased in DM-1 patients. The EM algorithm permitted the reconstruction of 116 of the 123 TNF and 129 of the 132 HLA haplotypes with a probability higher than 95% (data available from the corresponding author on request).

TABLE 1. Allelic distribution of TNF microsatellite and HLA-DR/DQ alleles in Brazilian type 1 diabetes (DM-1) patients (P) and controls (C)

	TNFa		TNFb		TNFc		TNFd		TNFe		HLA-DQB1		HLA-DRB1	
	P	C	P	C	P	C	P	C	P	C	P	C	P	C
01	*0.143	0.046	0.179	0.171	0.643	0.654	0.091	0.079	0.089	0.171	0.000	0.004	0.068	0.083
02	0.179	0.246	0.036	0.021	0.357	0.346	0.045	0.046	0.036	0.008	**0.571	0.229		
03	0.000	0.021	0.089	0.133			0.386	0.383	0.875	0.821	0.257	0.279	***0.364	0.146
04	0.089	0.121	0.286	0.308			0.477	0.325			0.000	0.058	0.159	0.125
05	0.071	0.054	0.357	0.312			0.000	0.142			0.057	0.179		
06	0.143	0.125	0.018	0.029			0.000	0.021			0.114	0.237		
07	0.161	0.075	0.036	0.025			0.000	0.004			0.000	0.013	0.182	0.104
08	0.000	0.004											0.023	0.046
09	0.000	0.021											0.045	0.004
10	0.143	0.158											0.000	0.021
11	0.054	0.062											0.023	0.096
12	0.000	0.038												
13	0.000	0.029											0.091	0.175
14	0.018	0.000											0.000	0.038
15													0.023	0.096
16													0.023	0.067
2*n*	56	240	56	240	56	240	44	240	56	240	35	240	44	240

*TNFa1 (P = 0.0138; RR = 3.1; EF = 0.10); **HLA-DQB1*02 allele group (P = 0.0001; RR = 2.5; EF = 0.34), ***HLA-DRB1*03 allele group (P = 0.0012; RR = 2.5; EF = 0.22).

Among the HLA and TNF reconstructed haplotypes, only the TNFa4-b5-c1-d4-e3 and TNFa10-b5-c1-d4-e3 haplotypes were overrepresented in T1DM patients.

DISCUSSION

In the present series, the TNFa1 allele conferred susceptibility to the development of T1DM, in agreement with the findings reported by Monos *et al.*,[4] who reported increased frequency of the TNFa1-b5 haplotype associated with the HLA-DRB1*0301 and B18 alleles. On the other hand, Pociot *et al.*[5] reported increased frequency of the TNFa2, TNFb2, and HLA-B15 haplotype in HLA-DR3 and DR4 positive T1DM patients. This allele combination was associated with increased TNF-α production, and was called diabetogenic haplotype.[6]

Regarding the HLA class II polymorphism, the allele groups HLA-DRB1*03 and -DRB1*04 as well as the haplotypes HLA-DRB1*04/DQB1*02 and HLA-DRB1*03/-DQB1*02 were overrepresented in T1DM patients. Both allele groups have been previously associated with T1DM. The association with HLA-DR and -DQ alleles corroborates the participation of these markers as previously reported by other authors in other populations.

Haplotypes encompassing *TNFa-e* microsatellites and HLA-DR-DQ alleles could not be reliably reconstructed by two reasons. First, due to the small number of patients completely genotyped for the seven genetic markers, and second, because of the presence of a recombination hotspot between these clusters of genes, located near the NOTCH-4 gene.[7] To establish extended haplotypes involving all the seven markers, a familial approach would be more effective; however, the presence of the NOTCH-4 hotspot[7] might result in biologically unreliable haplotypes, as long as these genes would not exhibit strong linkage disequilibrium in the whole population.

ACKNOWLEDGMENT

This work was supported by FAPESP–Fundação de Amparo a Pesquisa do Estado de São Paulo (Grant: 01/04101-9).

REFERENCES

1. Udalova, I.A., S.A. Nepospasov, G.C. Webb, *et al.* 1993. Highly informative typing of the human TNF locus using six adjacent polymorphic markers. Genomics **16:** 180–186.

2. TSUKAMOTO, K., N. OHTA, H. SHIRAI & M. EMI. 1998. A highly polymorphic (CA) repeat marker at in the human tumor necrosis factor alpha. J. Hum. Genet. **43:** 278–279.
3. EXCOFFIER, L. & M. SLATKIN. 1995. Maximum-likelihood estimation of molecular haplotype frequencies in a diploid population. Mol. Biol. Evol. **12:** 921–927.
4. MONOS, D.S., M. KAMOUN, I.A. UDALOVA, *et al.* 1995. Genetic polymorphism of the human tumor necrosis factor region in insulin-dependent diabetes mellitus. Linkage disequilibrium of TNF ab microsatellite alleles with HLA haplotypes. Hum. Immunol. **44:** 70–79.
5. POCIOT, F., L. BRIANT, C.V. JONGENEEL, *et al.* 1993. Association of tumor necrosis factor (TNF) and class II major histocompatibility complex alleles with the secretion of TNF-alpha and TNF-beta by human mononuclear cells: a possible link to insulin-dependent diabetes mellitus. Eur. J. Immunol. **23:** 224–231.
6. STENZEL, A. 2004. Patterns of linkage disequilibrium in the MHC region on human chromosome 6p. Hum. Genet. **114:** 377–385.
7. HAJEER, A.H., & I.V. HUTCHINSON. 2001. Influence of TNF alpha gene polymorphisms on TNF alpha production and disease. Hum. Immunol. **62:** 1191–1199.

Is HLA Class II Profile Relevant for the Study of Large-Scale Differentially Expressed Genes in Type 1 Diabetes Mellitus Patients?

DIANE M. RASSI,[a,b] CRISTINA M. JUNTA,[b] ANA L. FACHIN,[b] PAULA SANDRIN-GARCIA,[b] STEPHANO S. MELLO,[b] ANA P.M. FERNANDES,[c] NEIFE N.H.S. DEGHAIDE,[d] MARIA C. FOSS-FREITAS,[E] MILTON C. FOSS,[d,e] ELZA T. SAKAMOTO-HOJO,[b] GERALDO A.S. PASSOS,[b] AND EDUARDO A. DONADI[a,b,d]

[a]*Immunology Program—Faculty of Medicine of Ribeirão Preto, University of São Paulo, Brazil—14049-900*

[b]*Molecular Immunogenetics Group—Faculty of Medicine of Ribeirão Preto, University of São Paulo, Brazil—14049-900*

[c]*General and Specialized Nursing-Faculty of Medicine of Ribeirão Preto, University of São Paulo, Brazil—14049-900*

[d]*Division Clinical Immunology-Faculty of Medicine of Ribeirão Preto, University of São Paulo, Brazil—14049-900*

[e]*Division of Endocrinology-Faculty of Medicine of Ribeirão Preto, University of São Paulo, Brazil—14049-900*

ABSTRACT: We have previously identified 30 differentially expressed genes when comparing recently diagnosed type 1 diabetes mellitus (DM-1) patients and controls paired for sex, age, and ethnic background. In this article we performed the hierarchical clustering of these genes taking into account the human-leukocyte-antigen (HLA)-DRB1/DQB1 profile. The dendrogram obtained using the Cluster program grouped patients and controls into three clusters, one including individuals with no susceptibility alleles, another including individuals with at least three susceptibility alleles, and a third intermingling susceptibility/protective alleles. In addition to other variables, the results of the present article suggest that the major histocompatibility complex (MHC) class II profile may be of relevance for the study of a large-scale differentially expressed genes.

Address for correspondence: Dr. Eduardo A. Donadi, Divisão de Clínica Médica, Faculdade de Medicina de Ribeirão Preto, Universidade de São Paulo—USP, 14049-900, S.P., Brazil. Voice: +55-16-3602-2566; fax: +55-16-3633-6695.
e-mail: eadonadi@fmrp.usp.br

**Ann. N.Y. Acad. Sci. 1079: 305–309 (2006). © 2006 New York Academy of Sciences.
doi: 10.1196/annals.1375.046**

Keywords: type 1 diabetes mellitus; gene expression; microarrays; metabolism genes

INTRODUCTION

Approximately 20 groups of genes have been associated with susceptibility to type 1 diabetes mellitus (DM-1), however, the largest contribution comes from the major histocompatibility complex (MHC) region, located in chromosome 6p21.[1] The role of MHC class II genes has been extensively studied in several distinct populations. In the Caucasian populations, the DRB1*0405, DQB1*0302, DQB1*0201, and DQA1*0301 alleles have been primarily associated with susceptibility to DM-1, whereas the DRB1*0701, *1501, *1101, *1301 and DQB1*0301, *0303, *0601, *0602 have been associated with protection against the development of DM-1.[2] Although the Brazilian population is considered to be genetically highly diverse, with the contribution of genes from individuals of various ethnic groups,[3] the DQB1*0302 and DQB1*0201 alleles have also been associated with susceptibility to the disease.[3] In a previous study we evaluated the differential large-scale gene expression in total peripheral blood mononuclear cells obtained from recently diagnosed DM-1 patients.[4] Some of the differentially expressed genes, potentially associated with disease pathogenesis, were related to phosphate, protein, and lipid metabolism.[4] To further evaluate whether the human-leukocyte-antigen (HLA) class II profile of these patients may influence the hybridization signatures of the differentially expressed genes, we used a hierarchical clustering algorithm according to the HLA-DB1 and -DQB1 profiles, whose objective was to compute a dendrogram that would assemble all elements into a single tree.

MATERIALS AND METHODS

Six prepubertal (median age: 9 years) recently diagnosed (<6 months) DM-1 patients and six normal individuals presenting no family history of DM-1 or other autoimmune disorders and matched to the patients for sex and age were studied. All subjects were submitted to complete anamnesis and physical examination, and presented no infectious diseases. Patients were selected only after adequate insulin treatment leading to metabolic control of the disease, that is, normalization of glucose and glycate hemoglobin levels. Informed written consent was obtained from all individuals, and the local Ethics Committee approved the study protocol (Process No. 7945/99).

Total RNA obtained from peripheral blood mononuclear cells was extracted with Trizol (Invitrogen, Carlsbad, CA) according to manufacturer instructions. The gene expression profile was assessed using glass slide cDNA microarrays (IMAGE Consortium, available at http://image.llnl.gov). Differentially and

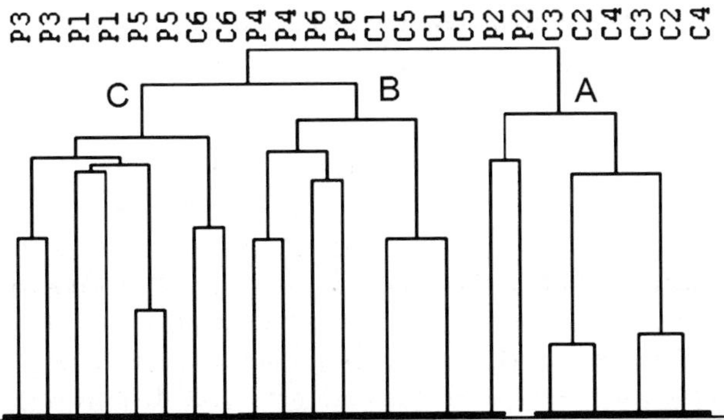

Patient and/or Control	HLA-DRB1	HLA-DQB1
P3	***0401** **0701*	***0201**, *0301
P1	**0701*, *1601	***0201**, *0502
P5	***0301, *0401**	***0201**, *0301
C6	***0301, *0405**	***0201,*0302**
P4	***0401**, *0701	***0201**, *0301
P6	**0701*, *0803	*0301, *0302
C1	**0701, *1301*	*0603, *0303
C5	**0701, *1101*	***0201**,*0301
P2	**0701, *1101*	***0201**, *0301
C3	**1501, *1303*	**0602*, *0301
C2	**1501, *1401*	**0602*
C4	**1502, *1301*	**0601*, *0603

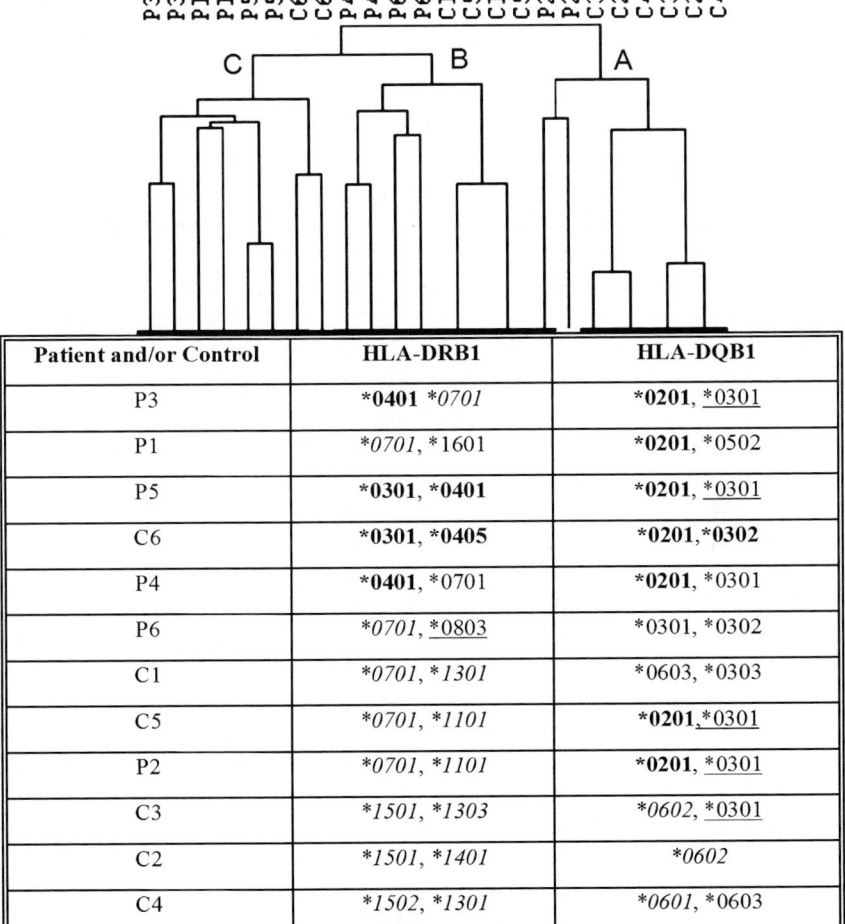

FIGURE 1. Hierarchical clustering of the significantly and differentially expressed genes observed in patients (P1–P6) with DM-1 and in controls (C1–C6). As the experiments were performed in duplicate, two numbers were assigned for each individual in the dendrogram, which has three major clusters A, B, and C. Cluster A (P2, C3, C2, C4) includes individuals with no susceptibility alleles, whereas cluster B (P4, P6, C1, C5) includes individuals with at least two susceptibility alleles, and cluster C (P3, P1, P5, C6) includes individuals with susceptibility/protective alleles. Susceptibility (in bold), protective (*in italics*), and neutral (underlined) DRB1 and DQB1 alleles[1] are also shown.

significantly expressed genes were obtained using the SAM (Significance Analysis of Microarrays) program (available at; http://www-stat.stanford.edu/~tibs/sam/). The hierarchical clustering algorithm was obtained using the Cluster software (available at http:rana.ibl.gov/EisenSoftware.htm) that applies the Pearson correlation and the average linkage for clustering organization from independent determinations of each patient studied. A total of 30 genes (21 induced and 9 repressed) were identified after applying the SAM program, as previously reported.[4]

RESULTS AND DISCUSSION

The dendrogram obtained by the Cluster program exhibited three major clusters (FIG. 1). Cluster A included three control individuals (C2, C3, and C4) and patient P2. Overall, the control individuals of cluster A did not exhibit DM-1 susceptibility alleles, whereas P2 possessed DQB1 alleles associated with susceptibility to the DQB1*0201 and *0301 and DRB1 alleles associated with protection against (*0701 and *1101) the disease development. On the other hand, cluster C included three patients (P1, P3, and P5) possessing two or three susceptibility alleles (DRB1*0401, *0301, and DQB1*0201). Clustered together with this group of patients, the control subject C6 exhibited four DM-1 susceptibility alleles (DRB1*0301, *0405, DQB1*0201, *0302) and exhibited no personal or family history of DM-1. Finally, cluster B included two patients (P4 and P6) who possessed two DM-1 susceptibility alleles (DQB1*0201, *0301) and at least one protective allele (DRB*0701), and the C1 and C5 controls exhibited more protective than susceptibility alleles. It is interesting to observe that patient P2 (cluster A) and control C5 (cluster B), who possessed identical DRB1 and DQB1, were clustered in distinct groups.

Considering that all patients had their disease diagnosed at closely similar times (<6 months), that the age and sex of the controls were closely similar, and that all patients were studied only after metabolic control of the disease, the results of the present study suggest that the HLA class II profile is another relevant variable to be controlled when differential gene expression is assessed.

Although the role of susceptibility/protective MHC class II alleles in differential gene expression has not been elucidated, the results of this study suggest that, in addition to sex, age, and ethnic background, the pairing of MHC class II alleles seems to be relevant for this type of study, and that further studies are needed to solve this question.

ACKNOWLEDGMENTS

This study was funded by FAPESP—Fundação de Amparo à Pesquisa do Estado de São Paulo (Grants No. 01/04101–9 and 99/12135-9) and CNPq (Brazil).

REFERENCES

1. ATKINSON, M.A. & G. EISENBARTH. 2001. Type 1 diabetes: new perspectives on disease pathogenesis and treatment. Lancet **358:** 221–229.

2. Boitard, C., J. Timsit, E. Larger & D. Dubois. 1997. Immune mechanisms leading to type 1 insulin-dependent diabetes mellitus. Horm. Res. **48**(Suppl 4): 58–63.
3. Fernandes, A.P.M., P. Louzada-Junior, M.C. Foss & E.A. Donadi. 2002. HLA-DRB1 and DQA1 allele profile in Brazilian patients with type 1 diabetes mellitus. Ann. N. Y. Acad. Sci. **958:** 305–308.
4. Rassi, D.M., C.M. Junta, A.L. Fachin, *et al.* 2006. Metabolism genes are amongst the differentially expressed ones observed in lymphomononuclear cells of recently diagnosed type 1 diabetes mellitus patients. Ann. N. Y. Acad. Sci. This volume.

Feasibility of a Type 1 Diabetes Primary Prevention Trial Using 2000 IU Vitamin D3 in Infants from the General Population with Increased HLA-Associated Risk

BRANDY A. WICKLOW AND SHAYNE P. TABACK

For the Winnipeg DVD Study Group, Departments of Pediatrics and Child Health and Community Health Sciences, University of Manitoba, Winnipeg, Manitoba, Canada R3E 0Z2

Abstract: Recent epidemiologic, immunologic, and NOD mouse studies suggest that intervention in the vitamin D system may be a successful method to prevent type 1 diabetes. Newborns at increased HLA-associated risk are randomized to receive either 400 or 2000 IU vitamin D3 by 1 month of age. We show that recruitment of babies from the general population for identification of HLA-associated risk status followed by enrollment to a randomized controlled prevention trial is feasible in Canada.

Keywords: type 1 diabetes; autoimmunity; prevention; vitamin D; pilot randomized controlled trial

INTRODUCTION

One approach to primary prevention of type 1 diabetes includes screening of newborn for genetic risk followed by intervention in high-risk infants. Recent epidemiologic,[1] immunologic,[2] and NOD mouse studies[3–5] suggest intervention in the vitamin D system may achieve primary prevention. Our objective is to conduct a pilot type 1 diabetes primary prevention trial using high-dose (2000 IU) vitamin D3 supplementation in newborns at-risk from the general population.

METHODS

Recruitment coordinators attended general obstetrics clinics. Cord blood or heel stick samples were collected postnatally. Following DNA isolation

Address for correspondence: Dr. Shayne P. Taback, 685 William Avenue, Winnipeg, MB, Canada R3E 0Z2. Voice: 204-787-1222; fax: 204-787-1655.
e-mail: tabacksp@cc.umanitoba.ca

**Ann. N.Y. Acad. Sci. 1079: 310–312 (2006). © 2006 New York Academy of Sciences.
doi: 10.1196/annals.1375.047**

and amplification, low-resolution HLA DQB1 typing was done using Dynal strip detection and pattern matching software. Babies with DQB1*02 and/or *03 genotypes were subsequently typed using high-resolution methodology. Those with DQB1*0201 and/or *0302 had HLA DRB1 low-resolution typing. DR4 positive high-resolution typing was performed to exclude *0403 and related alleles. Babies participating in the trial were randomized to receive either 400 or 2000 IU vitamin D3 by 1 month of age. Frequent follow-up visits in the first year of life were scheduled for measurements of auxology, bone densitometry, and biochemistry: serum calcium, phosphate, creatinine, 25-OH-vitamin D and 1,25-OH-vitamin D levels; and urine calcium, phosphate, and creatinine. Renal ultrasound is performed at 1 year of age.

RESULTS

Six hundred sixty-nine women were approached to date; 67% consented. The eligibility rates for the trial were: HLA genotype DRB1*03, DQB1*0201/DRB1*04, DQB1*0302 (where DRB1*04 is not equal to *0403 or related alleles): 7420 or 1.7% (95% CI: 0.8–3.4) and homozygous genotypes, either DRB1*03, DQB1*0201 or DRB1*04, DQB1*0302 (where DRB1*04 is not equal to *0403 or related alleles): 4230 or 1.7% (95% CI: 0.7–4.4). To date, 7 babies have been enrolled in the unblinded intervention trial; 4 babies randomized to receive 2000 IU per day have normal serum and urine calcium measurements, including 1 who has completed 12 months of treatment.

CONCLUSIONS

Recruitment of babies from the general population for identification of HLA-associated risk status followed by enrollment to a randomized controlled prevention trial is feasible in Canada. A prevention trial using 2000 IU per day of vitamin D3 is acceptable to families of infants at increased genetic risk. Early study results are in accord with the suggestion from medical literature that 2000 IU/day can be safely given.[6] The acceptability, low cost, and safety of the intervention suggest the possibility of definitively testing the hypothesis using a "large simple"[7] multi-institutional randomized controlled trial.

ACKNOWLEDGMENTS

Study funding was provided by: The Canadian Diabetes Association (operating grant), The Manitoba Medical Service Foundation (Clinical Research Professorship and research support to SPT), The Manitoba Institute of Child Health, and The Health Science Centre Medical Staff Council (resident research grant to BAW). The Winnipeg Diabetes-Vitamin D Study Group includes L. Berard RN, D. Black MD, E. Bloomfield, T. Blydt-Hansen MD, D. Catte RD, H.J. Dean MD, C. Greenberg MD, J. Laforte RD, J. Schellenberg RN, M.L. Schroeder MD, E.A.C. Sellers MD, S.P. Taback MD (PI), H.A. Weiler PhD, B. Wicklow MD, and C.K. Yuen MD.

REFERENCES

1. HYPPONEN, E., E. LAARA, A. REUNANEN, *et al.* 2001. Intake of vitamin D and risk of type 1 diabetes: a birth-cohort study. Lancet **9292:** 1500–1503.
2. GRIFFIN, M.D., N. XING & R. KUMAR. 2003. Vitamin D and its analogs as regulators of immune activation and antigen presentation. *In* Annual Review of Nutrition. McCormick D.B., D.M. Bier & R.J. Cousins, Eds.: 117–145. Annuals Reviews. Palo Alto.
3. MATHIEU, C., M. WAER, J. LAUREYS, *et al.* 1994. Prevention of autoimmune diabetes in NOD mice by 1,25 dihydroxyvitamin D3. Diabetologia **37:** 552–558.
4. ZELLA, J.B., L.C. MCCARY & H.F. DELUCA. 2003. Oral administration of 1,25-dihydroxyvitamin D3 completely protects NOD mice from insulin-dependent diabetes mellitus. Arch. Biochem. Biophys. **417:** 77–80.
5. GIULIETTI, A., C. GYSEMANS, K. STOFFELS, *et al.* 2004. Vitamin D deficiency in early life accelerates type 1 diabetes in non-obese diabetic mice. Diabetologia 2004; Published online January 31.
6. CALIKOGLU, A.S. & M.L. DAVENPORT. 2003. Prophylactic vitamin D supplementation. *In* Vitamin D and Rickets. Hochberg Z., Ed.: 233–258. Karger. Basel.
7. YUSUF, S., R. COLLINS & R. PETO. 1984. Why do we need some large, simple randomized trials? Stat. Med. **3:** 409–422.

Interleukin-10 Plasmid Construction and Delivery for the Prevention of Type 1 Diabetes

MINHYUNG LEE,[a] HYEWON PARK,[a,b] JEEHEE YOUN,[b] EUN TAEX OH,[a] KYUNGSOO KO,[c] SUNGWAN KIM,[a,d] AND YONGSOO PARK[a,b]

[a]*Department of Bioengineering, College of Engineering, Hanyang University, 471-020 Seoul, Korea*

[b]*Department of Internal Medicine and Cell Biology, College of Medicine, Hanyang University, Seoul, Korea*

[c]*Department of Internal Medicine, College of Medicine, Inje University, Seoul, Korea*

[d]*Department of Pharmaceutics and Pharmaceutical Chemistry, Center for Controlled Chemical Delivery, University of Utah, Salt Lake City, Utah 84112, USA*

ABSTRACT: Studies of animals with spontaneous autoimmune diabetes have revealed that autoreactive T cells that mediate islet β cell destruction can be manipulated by the administration of Th_2 cytokines. In this article, the effect of interleukin-10 (IL-10) gene delivery was evaluated *in vitro* and *in vivo* with a novel IL-10 plasmid, pSI-IL-10-NFκB. In pSI-IL-10-NFκB, the expression of the IL-10 gene was driven by the SV40 promotor/enhancer. The nuclear factor κB (NFκB) binding sites were also introduced to facilitate nuclear transport of the plasmid in the cell. *In vitro* transfection assay with pSI-IL-10-NFκB showed a similar expression level of IL-10 to the plasmid without NFκB binding sites (pSI-IL-10). pSI-IL-10-NFκB and pSI-IL-10 were intravenously injected into 5-week-old nonobese diabetic (NOD) mice using polyethylenimine (PEI) as a gene carrier. Both groups had persistent gene expression, longer than 5 weeks, and secreted the similarly high IL-10 serum levels. Interestingly, the degree of insulitis in the pSI-IL-10-NFκB group was improved over the pSI-IL-10 group, PEI-only group, and noninjected controls. The serum glucose levels showed that single injection of pSI-IL-10-NFκB prevented the development of diabetes in 100% of the pSI-IL-10-NFκB–injected animals (5/5), while that of pSI-IL-10 prevented diabetes in 40% of the treated animals (2/5). These results suggest that pSI-IL-10-NFκB with

Address for correspondence: Yongsoo Park, M.D., Department of Internal Medicine, Hanyang University Hospital, 249-1 Kyomun-dong, Kuri, Kyunggi-do 471-020, Korea. Voice: 82-31-560-2239; fax: 82-31-553-7369.
e-mail: parkys@hanyang.ac.kr

Ann. N.Y. Acad. Sci. 1079: 313–319 (2006). © 2006 New York Academy of Sciences.
doi: 10.1196/annals.1375.048

PEI can effectively reduce the incidence of insulitis and type 1 diabetes in NOD mice.

KEYWORDS: IL-10; nonviral gene delivery; NFκB binding sites; type 1 diabetes; NOD mouse

INTRODUCTION

Type 1 diabetes (T1D) is an autoimmune disease resulted from the destruction of the pancreatic β cell mediated by T lymphocytes that react specifically to one or more β cell proteins. Studies of animals with spontaneous T1D have indicated that autoreactive T cells that mediate β cell destruction can be manipulated by the administration of cytokines, especially Th_2 cytokines such as interleukin-10 (IL-10). In spite of their known efficacies as therapeutic agents, the cytokines are not clinically applicable because of their short half-lives. One way to overcome this drawback is to deliver a gene that enables the production of cytokine in the body. If a plasmid encoding IL-10 is delivered and processed effectively, therapeutic level of IL-10 can be achieved in the body for the modulation of immunologic triggering.

Nonviral gene delivery system is more desirable than the viral gene delivery system in terms of safety and ability carrying large amounts of DNA.[1,2] Nonviral gene delivery is typically composed of liposomes, polymers, and polymer-lipid hybrids.[1] In our previous report, an IL-10 gene delivery was tried using a degradable polymeric carrier.[3] The results showed that the IL-10 expression by the gene delivery prevented the development of insulitis in nonobese diabetic (NOD) mice effectively.[3] However, the mice eventually developed diabetes with increased serum glucose level by the single injection of the IL-10 gene.[4] This suggests that more efficient gene delivery system may be beneficial in the IL-10 gene delivery for T1D gene therapy. In the present study, the effect of IL-10 gene delivery was evaluated both *in vitro* and *in vivo* using a novel plasmid, pSI-IL-10-NFκB. In pSI-IL-10-NFκB, the expression of the IL-10 gene was controlled under the SV40 promotor/enhancer. In addition, nuclear factor κB (NFκB) binding sites were introduced to increase the nuclear transport of the plasmid in a cell. NFκB is a ubiquitous transcription factor which is localized in the cytoplasm in the absence of stimulation. Under stimulatory condition, NFκB is actively transported into the nucleus. Therefore, a plasmid with NFκB binding sites bound to NFκB and was cotransported into the nucleus under stimulation. However, the transfection was enhanced by 2.6- to 5.8-fold by the insertion of NFκB binding sites into plasmids even under nonstimulatory condition, because of basal transport of NFκB. In this study, pSI-IL-10-NFκB was constructed and evaluated *in vitro* and *in vivo* using polyethylenimine (PIE) as a gene carrier.

METHODS

Construction of IL-10 Plasmid with NFκB Binding Sites

pSI was purchased from Promega (Madison, WI). The IL-10 cDNA was isolated from pCAGGS-IL10 and inserted at XhoI site of pSI, resulting in the construction of pSI-IL-10 (FIG. 1). The NFκB binding sites were synthesized chemically. The sequence of the NFκB binding site is as follows: 5′-GGGGACTTTCC-3′. Five copies of the NFκB binding sites were inserted upstream of the SV40 promotor/enhancer at BglII site of pSI-IL-10, resulting in the construction of pSI-IL-10-NFκB (FIG. 1). The constructed plasmids were confirmed by restriction enzyme reactions and direct sequencing.

In Vitro Study

Polymer/DNA complexes were prepared by self-assembly. PEI (25,000 Da) was dissolved in 5% glucose solution. The diluted polymer solution was slowly dropped into the prepared DNA plasmid and left for 30 min for formation of complex. PEI/DNA complex was prepared at a 5/1 N/P (nitrogen of polymer/phosphate of DNA) ratio. HepG2 cells were cultured and transfected with PEI/pSI-IL-10-NFκB or PEI/pSI-IL-10 complex as previously described.[5] After transfection, the medium was collected and the amount of IL-10 was determined by using an optE1A mouse IL-10 ELISA set (Pharmingen, San Diego, CA).

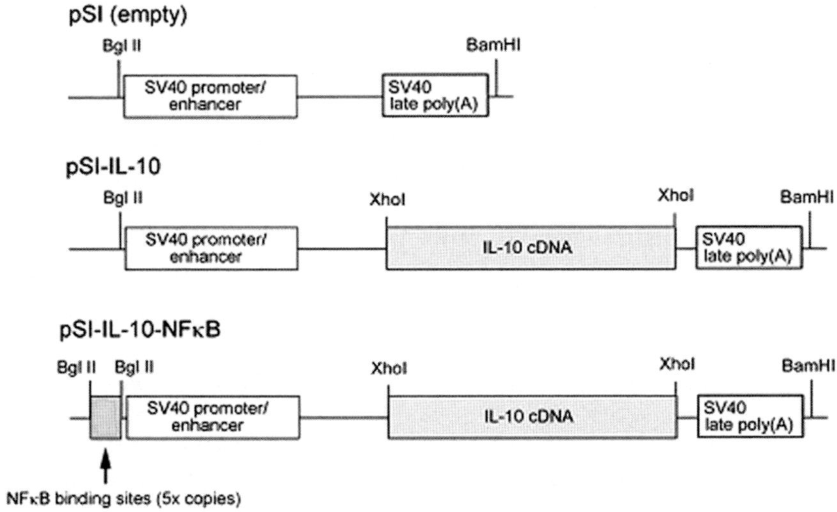

FIGURE 1. The schematic presentation of the structure of pSI (empty), pSI-IL-10, and pSI-IL-10-NFκB.

In Vivo Study

Four-week-old female NOD mice were purchased from Jackson Laboratory (Bar Harbor, ME) and kept under pathogen-free conditions. PEI/DNA complex was intravenously injected at a 5 weeks of age via tail vein at a dose of 50 μg of DNA per mouse. Mice were sacrificed at the scheduled times. The blood was collected, centrifuged at 3500 rpm for 10 min and stored at −70°C (n = 8 in each group; pSI-IL-10-NFκB group, pSI-IL-10 group, PEI-only group, and noninjected controls; total $n = 32$). The pancreas was harvested and stored at −70°C until use. The amount of IL-10 in the serum was also determined by the same mouse IL-10 ELISA kit. The pancreas sections (5μm) were cut and stained with hematoxyline-eosin. More than 20 islets from each pancreas were examined using double-blinded methods from four animal groups. Each islet was graded into five grades as previously described.[6] We obtained blood glucose levels weekly and analyzed glucose levels with an Accu-Check Instant glucometer (Roche Diagnostics Co., Indianapolis, IN). Two consecutive glucose levels ≥13.9 mmol/L were considered as hyperglycemia.

Statistical Analysis

Comparison of IL-10 levels were made by Student's t-test. The comparison of the effect on the suppression of insulitis or on the T1D development was made by χ^2 test.

RESULTS

Production of IL-10 in Transfected HepG2 Cells

To evaluate the expression levels of IL-10 *in vitro*, pSI-IL-10-NFκB and pSI-IL-10 were transfected to HepG2 cells. ELISA for IL-10 was performed 48 h after transfection. The results showed that pSI-IL-10-NFκB and pSI-IL-10 expressed much higher level of IL-10 than pSI. However, the pSI-IL-10-NFκB–transfected cells secretes similar amount of IL-10 to the pSI-IL-10–transfected cells.

In Vivo Transfection of PEI/pSI-IL-10-NFκB Complex

The PEI/pSI-IL-10 and PEI/pSI-IL-10-NFκB complexes were injected into 5-week-old NOD mice and compared with the PEI-only group. Noninjected group served as the negative control. The expression levels of IL-10 were evaluated by ELISA with serum at various time points. The expression of IL-10 was highest 1 day after the injection and the level continuously decreased with time. Both groups had persistent gene expression longer than 5 weeks, and secreted the similarly high IL-10 serum levels.

Prevention of Autoimmune Insulitis and Diabetes Development

The insulitis level of each injection group was evaluated 9 weeks after the injection. The degree of insulitis in the pSI-IL-10-NFκB group was improved over that in the pSI-IL-10 group, PEI-only group, and noninjected controls (FIG. 2). We measured glucose levels weekly up to the age of 32 weeks, revealing that a single injection of pSI-IL-10-NFκB prevented the development of diabetes in 100% of the treated animals (0/5 develop diabetes). In contrast, the pSI-IL-10 group, PEI-only group, and noninjected control group develop diabetes in 60% (3/5), 75% (3/4), and 60% (3/5) of the treated animals, respectively. These results suggest that a single injection of the novel plasmid with NFκB binding sites along with PEI can effectively reduce the incidence of insulitis and T1D in NOD mice.

DISCUSSION

In spite of its remarkable advantages as a therapeutic agent for T1D development, Th_2 cytokines are not immediately clinically applicable because of their short half-lives. To overcome this drawback, a new IL-10 gene delivery was constructed and evaluated *in vitro* and *in vivo*. It was previously suggested

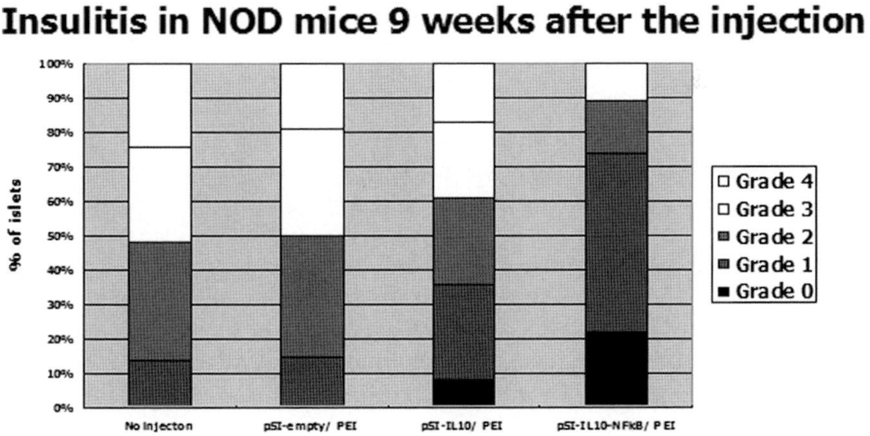

FIGURE 2. Suppression of insulitis after intravenous injection of PEI/pSI-IL-10-NFκB plasmid complexes in NOD mice. Insulitis was evaluated 9 weeks after the injection by hematoxylin-eosin staining of islets from each pancreas. More than 20 islets from each pancreas were examined using double-blind methods from four animal groups ($n = 2$ in each group).

that there are three barriers in the intracellular delivery of DNA.[7] The three barriers are cellular membrane, endosomal membrane, and nucleus membrane. For conventional gene therapy, polymer/DNA complex is internalized into the cells by endocytosis. After endocytosis, the polymer/DNA complex must escape from the endosomal compartment before fusion to lysosome to avoid enzymatic degradation in lysosome. Then, DNA must be delivered to the nucleus for transcription. One way to enhance gene expression efficiency is to increase nuclear transport of plasmid into cells. NFκB is a family of transcription factors present in every cell type.[8] The previous report suggests that the incorporation of the NFκB binding sites into the delivered DNA facilitated the intracellular trafficking of the DNA and eventually increased the gene expression level.[9] In this study, pSI-IL-10-NFκB was constructed with five copies of the NFκB binding sites. The *in vitro* and *in vivo* transfection showed that the IL-10 expression level was not induced significantly. However, the injection of pSI-IL-10-NFκB was therapeutically effective, compared to other plasmids. A single systemic injection of pSI-IL-10-NFκB using PEI expressed IL-10 effectively for up to 5 weeks and decreased the degree of insulitis dramatically. A total of 74% of observed islets were intact in the pSI-IL-10-NFκB group, compared with 14% in the control group. Moreover, in the pSI-IL-10-NFκB group, no mouse out of five developed diabetes until 32 weeks of age. The effect on the suppression of insulitis and diabetes in this study was greater than that in our previous studies applying different strategies.[3,4,6] This result indicates that complete prevention of T1D can be achieved by a single injection of the cytokine gene with polymeric gene carrier.

It is unclear why pSI-IL-10-NFκB was effective in the prevention of T1D, although it showed similar level of the IL-10 expression to pSI-IL-10. We speculate that the nuclear transport of DNA might have some inhibitory effect on the development of T1D. It has been suggested that the activation of NFκB participates in chronic inflammatory disorders including diabetes. As each pSI-IL-10-NFκB has five copies of the NFκB binding sites, active NFκBs may bind to these sites and not be available to other promotor sites, resulting in the alteration of the gene expression profile. This hypothesis is to be tested yet.

We started the intervention using 5-week-old mice as most reports of immune intervention in NOD mice showed that treatment should be initiated at the early stage of insulitis.[10] Although the local delivery of cytokines to sites of inflammation for a rational and effective immunotherapy might be plausible, most reports of systemically administered IL-4 or IL-10 have demonstrated the benefits of this strategy.[3,4,6,11]

In conclusion, systemic delivery of pSI-IL-10-NFκB using polymeric gene carrier was effective in the gene therapy to prevent T1D in NOD mice. Although the mechanism of the system is not evident, the pSI-IL-10-NFκB/PEI system may be useful to eventually develop an effective and safe gene therapy system for T1D.

ACKNOWLEDGMENTS

This work was supported by the grants from Korea Science & Engineering Foundation (R01-2001-00177 and R01-2005-10075).

REFERENCES

1. Han, S. *et al.* 2000. Development of biomaterials for gene therapy. Mol. Ther. **2:** 302–317.
2. Lee, M. & S.W. Kim. 2005. Polyethylene glycol-conjugated copolymers for plasmid DNA delivery. Pharm. Res. **22:** 1–10.
3. Koh, J.J. *et al.* 2000. Degradable polymeric carrier for the delivery of IL-10 plasmid DNA to prevent autoimmune insulitis of NOD mice. Gene. Ther. **7:** 2099–2104.
4. Ko, K. *et al.* 2001. Combined administration of plasmids encoding IL-4 and IL-10 prevents the development of autoimmune diabetes in nonobese diabetic mice. Mol. Ther. **4:** 313–316.
5. Oh, S. *et al.* 2003. GLP-1 gene delivery for the treatment of type 2 diabetes. Mol. Ther. **7:** 478–483.
6. Lee, M. *et al.* 2003. Prevention of autoimmune insulitis by delivery of a chimeric plasmid encoding interleukin-4 and interleukin-10. J. Control Release **88:** 333–342.
7. Nishikawa, M. & L. Huang. 2001. Nonviral vectors in the new millennium: delivery barriers in gene transfer. Hum. Gene Ther. **12:** 861–870.
8. Barnes, P.J. & M. Karin. 1997. Nuclear factor-κB-a pivotal transcription factor in chronic inflammatory diseases. N. Engl. J. Med. **336:** 1066–1071.
9. Mesika, A. *et al.* 2001. A regulated, NFκB-assisted import of plasmid DNA into mammalian cell nuclei. Mol. Ther. **3:** 653–657.
10. Leiter, E.H. 1996. Lessons from the animal models: the NOD mouse. *In* Prediction, Prevention and Genetic Counseling in IDDM. J.P. Palmer, Ed.: 201–226. John Wiley & Sons. Chichester.
11. Cameron, M.J. *et al.* 2000. Immunotherapy of spontaneous type 1 diabetes in nonobese diabetic mice by systemic interleukin-4 treatment employing adenovirus vector-mediated gene transfer. Gene Ther. **7:** 1840–1846.

TEDDY–The Environmental Determinants of Diabetes in the Young

An Observational Clinical Trial

WILLIAM A. HAGOPIAN,[a] ÅKE LERNMARK,[b] MARIAN J. REWERS,[c] OLLI G. SIMELL,[d] JIN-XIONG SHE,[e] ANETTE G. ZIEGLER,[f] JEFFREY P. KRISCHER,[g] AND BEENA AKOLKAR[h]

[a]*Pacific Northwest Research Institute, Seattle, Washington 98122, USA*

[b]*University Hospital MAS, 20522 Malmö, Sweden*

[c]*University of Colorado, Denver, Colorado 80162, USA*

[d]*Turku University Central Hospital, Turku, 20520 Finland, USA*

[e]*Medical College of Georgia, Augusta, Georgia 30912, USA*

[f]*Diabetes Research Institute, 80804 Munich, Germany*

[g]*University of South Florida, Tampa, Florida 33612, USA*

[h]*National Institutes of Health, Bethesda, Maryland 20892, USA*

ABSTRACT: The aim of the TEDDY study is to identify infectious agents, dietary factors, or other environmental agents, including psychosocial factors, which may either trigger islet autoimmunity, type 1 diabetes mellitus (T1DM), or both. The study has two end points: (*a*) appearance of islet autoantibodies and (*b*) clinical diagnosis of T1DM. Six clinical centers screen newborns for high-risk HLA genotypes. As of December 2005 a total of 54,470 newborns have been screened. High-risk HLA genotypes among 53,560 general population (GP) infants were 2576 (4.8%) and among 910 newborns with a first-degree relative (FDR) were 194 (21%). A total of 1061 children have been enrolled. The initial enrollment results demonstrate the feasibility of this complex and demanding a prospective study.

KEYWORDS: type 1 diabetes; islet autoantibodies; HLA; virus

INTRODUCTION

The incidence of type 1 diabetes mellitus (T1DM), one of the most common and serious chronic diseases in children is increasing worldwide.[1,2] While

Address for correspondence: Åke Lernmark, Ph.D., CRC Lund University, Department of Clinical Sciences, University Hospital MAS, SE-205 02 Malmö, Sweden. Voice: +46 40 391901; fax: +46 40 39 19 19.
e-mail: Ake.lernmark@med.lu.se

Ann. N.Y. Acad. Sci. 1079: 320–326 (2006). © 2006 New York Academy of Sciences.
doi: 10.1196/annals.1375.049

the incidence is highest in Scandinavia (30–50/100,000), intermediate in the United States (15–25/100,000 in 1998), and somewhat lower in Central and Eastern Europe (5–15/100,000), it is unclear to what extent these geographic differences may reflect variation in genetic susceptibility, in prevalence of causal environmental factors, or both; although major advances have been made in the identification of genetic factors that confer susceptibility or resistance to T1DM.[3,4] The dissection of the etiology of T1DM is further complicated by epidemiological observations that approximately 85–90% of new onset patients have no first degree relative (FDR) with T1DM despite a strong familiar clustering of patients.[5] Genetic variability in the HLA region explains ~50% of the familiar clustering[6] but other genes identified so far provide more modest contributions to risk.[3,4] Additional factors are important, because only 1 out of 15 people in the general population (GP) with the highest risk HLA genotypes develops T1DM.

The mechanisms by which environmental factors may trigger either islet autoimmunity, T1DM, or both in susceptible subjects are not understood. The aim of the present multicenter study is to examine from birth high-risk GP children and FDR and systematically screen them for candidate environmental and genetic factors. Identification of such factors will lead to a better understanding of disease pathogenesis and result in new strategies to prevent, delay, or reverse T1DM.

SUBJECTS AND METHODS

Subjects

A cohort of children with elevated genetic risk for T1DM is established by screening newborns from the GP and from families with FDR diagnosed with T1DM. A total of six clinical centers from Seattle, WA, Denver, CO, Augusta, GE, Munich, Germany, Turku, Finland, and Malmö, Sweden participate.

HLA Typing and Genetic Risk

Genetically susceptible children are identified through newborn HLA-DR/DQ screening. Genotype screening is performed using either a dried blood spot (DBS) punch or a small volume whole blood lysate (WBL) specimen. A screening blood sample is obtained either at birth as a cord blood sample or using heel stick capillary sample up to the age of 3 months. This exception is made to maximize the number of newborn relatives participating in this study. After polymerase chain reaction (PCR) amplification of exon 2 of the HLA Class II gene (DRB1, DQA1 or DQB1), alleles will be identified either by direct sequencing, oligonucleotide probe hybridization, or other genotyping techniques (TABLE 1).

TABLE 1. HLA genotypes used to enroll newborns in the TEDDY study

TEDDY genotype
DR4- DQA1*0301-DQB1*0302@ / DR3- DQA1*0501-DQB1*0201
DR4- DQA1*0301-DQB1*0302 / DR4- DQA1*0301-DQB1*0302
DR4- DQA1*0301-DQB1*0302@ / DR8- DQA1*0401-DQB1*0402
DR3-DQA1*0501-DQB1*0201 / DR3-DQA1*0501-DQB1*0201
DR4- DQA1*0301-DQB1*0302@ / DR4- DQA1*0301-DQB1*0201
DR4- DQA1*0301-DQB1*0302@ / DR1#- DQA1*0101-DQB1*0501
DR4- DQA1*0301-DQB1*0302@ /DR13-DQA1*0102-DQB1*0604
DR4- DQA1*0301-DQB1*0302 / DR4- DQA1*0301-DQB1*0304
DR4- DQA1*0301-DQB1*0302@ / DR9- DQA1*0301-DQB1*0303
DR3- DQA1*0501-DQB1*0201 / DR9- DQA1*0301-DQB1*0303

Genotypes a–d are eligible from the GP and genotypes a–j for FDR.
@Acceptable alleles in this haplotype include both DQB1*0302 and *0304.
#In this DQB1*0501 haplotype, DR10 must be excluded. Only DR1 is eligible.

Follow-Up Schedule for Children with Increased Genetic Risk

Children with increased genetic risk are followed for environmental exposures and diet with a clinic visit every 3 months for the first 4 years of life and then biannually until age the 15 years. Stool samples are collected to assess viral exposures at monthly intervals for the first 4 years of life and then biannually until the age 15. In addition, dietary, infectious, and psychosocial assessments are completed at each visit to the clinic.

RESULTS

The TEDDY study was initiated September 1, 2004 with the aim to screen 220,800 newborn children over a total of 4 years. After an initial start-up phase all six clinical centers have been recruiting newborns for about 1 year. As of December 2005 the data show that a total of 54,470 (98% of expected) newborns have been screened. High-risk HLA genotypes among 53,560 GP infants were 2576 (4.8%) and among 910 FDR newborns were 194 (21%). The HLA distribution of these children demonstrate that the 97% of the 2528 eligible children typed so far represents the high-risk genotypes a, b, c, and d (TABLE 2). A total of 1061 children have been enrolled at the end of December 2005. The first group of children has been followed for 1 year and the prospective analysis has continued successfully with only a few families leaving the study. One TEDDY infant has developed T1DM at 8 months of age.

DISCUSSION

The present report represents about 1-year experience in screening newborn children to be enrolled in the TEDDY study. The target to screen 55,200

TABLE 2. HLA genotypes among eligible and enrolled newborns in the TEDDY study

TEDDY genotype	Eligible *n*	%	Enrolled *n*	%
a	977	38.4	403	41.8
b	503	19.7	186	19.2
c	444	17.4	157	16.2
d	555	21.8	188	19.5
e	2	0.1	2	0.2
f	40	1.6	18	1.8
g	7	0.3	3	0.3
h	3	0.1	3	0.3
i	4	0.2	2	0.2
j	8	0.3	2	0.2
Total	2,543		964	

newborn children per year to reach 220,800 children over a 4-year period was reached. Consistent with the observations that only 10–15% of newly diagnosed T1DM children have an FDR with the disease,[5] it is noted that 910 (1.7%) of 54,470 screened newborns belong to this group. This frequency is far from a true reflection of the prevalence rate of T1DM in participating GPs but rather reflects our planned effort to screen children born in families with a father, mother, or sibling with T1DM. The rationale for a focus on FDR is the well-known risk for a child to develop T1DM if the father, mother, or a sibling (in this order) is affected as compared to the GP. The average increase is three- to eightfold which means that a higher proportion of newborns in the FDR group will not only reach the first end point of islet autoantibody positivity but also the second end point of T1DM during 15 years of follow up.

The HLA genotypes selected as TEDDY inclusion criteria (TABLE 1) represent both genotypes that confer the highest risk in population-based studies[7,8] as well as in family studies.[8,9] The a, b, c, and d TEDDY genotypes are also the genotypes that predominate subjects with T1DM regardless of whether they represent the GP or FDR. It is noted that the two most critical haplotype for T1DM risk is the DR4-DQA1*0301-B1*0302 and the DR3-DQA1*0501-B1*0201 haplotypes. In particular, the DR4-DQA1*0301-B1*0302 haplotype predominates and is present in 8 out of 10 of the TEDDY genotypes. Only the "d" and "j" haplotypes are non-DR4-DQA1*0301-B1*0302 and after 1 year of screening 20% of eligible children were DR3-DQA1*0501-B1*0201 homozygous. This group will serve as an important immunogenetics reference group with respect to trigger exposures and the development of islet autoantibodies.

The TEDDY study will provide an important opportunity to improve our understanding of the events leading to T1DM by studying from birth high-risk GP children and FDR and by systematic screening of candidate environmental and genetic factors. In addition, samples collected by TEDDY will create a valuable resource for investigators proposing innovative hypotheses concerning candidate environmental and genetic factors.

The long-term goal of the TEDDY study is the identification of infectious agents, dietary factors, or other environmental agents, including psychosocial factors, which trigger beta cell autoimmunity, T1DM, or both, in genetically susceptible individuals or which protect against the disease. Identification of such factors will lead to a better understanding of disease pathogenesis and result in new strategies to prevent, delay, or reverse T1DM.

ACKNOWLEDGMENT

The TEDDY Study Group (Appendix) is Funded by the National Institute of Diabetes and Digestive and Kidney Diseases (NIDDK), National Institute of Allergy and Infectious Diseases (NIAID), National Institute of Child Health and Human Development (NICHD), National Institute of Environmental Health Sciences (NIEHS), Juvenile Diabetes Research Foundation (JDRF), and Centers for Disease Control and Prevention (CDC).

APPENDIX

The Teddy Study Group

Colorado Clinical Center: Marian Rewers, M.D., Ph.D., PI,[1,4,6,10,11] Katherine Barriga,[12] Judith Baxter,[9,12] Ann Deas, George Eisenbarth, M.D., Ph.D., Lisa Emery, Patricia Gesualdo,[2,12] Michelle Hoffman,[12] Jill Norris, Ph.D.,[2,12] Kathleen Waugh,[7,12] Stacey Weber. University of Colorado at Denver and Health Sciences Center, Barbara Davis Center for Childhood Diabetes.

Georgia/Florida Clinical Center: Jin-Xiong She, Ph.D., PI,[1,3,4,11] Andy Muir, M.D.,[7] Desmond Schatz, M.D.,[*4,5,7,8] Diane Hopkins,[12] Leigh Steed,[12] Angela Choate,[*12] Katherine Silvis,[2] Meena Shankar,[*2] Yi-Hua Huang, Ph.D., Ping Yang, Wei-Peng Zheng, Hong-Jie Wang, Kim English and Richard McIndoe, Ph.D. Medical College of Georgia, *University of Florida.

Germany Clinical Center: Anette G. Ziegler, M.D., PI,[1,3,4,11] Ezio Bonifacio, Ph.D.,[*5] Andrea Baumgarten,[12] Sandra Hummel, Ph.D.,[2] Mathilde Kersting,[2] Stephanie Koenig,[2] Annette Knopff,[7] Angelika Locher,[12] Roswith Roth, Ph.D.,[9] Stefanie Schoen,[2] Petra Schwaiger,[7] Wolfgang Sichert-Hellert, Ph.D.,[2] Christiane Winkler,[2,12] Diana Zimmermann, Ph.D.[7,12] Diabetes Research Institute, *San Raffaele Institute.

Finland Clinical Center: Olli G. Simell, M.D., Ph.D., PI,[¥1,4,11] Kirsti Nanto-Salonen, M.D., Ph.D.,[¥12] Jorma Ilonen, M.D., Ph.D.,[¥3] Mikael Knip, M.D., Ph.D.,[*±] Riitta Veijola, M.D., Ph.D.,[µ¤] Tuula Simell, Ph.D.,[¥9,12] Ulla Uusitalo, Ph.D.,[§2] Heikki Hyöty, M.D., Ph.D.,[*±6] Suvi

M. Virtanen, M.D., Ph.D.,[*§2] Carina Kronberg-Kippilä,[§2] Maija Torma,[¥] Eeva Ruohonen,[¥] Minna Romo,[¥] Elina Mantymaki,[¥] Tiina Niininen,[*±] Mia Nyblom,[*±] Aino Stenius.[μ¤] [¥]University of Turku, [*]University of Tampere, [μ]University of Oulu, Turku University Hospital, [±]Tampere University Hospital, [¤]Oulu University Hospital, [§]National Public Health Institute, Finland.

Sweden Clinical Center: Åke Lernmark, Ph.D., PI,[1,3,4,5,8,10,11] Peter Almgren, Carin Andrén-Aronsson,[2] Eva Andersson, Sylvia Bianconi-Svensson,[2] Ulla-Marie Carlsson, Corrado Cilio, M.D., Ph.D., Joanna Gerardsson, Barbro Gustavsson, Anna Hansson,[2] Gertie Hansson,[12] Ida Hansson, Sten Ivarsson, M.D., Ph.D.,[6,7] Helena Larsson M.D., Elli Karlsson, Anastasia Katsarou M.D., Barbro Lernmark, Ph.D.,[9,12] Thea Massadakis, Anita Nilsson, Monica Sedig Järvirova, Birgitta Sjöberg, Anne Wallin, Åsa Wimar. Lund University.

Washington Clinical Center: William A. Hagopian, M.D., Ph.D., PI,[1,3,4,7,11] Michael Brantley,[7,12] Claire Cowen, Peng Hui, M.D., Ph.D., Kristen M. Hay,[2] Melissa Jackson, Viktoria Stepikova, Jennifer Ugale.[2,12] Pacific Northwest Research Institute.

Data Coordinating Center: Jeffrey P. Krischer, Ph.D., PI,[1,4,5,10,11] Carole Bray,[12] David Cuthbertson, Veena Gowda, Kimberly Hunt,[12] Shu Liu, Jamie Malloy, Cristina McCarthy,[12] Wendy McLeod,[2,9] Susan Moyers, Ph.D.,[2,10] Lavanya Nallamshetty, Susan Smith.[12] University of South Florida.

Project officer: Beena Akolkar, Ph.D.,[1,3,4,5,7,10,11] National Institutes of Diabetes and Digestive and Kidney Diseases.

Other contributors: Thomas Briese,[6] Columbia University, Henry Erlich,[3] Children's Hospital Oakland Research Institute, Suzanne Bennett Johnson,[9,12] Florida State University, Steve Oberste,[6] Centers for Disease Control and Prevention.

Committees:

[1]Ancillary Studies, [2]Diet, [3]Genetics [4]Human Subjects/Publicity/Publications, [5]Immune Markers, [6]Infectious Agents, [7]Laboratory Implementation, [8]Maternal Studies, [9]Psychosocial, [10]Quality Assurance, [11]Steering, [12]Study Coordinators.

REFERENCES

1. Green, A. & C.C. Patterson. 2001. Trends in the incidence of childhood-onset diabetes in Europe 1989–1998. Diabetologia **44**(Suppl 3): B3–B8.
2. Onkamo, P. *et al.* 1999. Worldwide increase in incidence of type I diabetes–the analysis of the data on published incidence trends. Diabetologia **42:** 1395–1403.

3. Concannon, P. *et al.* 2005. Type 1 diabetes: evidence for susceptibility loci from four genome-wide linkage scans in 1,435 multiplex families. Diabetes **54:** 2995–3001.
4. Rich, S.S. & P. Concannon. 2002. Challenges and strategies for investigating the genetic complexity of common human diseases. Diabetes **51**(Suppl 3): S288–S294.
5. Dahlquist, G. *et al.* 1989. The Swedish Childhood Diabetes Study—results from a nine year case register and one year case-referent study indicating that type 1 (insulin-dependent) diabetes mellitus is associated with both type 2 (non-insulin-dependent) diabetes mellitus and autoimmune disorders. Diabetologia **32:** 2–6.
6. Davies, J.L. *et al.* 1994. A genome-wide search for human type 1 diabetes susceptibility genes. Nature **371:** 130–136.
7. Graham, J. *et al.* 2002. Genetic effects on age-dependent onset and islet cell autoantibody markers in type 1 diabetes. Diabetes **51:** 1346–1555.
8. Veijola, R. *et al.* 1996. HLA-DQB1-defined genetic susceptibility, beta cell autoimmunity, and metabolic characteristics in familial and nonfamilial insulin-dependent diabetes mellitus. J. Clin. Invest. **98:** 2489–2495.
9. Baisch, J.M. *et al.* 1990. Analysis of HLA-DQ genotypes and susceptibility in insulin-dependent diabetes mellitus. N. Engl. J. Med. **322:** 1836–1882.

Protection From Type 1 Diabetes by Vitamin D Receptor Haplotypes

ELIZABETH RAMOS-LOPEZ,[a] THOMAS JANSEN,[a] VYTAUTAS IVASKEVICIUS,[b] HEINRICH KAHLES,[a] CHRISTIAN KLEPZIG,[a] JOHANNES OLDENBURG,[b] AND KLAUS BADENHOOP[a]

[a]*Department of Internal Medicine I, Division of Endocrinology, University Hospital Frankfurt, 60590 Frankfurt am Main, Germany*

[b]*Red Cross Blood Transfusion Center, Institute of Transfusion Medicine and Immunohaematology, 60590 Frankfurt am Main, Germany*

ABSTRACT: Vitamin D has been involved in the modulation of calcium and bone metabolism as well as in the immune system, where it suppresses the proliferation of activated T cells. These effects are exerted via the vitamin D receptor (VDR). Polymorphisms within this gene have been exhaustively studied in diverse autoimmune diseases but with inconsistent results. We previously reported a positive association of polymorphisms within the VDR gene (Apa I, Taq I, Bsm I, and Fok I). In the present article we extended our previous reports to seven additional polymorphisms (rs757343, rs9729, rs2853559, rs1989969, rs3847987, rs2238135, and rs4516035) in a larger set of German simplex type 1 diabetes families. Additionally we correlated serum levels of 25(OH)D_3 and 1,25$(OH)_2D_3$ with VDR genotypes and haplotypes. The haplotypes "CG" (Taq I-Apa I), "CGG" (Taq I-Apa I-Tru I), "CGC" (Taq I-Apa I-Fok I), "GCTG" (rs9729-Taq I-Apa I-Tru I), and "CGGC"(Taq I-Apa I, Tru I, Fok I) were less often transmitted, thus negatively associated with type 1 diabetes. Patients who carried the genotype "CC" of the rs3847987 polymorphism had higher median serum levels of 25(OH)D_3. Furthermore, the majority of patients with this genotype possessed normal serum levels of 25(OH)D_3. We conclude that variants of the VDR may confer a genetic protection from type 1 diabetes. Furthermore, normal serum levels of 25(OH)D_3 appear to correlate with a VDR genotype. This supports a role of vitamin D in the immune pathogenesis of type 1 diabetes.

KEYWORDS: vitamin D; vitamin D receptor; type 1 diabetes

Address for correspondence: Prof. K. Badenhoop, Department of Internal Medicine I, Division of Endocrinology, University Hospital Frankfurt, Theodor-Stern-Kai 7, 60590 Frankfurt am Main, Germany. Voice: +49-69-6301-5396; fax: +49-69-6301-6405.
e-mail: badenhoop@em.uni-frankfurt.de

Ann. N.Y. Acad. Sci. 1079: 327–334 (2006).
doi: 10.1196/annals.1375.050

INTRODUCTION

The vitamin D system has been involved in a wide variety of biological processes including the calcium and bone metabolism as well as the immune system. The most active form of vitamin D, $1{,}25(OH)_2D_3$, prevents spontaneous autoimmune diabetes in nonobese diabetic (NOD) mice.[1] Additionally there is evidence that the supplementation of vitamin D in early life reduces the risk for type 1 diabetes.[2]

$1{,}25(OH)_2D_3$ showed to inhibit antigen-induced T cell proliferation, cytokine production, and selective development of Th1 cells.[3,4] These effects are mediated via the vitamin D receptor (VDR), that is found in high concentrations on T lymphocytes and macrophages.[5]

In humans, the VDR gene has been mapped to chromosome 12q12-q14 consisting of 14 exons spanning a region of approximately 75 kb of genomic DNA.[6] The VDR can regulate expression of genes by interaction with specific response elements in the promotor region of hormone-sensitive target genes.[7]

Polymorphisms or haplotypes within the VDR have been suggested to play a role in the pathogenesis of diverse autoimmune endocrine diseases including type 1 diabetes.[8,9] Nevertheless a recent study could not confirm an association between VDR polymorphisms and type 1 diabetes.[10,11]

Given the controversial association between polymorphisms within the VDR gene and type 1 diabetes, we extended our previous report[9] of the polymorphisms Apa I (rs7975232), Taq I (rs731236), Bsm I (rs1544410), and Fok I (rs10735810) to a larger set of type 1 simplex diabetes families. Furthermore, we investigated the role of the polymorphisms rs757343 (Tru I), rs9729, rs2853559, rs1989969, rs3847987, rs2238135, and rs4516035 in order to confirm VDR genotypes or haplotypes as markers for type 1 diabetes in our population.

Additionally the influence of the above mentioned single nucleotide polymorphism (SNPs) on the serum levels of the vitamin D metabolites $25(OH)D_3$ and $1{,}25(OH)_2D_3$ was evaluated.

SUBJECTS AND METHODS

Subjects

Type 1 diabetes was diagnosed according to the World Health Organization criteria. All families were recruited from the endocrine outpatient clinics at the University Hospital Frankfurt am Main, Germany. The female–male ratio of the affected siblings was 1:1.03 and the median age at the diagnosis was 11.5 years. All participants were of German origin.

The study protocol was approved by the Ethics Committee of the University Hospital Frankfurt am Main and written informed consent was obtained of all subjects.

Genotyping

Genomic DNA was amplified using polymerase chain reaction (PCR). Amplified DNA was digested with restriction enzymes (purchased from New England Biolabs Beverly, MA) according to manufacturer's instructions. Digestions products were separated in a 3% agarose gel stained with ethidiumbromide.

The number of families analyzed for each SNP, primers sequences, length of the PCR products, annealing temperature T (°C), restriction enzymes, and sizes of the obtained fragments as well as the cut alleles are listed in TABLE 1. rs9729 and rs4516035 polymorphisms were genotyped using real time PCR (ABI 7300; Applied Biosystems Darmstadt, Germany) according to manufacturer's instructions.

Apa I, Taq I, Bsm I, Fok I, and Tru I were genotyped as previously reported[9]and the alleles were denominated by a lower case letter in the presence of a restriction site and by a capital letter in its absence. The remaining polymorphisms were designated according to the allele that was cut by the restriction enzyme.

Measurement of $25(OH)D_3$ and $1,25(OH)_2D_3$ Serum Level

Serum samples were obtained for measurement of the $25(OH)D_3$ (n = 158) and for the $1,25(OH)_2D_3$ (n = 149) concentrations in type 1 diabetes patients.

Serum concentrations of $25(OH)D_3$ and $1,25(OH)_2D_3$ were measured by radioimmunoassay (I^{125} RIA Kit, [DiaSorin, Stillwater, MN] and Gamma-B 1,25-Dihydroxy Vitamin D RIA [Immunodiagnostic Systems, Boldon, UK], respectively). Concentrations of $25(OH)D_3$ <10 ng/mL were defined as vitamin D deficiency and <20 ng/mL as insufficiency,[12,13] while concentration of the most active vitamin D metabolite, $1,25(OH)_2D_3$ of 19.9–67 pmol/ML were considered normal according to the.

Statistical Analysis

SNPs frequencies and haplotypes frequencies were estimated by using Unphased software available from the website www.mrc-bsu.cam.ac.uk/personal/frank/software/unphased.[14] P values were corrected by multiplying for the number of different alleles or haplotypes tested. A corrected P (Pc) <0.05 was considered significant.

Differences of vitamin D levels, $25(OH)D_3$, and $1,25(OH)_2D_3$ were evaluated by t-test and the χ^2 test, respectively, using Bias Statistical package 7.01 (Epsilon, Weinheim, Germany).

TABLE 1. Primers, probes, and PCR's conditions

SNP	Families	Primers	T (°C)	Enzyme	Fragments (bp)	Allele
rs7975232 (Apa I)*	217	5′-AGTAAGAGTCTGGCAAAGATAGC-3	58	Apa I	290216,6,104	G
rs731236 (TaqI)*	222	5′-AAACACTTCGAGCACAAGG-3		Taq I	400,210	C
rs1544410 (Bsm I)**	254	5-′GGCAACCTGAAGGGAGACGTA-3′	60	Bsm I	258, 203	G
rs757343 (Tru I)**	238	5′-CTCTTTGGACCTCATCACCGAC-3′		Tru I	363, 98	A
rs10735810 (Fok I)	245	5′-AGCTGGCCCTGGCACTGACTCTGCTCT-3′	60	Fok I	207,60	T
		5′-ATGGAAACACCTTGCTTCTTCTCCCTC-3′				
rs9729	208	Assay No. C_8716058				
rs2853559	165	5′-TACCCCACACCACATCCTCG-3′	69	Nde I	288197	T
		5′-TTCTGGTTTTCTGCAACACTGC-3′				
rs1989969	184	5′-GTGAAGTGAGTGAGGACACAGG-3′	65	Acc I	335,75	C
		5′GGT GGA TGC AGA AAG GAG C-3′				
rs3847987	184	5′-CTCAACCAACCCCTTAGACC-3′	65	Hae III	220,46	C
		5′-AACCTAACCCCTTTCCTGC-3′				
rs2238135	150	5′-GAAGTGAGTGAGGACACAGG-3′	65.4	BsI I	253154	C
		5′-GTGGATGCAGAAAGGAGC-3′				
rs4516035#	123	Assay No. C_2880805				

*rs7975232 (Apa I) and rs731236 (Taq I) were genotyped with the same primer set.
**rs 1544410 (Bsm I) and rs757343 (Tru I) were genotyped with the same primer set.
#rs4516035 was found only as mono allelic.

RESULTS

Single Nucleotide Polymorphisms

None of the polymorphisms showed any significant association with type 1 diabetes (data not shown).

Haplotypes

The haplotypes "CG" (Taq I-Apa I), "CGG" (Taq I-Apa I-Tru I), "CGC" (Taq I-Apa I-Fok I), "GCTG" (rs9729-Taq I-Apa I-Tru I), and "CGGC"(Taq I-Apa I, Tru I, Fok I) were negatively associated with type 1 diabetes after correction for multiple testing. They were less often transmitted from parents to the affected sibling (5.0 versus 25.2 times, $P = 0.0001$, $Pc = 0.0004$; 5.2 versus 22.0 times, $P = 0.0007$, $Pc = 0.0049$; 2.0 versus 17.2 times, $P = 0.0001$, $Pc = 0.0008$; 4.0 versus 19.0 times, $P = 0.0009$, $Pc = 0.0099$; 2.4 versus 15.2 times, $P = 0.0004$, $Pc = 0.0044$, respectively, TABLE 2).

25(OH)D_3 and 1,25(OH)$_2D_3$ Serum Levels

Patients, who carried the genotype "CC" of the rs3847987 polymorphism had higher levels of the median of 25(OH)D_3 than those with the genotype "GG" or "GC" (21 ng/mL versus 12 ng/mL; $P = 0.0234$, data not shown). The genotype distribution of this polymorphism according to the 25(OH)D_3 status revealed that the majority of the patients, who carried the genotype "CC" were found in the group with normal 25(OH)D_3 serum levels (78.5% versus 68%, $P = 0.0192$; data not shown). No association of the rs3847987 with 1,25 (OH)$_2D_3$ was found.

Analysis of the other polymorphisms did not reveal any association (data not shown).

DISCUSSION

VDR polymorphisms have been associated with susceptibility to type 1 diabetes in diverse populations and autoimmune diseases.[8,9]

In contrast to our earlier findings[9] recent studies revealed no association of genotypes or haplotypes of the 3′ untranslated region (UTR) polymorphisms with type 1 diabetes.[10,11]

In our present study we have failed to reproduce our previous findings concerning the haplotypes from the polymorphisms Apa I, Taq I, and Bsm I,[9] which were found in other populations.[15] However these studies were performed in relatively small cohorts.

TABLE 2. Distribution of the VDR haplotypes in type 1 diabetes families

Haplotype*	Frequency	T	NT	*P*	*Pc*
rs9729, Taq I, Apa I, Tru I ($n = 151$)					
TCTG	35.1	129.8	96.0	0.0055	
GTGG	33.7	118.9	98.0	0.0851	
TTTA	9.2	31.1	28.0	0.6907	
TTTG	4.8	13.1	18.0	0.3725	
GCTG	3.6	4.0	19.0	0.0009	0.0099
GTTG	3.2	5.0	15.9	0.0139	
TTGG	3.1	9.0	11.0	0.6719	
GCGG	1.9	2.0	10.0	0.0153	
TCGG	1.1	1.2	6.0	0.0503	
GTTA	1.1	2.0	5.1	0.2229	
TTGA	1.1	2.8	4.0	0.6596	
Taq I, Apa I, Tru I ($n = 177$)					
CTG	38.4	162.8	129.2	0.0136	
TGG	36.0	144.7	129.0	0.2465	
TTA	10.2	36.9	40.3	0.6278	
TTG	8.6	23.3	41.8	0.0200	
CGG	3.6	5.2	22.0	0.0007	0.0049
TGA	2.0	4.1	11.0	0.0730	
CTA	1.3	3.0	6.8	0.2589	
Taq I, Apa I ($n = 209$)					
CT	40.2	199.0	173.8	0.0939	
TG	37.9	184.0	167.8	0.2787	
TT	18.7	76.0	97.2	0.0763	
CG	3.3	5.0	25.2	0.0001	0.0004
Taq I, Apa I, Tru I, Fok I ($n = 166$)					
CTGC	25.9	95.7	89.0	0.4190	
TGGC	22.5	88.2	72.3	0.1500	
TGGT	14.3	52.5	49.7	0.7907	
CTGT	12.6	53.0	36.8	0.1183	
TTAC	6.3	23.6	21.5	0.9784	
TTGC	5.3	16.1	21.9	0.3519	
TTAT	3.4	10.4	13.8	0.6259	
TTGT	2.7	5.2	13.7	0.0508	
CGGC	2.5	2.4	15.2	0.0004	0.0044
CGGT	1.2	3.0	5.4	0.5758	
TGAC	1.1	3.1	4.7	0.4905	
Taq I, Apa, Fok I ($n = 196$)					
CTC	26.5	114.7	115.0	0.8580	
TGC	23.0	110.6	89.0	0.0880	
TGT	15.8	66.4	70.9	0.7249	
CTT	13.5	67.3	49.9	0.1235	
TTC	11.7	49.7	51.9	0.7249	
TTT	6.2	20.4	33.2	0.0827	
CGC	2.2	2.0	17.2	0.0001	0.0008
CGT	1.2	3.0	7.0	0.2423	

*Only haplotypes with a frequency >1% are listed.
T = transmitted; NT = not transmitted; *Pc* = corrected *P* value.

Nevertheless, we confirm the association of the haplotypes "CG" (Apa I-Taq I), as we previously reported[9] as well as the haplotypes "CGG" (Taq I-Apa I-Tru I), "CGC" (Taq I-Apa I-Fok I), "TCTG" (rs9729-Taq I-Apa I-Tru I), and "CGGC" (Apa I-Fok I-Taq I-Tru I). These haplotypes could be considered as protective markers in the susceptibility to type 1 diabetes in the German population; because of their reduced transmission. Why and how these infrequent haplotypes confer protection is unclear at present. However they may also be related to vitamin D metabolism.

Taq I and Fok I polymorphisms were reported previously as the best-fit model for VDR mRNA expression.[16] Nevertheless, we failed to find a correlation between these polymorphisms and $25(OH)D_3$ or $1,25(OH)_2D_2$ levels. On the other hand we found a correlation between $25(OH)D_3$ and the rs3847987 polymorphism, where the majority of the patients with the genotype "CC" possessed a higher serum level of $25(OH)D_3$. This may explain that vitamin D deficiency or insufficiency has a genetic basis.

In conclusion, although the role of polymorphisms within the VDR as marker for type 1 diabetes remains controversial, our work points to a protective role of VDR haplotypes in type 1 diabetes.

REFERENCES

1. MATHIEU, C., J. LAUREYS, H. SOBIS, *et al.* 1992. 1,25-Dihydroxyvitamin D3 prevents insulitis in NOD mice. Diabetes **41:** 1491–1495.
2. GIULIETTI, A., C. GYSEMANS, K. STOFFELS, *et al.* 2004. Vitamin D deficiency in early life accelerates Type 1 diabetes in non-obese diabetic mice. Diabetologia **47:** 451–462.
3. MATTNER, F., S. SMIROLDO, F. GALBIATI, *et al.* 2000. Inhibition of Th1 development and treatment of chronic-relapsing experimental allergic encephalomyelitis by a non-hypercalcemic analogue of 1,25-dihydroxyvitamin D(3). Eur. J. Immunol. **30:** 498–508.
4. D'AMBROSIO, D., M. CIPPITELLI, M.G. COCCIOLO, *et al.* 1998. Inhibition of IL-12 production by 1,25-dihydroxyvitamin D3. Involvement of NF-kappaB down-regulation in transcriptional repression of the p40 gene. J. Clin. Invest. **101:** 252–262.
5. VELDMAN, C.M., M.T. CANTORNA & H.F. DELUCA. 2000. Expression of 1,25-dihydroxyvitamin D(3) receptor in the immune system. Arch. Biochem. Biophys. **374:** 334–338.
6. MIYAMOTO, K., R.A. KESTERSON, H. YAMAMOTO, *et al.* 1997. Structural organization of the human vitamin D receptor chromosomal gene and its promoter. Mol. Endocrinol. **11:** 1165–1179.
7. KOSZEWSKI, N.J., S. KIESSLING & H.H. MALLUCHE. 2001. Isolation of genomic DNA sequences that bind vitamin D receptor complexes. Biochem. Biophys. Res. Commun. **283:** 188–194.
8. ANGEL, B., J.L. SANTOS, E. CARRASCO, *et al.* 2004. Vitamin D receptor polymorphism and susceptibility to type 1 diabetes in Chilean subjects: a case-parent study Eur. Eur. J. Epidemiol. **19:** 1085–1087.

9. PANI, M.A., M. KNAPP, H. DONNER, *et al.* 2000. Vitamin D receptor allele combinations influence genetic susceptibility to type 1 diabetes in Germans. Diabetes **49:** 504–507.
10. TURPEINEN, H., R. HERMANN, S. VAARA, *et al.* 2003. Vitamin D receptor polymorphisms: no association with type 1 diabetes in the Finnish population. Eur. J. Endocrinol. **149:** 591–596.
11. NEJENTSEV, S., J.D. COOPER, L. GODFREY, *et al.* 2004. Analysis of the vitamin D receptor gene sequence variants in type 1 diabetes. Diabetes **53:** 2709–2712.
12. MALABANAN, A., I.E. VERONIKIS & M.F. HOLICK. 1998. Redefining vitamin D insufficiency. Lancet **351:** 805–806.
13. OGUNKOLADE, B.W., B.J. BOUCHER, P.D. FAIRCLOUGH, *et al.* 2002. Expression of 25-hydroxyvitamin D-1-alpha-hydroxylase mRNA in individuals with colorectal cancer. Lancet **359:** 1831–1832.
14. DUDBRIDGE, F. 2003. Pedigree disequilibrium tests for multilocus haplotypes. Genet. Epidemiol. **25:** 115–121.
15. BAN, Y., M. TANIYAMA & Y. BAN. 2000. Vitamin D receptor gene polymorphism is associated with Graves' disease in the Japanese population. J. Clin. Endocrinol. Metab. **85:** 4639–4643.
16. OGUNKOLADE, B.W., B.J. BOUCHER, J.M. PRAHL, *et al.* 2002. Vitamin D receptor (VDR) mRNA and VDR protein levels in relation to vitamin D status, insulin secretory capacity, and VDR genotype in Bangladeshi Asians. Diabetes **51:** 2294–2300.

Living Donor Islet Transplantation, the Alternative Approach to Overcome the Obstacles Limiting Transplant

YASUHIRO IWANAGA,[a,b] SHINICHI MATSUMOTO,[b,c] TERU OKITSU,[a,b] HIROFUMI NOGUCHI,[a,b] HIDEO NAGATA,[a,b] YUKIHIDE YONEKAWA,[a,b] YUICHIRO YAMADA,[d] KAZUHITO FUKUDA,[d] KATSUSHI TSUKIYAMA,[d] AND KOICHI TANAKA[e]

[a]*Department of Transplantation and Immunology, Kyoto University Graduate School of Medicine, Kyoto, Japan 606-8507*

[b]*Diabetes Research Institute Kyoto, Kyoto, Japan 606-8507*

[c]*Kyoto University Hospital Transplantation Unit, Kyoto, Japan 606-8507*

[d]*Department of Diabetes and Clinical Nutrition, Kyoto University Graduate School of Medicine, Kyoto, Japan 606-8507*

[e]*Kobe Frontier Medical Center, Kobe, Japan 650-0047*

ABSTRACT: We performed the world's first successful living donor islet transplantation for unstable diabetes. A total of 408,114 islet equivalents were isolated from half a living pancreas and transplanted immediately to the recipient who was a 27-year-old female. The donor was a 56-year-old female in good health, mother of the recipient. The islets functioned immediately, and the recipient was weaned completely from insulin on the 22nd posttransplant day, and has maintained excellent glycemic control since. The donor was discharged on the 18th postoperative day with normal oral glucose tolerance test and without complications. Living donor islet transplantation could cure one insulin-dependent diabetes mellitus patients with a single donor. There are some advantages in the living donor islet transplantation: (*a*) living donor can alleviate the issue of donor shortage; (*b*) highly potent islets can be isolated from a living donor; and (*c*) the recipient can be treated with immunosuppressant and controlled blood glucose level tightly prior to the transplantation. These are important factors in overcoming the obstacles limiting islet transplantation. We believe that the living donor islet transplantation may become an additional option in treating insulin-dependent diabetes.

Address for correspondence: Yasuhiro Iwanaga, M.D., Ph.D., Department of Transplantation and Immunology, Kyoto University Graduate School of Medicine, 54 Kawara-cho Shogoin, Sakyo-ku, Kyoto, Japan 606-8507. Voice: 81-75-751-4699; fax: 81-75-751-3896.
e-mail: iwanaga@kuhp.kyoto-u.ac.jp

Ann. N.Y. Acad. Sci. 1079: 335–339 (2006).
doi: 10.1196/annals.1375.051

Keywords: living donor islet transplantation; insulin-dependent diabetes mellitus; living donor

After the success of islet transplantation reported by the University of Alberta group in 2000,[1] the demand for islet transplantation has significantly increased. There are still obstacles limiting islet transplantation including supplies of donor pancreata, the quality of isolated islets, side effects of immunosuppressants, and long-term outcomes.

To alleviate the donor shortage, living donor islet transplantation represents an alternative approach to expand the potential donor pool, particularly in countries such as Japan where access to cadaveric organ donors is especially limited.[2] We performed the living donor islet transplantation for unstable diabetes and could cure the patient with islets from half a living donor pancreas. As islet transplantation usually requires two or more cadaveric donors to cure one recipient, islets isolated from half a living donor pancreas may have high potency of engraftment. There are advantages in the living donor islet transplantation from the isolated islet's and the recipient's viewpoints.

In this study, we describe the advantages of the living donor islet transplantation for unstable diabetes.

METHOD

The recipient was a 27-year-old female who had pancreatic diabetes for 12 years. Her blood glucose was very unstable before transplantation. Blood C-peptide levels were negative (<0.1 ng/mL) after glucagon stimulation and HbA1c was 9.9%. Her daily insulin requirement was a mean of 28 units (0.56 U/kg per day). She had no renal and retinal complications. She was admitted to our hospital 2 weeks prior to the transplantation and her blood glucose was controlled tightly. In order to achieve the stable target trough levels of immunosuppressants at the time of transplantation, sirolimus and tacrolimus were given to the recipient 7 days before transplant. Basiliximab (20 mg) was administered 4 days before and repeated on the day of transplantation. Infliximab (5 mg/kg) was administered 1 day before the transplant.

The donor was a healthy 56-year-old female, mother of the recipient. To minimize the risk of inducing impaired glucose tolerance in the donor, and following the lessons learned previously by the Minnesota Group in 130 living donor pancreas transplants, we confirmed that our donor was not obese (criteria for body mass index <25 kg/m^2), had an entirely normal oral glucose tolerance test, and that the autoantibody levels for glutamate decarboxylase and insulin were negative.[3] We also evaluated the donor's remnant and resected pancreas volume after hemipancreatectomy preoperatively using three-dimensional computed tomography (3D-CT) volumetry. The donor underwent an open distal pancreatectomy, with the pancreatic transection plane to the left of the superior mesenteric vein. To avoid the warm ischemic injury of the graft, the splenic artery and vein were ligated and resected immediately before the tail of pancreas was removed. The resected pancreas graft was flushed immediately on the back-table with chilled solution, transferred to the islet isolation facility followed by processing of the islet isolation. The isolated islets were transplanted into the liver via percutaneous portal venous access under local anesthesia.

RESULTS

The donor's insulinogenic index was 1.43 (>0.5 by criteria), and the HbA1c was 5.0% (<5.6% by criteria). The remnant and resected pancreas volume was 43% and 57% of the total pancreas, respectively, as measured preoperatively using 3D-CT volumetry. The donor surgery was performed safely. The resected pancreas weight was 38 g after trimming. The cold ischemic time was 44 min. The total islet yield was 408,114 islet equivalents and the islet viability was 99%. The insulin stimulation index after glucose challenge test was 27.4. The recipient has been insulin-independent since day 22 posttransplant. The donor's postoperative clinical course was uneventful. She was discharged on the 18th postoperative day. Their blood C-peptide levels and HbA1c have been normal to date (FIG. 1).

DISCUSSION

The possibility of living donor islet transplantation provides an alternative approach to help meet the increasing disconnect between supply and demand for clinical islet transplantation. Furthermore, islets derived from living donors have the potential for considerably improved functional viability compared to cadaveric pancreas donation. The metabolic outcome of the recipient after this living donor islet transplant, using half a living pancreas appears similar to those after islet transplants, using two or more cadaveric whole pancreas in our program.[4–6] It is thought that the islets derived from living donor have the potential of nearly perfect quality due to no exposure to islet-toxic proinflammatory cytokines injury resulting from brain death[7] and the ability to reduce cold ischemic injury. In addition, the good pancreas for the islet isolation can be selected by the preoperative assessment of insulin secretory ability on the living donor. From the recipient's viewpoint, immunosuppressants can be initiated before transplant and the stable target trough levels can be achieved at the time of transplantation. In our case, the immunosuppressants were given to the recipient 7 days before transplant. Additionally, blood glucose can be controlled tightly prior to the transplantation which should help to improve the efficacy of islet engraftment.

On the other hand, disadvantage in the living donor islet transplantation is that donor's risk related to surgery is accompanied as in all forms of living donor

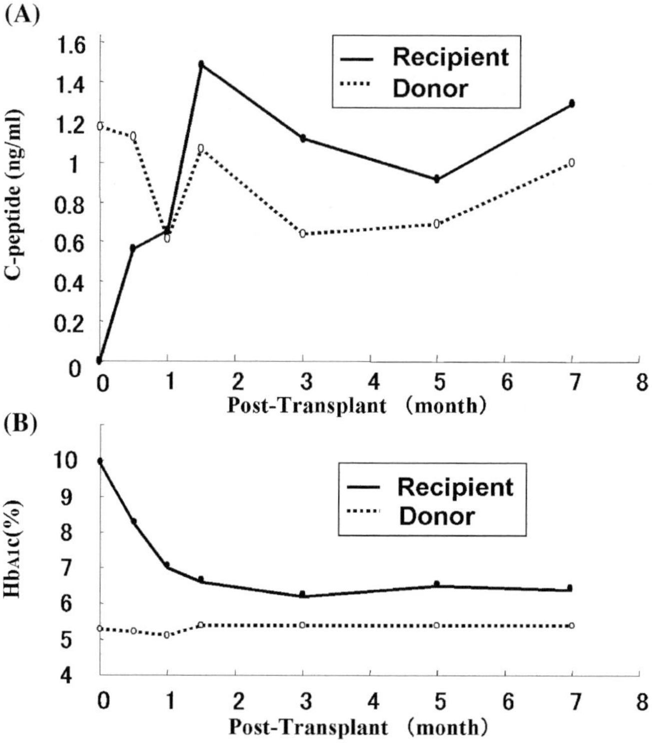

FIGURE 1. Change of the blood C-peptide level (**A**) and HbA1c (**B**) of the recipient and the donor after islet transplantation. The blood C-peptide levels and HbA1c of the recipient have been improved after transplantation. Those of the donor have been kept normal.

transplantation. There is the potential to induce new diabetes in a healthy donor. The pancreas donation for the living donor islet transplantation was performed safely according to the stringent selection criteria.

In conclusion, we describe the advantages of living donor islet transplantation for the treatment of unstable diabetes which are important factors in overcoming the obstacles limiting islet transplantation. We believe that the living donor islet transplantation may become an additional option in the treatment of insulin-dependent diabetes.

ACKNOWLEDGMENTS

This work was supported in part by the Ministry of Education, Science, and Culture, the Ministry of Health, Labour and Welfare, and the 21st Century Center of Excellence Program, Japan. We thank Yusuke Nakai, Michiko Ueda, and Akemi Ishii for their technical support.

REFERENCES

1. SHAPIRO, A.M.J., J.R.T. LAKEY, E.A. RYAN, *et al.* 2000. Islet transplantation in seven patients with type1 diabetes mellitus using a glucocorticoid-free immunosuppressive regimen. N. Engl. J. Med. **343:** 230–238.
2. MATSUMOTO, S., K. TANAKA, D.M. STRONG, *et al.* 2004. Efficacy of human islet isolation from the tail section of the pancreas for the possibility of living donor islet transplantation. Transplantation **78:** 839–843.
3. GRUESSNER, R.W.G. & D.E.R. SUTHERLAND. 2002. Living donor pancreas transplantation. Transplant Rev. **16:** 108–119.
4. MATSUMOTO, S. & K. TANAKA. 2005. Pancreatic islet cell transplantation using non-heart-beating-donors. J. Hepatobiliary Pancreat. Surg. **12:** 227–300.
5. MATSUMOTO, S., T. OKITSU, Y. IWANAGA, *et al.* Successful islet transplantation from non-heart-beating donor pancreata using modified Ricordi islet isolation method. Transplantation. In press.
6. MATSUMOTO, S., T. OKITSU, Y. IWANAGA, *et al.* 2005. Insulin independence after living donor distal pancreatectomy and islet allotransplantation. Lancet **365:** 1642–1644.
7. CONTRERAS, J.L., C. ECKSTEIN, C.A. SMYTH, *et al.* 2003. Brain death significantly reduces isolated pancreatic islet yields and functionality *in vitro* and *in vivo* after transplantation in rats. Diabetes **52:** 2935–2942.

DiaPep277® Preserves Endogenous Insulin Production by Immunomodulation in Type 1 Diabetes

DANA ELIAS,[a] ANN AVRON,[a] MERANA TAMIR,[a] AND ITAMAR RAZ[b]

[a]*DeveloGen Israel Ltd., Kiryat Weizmann, Rehovot 76326, Israel*

[b]*Hadassah Medical Center, Jerusalem 91120, Israel*

ABSTRACT: DiaPep277 is an immunomodulatory peptide that arrests β cell destruction in mouse models of type 1 diabetes mellitus (T1DM). This article extends an original pilot observation to two studies of 61 patients (age > 16 years), diagnosed with T1DM within 6 months, and with measurable β cell function. Patients were treated with placebo (*n* = 27) or 1.0 mg DiaPep277 (*n* = 34). After 13 months, 1.0 mg DiaPep277 treatment significantly (*P* = 0.02) preserved β cell function as compared to the control with a trend for reduced HbA1c. This was achieved without an increase in insulin dose in the DiaPep277 group and with excellent safety. DiaPep277-treated patients also had fewer Th1 DiaPep277-specific T cells.

KEYWORDS: hsp60; immunomodulation; β cells; clinical study

INTRODUCTION

The NOD mouse model has been useful in exposing the underlying autoimmune pathogenesis of type 1 diabetes mellitus (T1DM) that results in the specific destruction of the insulin-producing β cells. Heat shock protein 60 (hsp60) is a potent modulator of immune responses, acting through toll receptors (TLR2 and TLR4).[1,2] DiaPep277 is a 24-amino acid peptide analog of the positions 437–460 of hsp60 with the two original cysteines in the sequence replaced by valines for stability. In the NOD mouse model treatment with DiaPep277 has been shown to arrest disease even after clinical symptoms have appeared.[3,4] We have previously reported[5] the results of a 10-month follow-up of a clinical trial in which 35 patients, newly diagnosed (<6 months) were treated with either 1 mg DiaPep277 or placebo. This article extends the previous observations and increases the studied sample to 61 patients and the follow-up time to 13 months.

Address for correspondence: D. Elias, DeveloGen Israel Ltd., Kiryat Weizmann, Rehovot 76326, Israel. Voice: +972-8-9387777; fax: +972-8-9300083.
e-mail: Elias@Develogen.com

Ann. N.Y. Acad. Sci. 1079: 340–344 (2006).
doi: 10.1196/annals.1375.052

Study Designs

Patients were treated at a single center using the same methodology and all blood samples were tested in a central laboratory. Sixty-one patients over 16 years of age, diagnosed with T1DM within the last 6 months and with measurable fasting C-peptide (over 0.166 nmol/L) were treated with placebo (25 male and 2 female) or 1.0 mg DiaPep277 (27 male and 7 female) given subcutaneously as either 4 injections (Study 1)[5] at base line, at 1, 6, and 12 months or 7 injections, with the first 4 monthly and the next 3 at 3-monthly intervals (Study 2). Final results were obtained at 13 months of follow-up from base line. Clinical efficacy end points were the preservation of β cell function as measured by the change from base line in glucagon-stimulated C-peptide secretion, the change from base line in metabolic control as measured by the %HbA1c, and the insulin requirement as measured by the change from base line in the daily insulin dose expressed as units of insulin per kg body weight per day. Peripheral blood lymphocytes were isolated from fresh blood and reacted in culture with hsp60 and hsp60-derived peptides including DiaPep277. Bacterial recall antigens (tetanus toxoid and Tuberculin purified protein derivative [PPD]) were also used as lymphocyte stimulants, to test whether nonspecific modification of T cell responses was caused. The T cell responses were monitored by uptake of [^{3}H]-thymidine in a proliferation response and by cytokine secretion in an ELISPOT assay.[5] The ELISPOT assay measures the number of cells producing the measured cytokines and cells were assayed for interferon-γ (IFN-γ) (T helper cell type 1 [Th1]), or interleukin-13 (IL-13), IL-4, IL-10, and IL-5 (Th2 type). After 13 months of treatment, the type of T cell response to DiaPep277 was characterized according to whether the response included the inflammatory cytokine IFN-γ or exclusively the other, Th2 type of cytokines measured. A response was considered positive if there were three or more spots over the unstimulated background value.

Antibodies to DiaPep277 were measured in the sera of the patients by a classical enzyme-linked immunosorbent assay (ELISA) to test for the possible production of neutralizing antibodies to the peptide.

RESULTS

Clinical End Points

There was no significant difference between the baseline values of the DiaPep277-treated and placebo group patients at the start of the trial in body mass index, age, time from diagnosis, or any of the clinical end point parameters. After 13 months of follow-up, there were 54 patients that completed the analysis (24 placebo-treated patients and 30 DiaPep277-treated patients). The results are depicted in FIGURE 1. At this time, the β cell function had decreased

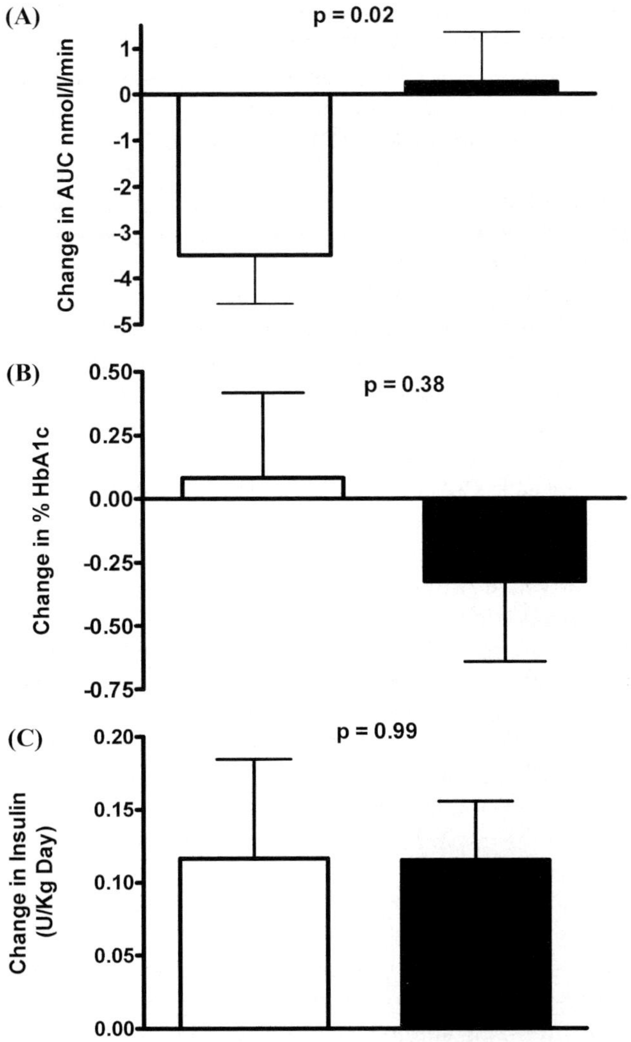

FIGURE 1. Efficacy end points. The change from baseline values at 13 months of follow-up are shown as mean and SEM for the placebo (□) and DiaPep277 (■) treated groups. (**A**) Stimulated C-peptide expressed as AUC, (**B**) % HbA1c, and (**C**) daily insulin dose. *P* values are shown for the difference between the two treatment arms.

in the placebo group but was fully preserved in the group treated with DiaPep277 (FIG. 1 A), change from base line in stimulated C-peptide area under the curve (AUC): -3.5 ± 1 versus 0.26 ± 1 nmol/min/L, respectively ($P = 0.02$, $N = 52$). Concurrently, the mean change from base line in %HbA1c fell by 0.3% in the DiaPep277-treated group while increasing by 0.1% in the placebo group

(FIG. 1 B). The improved metabolic control was achieved with no difference between the groups in the increase in daily insulin dose (FIG. 1 C, $P = 0.99$).

Immunological Monitoring

The treatment affected the type of T cell immune response to DiaPep277. Fewer patients in the 1.0 mg DiaPep277-treated group produced an IFN-γ response to DiaPep277 after 13 months than in the placebo group, 39% versus 93%, respectively. The Th2 type response, on the other hand, was increased in the DiaPep277-treated group, so that the average IL-10 response to DiaPep277 increased from a base line of 2 to 14 cells per 100,000 lymphocytes at 13 months, after the last administration. In the lymphocyte proliferation test the placebo group showed an increase over time in the number of patients that responded to three or more peptide epitopes derived from hsp60, including DiaPep277. In the DiaPep277 group there was reduced epitope spreading in the patients.

There was, however, no evidence of a change in the T cell immune responses to the bacterial recall antigens (PPD and tetanus toxoid) as all responses both by ELISPOT and proliferation remained positive throughout, without any significant quantitative change. There was also no evidence for neutralizing antibodies with the overwhelming majority of the patients maintaining a constant titer of antibodies to DiaPep277 throughout the study period (17% of DiaPep277-treated patients showed a decrease in titer while 3% showed an increase, in the placebo group 12.5% of patients showed a decrease in titer).

Safety was very similar between the two groups. Adverse events (AEs) were reported by 67% of the placebo patients as compared to 79% of the DiaPep277-treated patients at an average rate of 2.4 and 2.8 AEs per patient, respectively. Treatment-related AEs (6 AEs in 5 placebo patients and 12 AEs in 11 DiaPep277-treated patients) were exclusively related to the injection site, so they are probably related to the lipid solvent and not to the active peptide ingredient (except for one AE reported by a placebo patient). The injection site pain and edema were limited and resolved spontaneously.

CONCLUSIONS

DiaPep277 treatment fulfilled its expected effect, confirming the earlier observations in NOD mice[3,4] and newly diagnosed T1DM patients.[5] The treatment affected the specific immune responses, so that proinflammatory and pathogenic Th1 cells were downregulated, possibly by the IL-10 secreting T cells specific to DiaPep277, which were increased by the treatment. Whether these cells are Th2 or Tregulatory cells (Treg) in phenotype still needs to be clarified in further studies. Be that as it may, the immunological modulation was antigen-specific, as T cell responses to bacterial antigens were not suppressed or modified.

The immunological shift was accompanied by a significant preservation of endogenous insulin secretion, as determined by the stimulated C-peptide levels, which did not decrease from base line in the DiaPep277-treated group, unlike the placebo group that lost part of the β cell function. Since the duration of the studies' treatment and follow-up were restricted to 13 months, the decrease in endogenous insulin secretion by the placebo group was limited, yet the difference was statistically significant. A longer treatment and follow-up period would be necessary to show the long-term effects of DiaPep277 treatment on preservation of β cell function.

These studies were not designed with a treat to target value of less than 7% HbA1c for good metabolic control, therefore they were not ideal for assessing the impact of treatment on insulin dependence. Indeed, both groups showed a similar increase over time in the daily insulin dose. However, at the same insulin dose, the DiaPep277 group showed an improved metabolic control that was not reached by the placebo group. Although the difference was not statistically significant, it suggests that the better preservation of β cell function was effective in improving metabolic control. Since the safety profile of DiaPep277 is very good, the next step would be the staging of a conclusive study, powered to show significant clinical improvement.

REFERENCES

1. Zanin-Zhorov, A., G. Nussbaum, S. Franitza, *et al.* 2003. T cells respond to heat shock protein 60 via TLR2: activation of adhesion and inhibition of chemokine receptors. FASEB J. **17:** 1567–1569.
2. Flohe, S.B., J. Bruggemann, S. Lendemans, *et al.* 2003. Human heat shock protein 60 induces maturation of dendritic cells versus a Th1-promoting phenotype. J. Immunol. **170:** 2340–2348.
3. Elias, D., I.R. Cohen, D. Markovits, *et al.* 1994. Peptide therapy for diabetes in NOD mice. Induction and therapy of autoimmune diabetes in the non-obese diabetic (NOD/Lt) mouse by a 65-kDa heat shock protein. Lancet **343:** 704–706.
4. Elias, D. & I.R. Cohen. 1995. Treatment of autoimmune diabetes and insulitis in NOD mice with heat shock protein 60 peptide p277. Diabetes **44:** 1132–1138.
5. Raz, I., D. Elias, A. Avron, *et al.* 2001. Beta-cell function in new-onset type 1 diabetes and immunomodulation with a heat-shock protein peptide (DiaPep277): a randomised, double-blind, phase II trial. Lancet **358:** 1749–1753.

Cord Blood Islet Autoantibodies Are Related to Stress in the Mother during Pregnancy

BARBRO LERNMARK, KRISTIAN LYNCH, ÅKE LERNMARK, AND THE DiPiS STUDY GROUP

Department of Clinical Sciences Malmö, Lund University, CRC 214 02 Malmö, Sweden

ABSTRACT: A 2-month psychological questionnaire concerning pregnancy was answered by 20,920 nondiabetic mothers of singletons. Retrospective analysis showed increased levels of islet autoantibodies (IA) in 290 (1.4%) newborns. High IA levels in the child's cord blood correlated strongly with IA levels in the mother (GADA $r = 0.91, P < 0.0001$; IA-2A $r = 0.75, P = 0.0001$). High IA levels were found in newborns whose mothers during pregnancy had been more worried than usual ($P = 0.04$), had worried that the child would be sick ($P = 0.01$) or not survive ($P = 0.002$), or had experienced serious life events, like "serious accident in the family" ($P < 0.0001$) or "experienced violence" ($P = 0.02$). Associations with increased worries by the mother remained in newborns with high type 1 diabetes mellitus (T1DM)-human leukocyte antigen (HLA) risk, but not in non-HLA risk children. The prospective follow-up of these children will determine the importance of this early IA for postnatal islet autoimmunity, type 1 diabetes, or both.

KEYWORDS: stress; autoantibodies; type 1 diabetes

INTRODUCTION

Psychological stress and severe life events have been associated with islet autoimmunity[1–3] and type 1 diabetes (T1DM).[4,5] The aim of this article was to examine if stress and severe life events during pregnancy in nondiabetic mothers were related to increased levels of islet autoantibodies (IA) in their child's cord blood and to investigate if associations were stronger when the child had human leukocyte antigen (HLA)-T1DM risk genotypes.

Address for correspondence: Barbro Lernmark, Department of Clinical Sciences, Lund University, CRC, 214 02 Malmö, Sweden. Voice: +46-40-391908; fax: +46-40-391919.
e-mail: Barbro.Lernmark@med.lu.se

Ann. N.Y. Acad. Sci. 1079: 345–349 (2006).
doi: 10.1196/annals.1375.053

SUBJECTS AND METHODS

A total of 31,924 singletons born to nondiabetic mothers were included in the Diabetes Prediction in Skåne (DiPiS) Study. At delivery, cord blood was obtained from newborns and serum from mothers.

Newborns were HLA typed on dried blood spots (DBS) for high-risk DQA1*0501-DQB1*02, DQB1*0302 and protective DQB1*0301, 0602, and 0603 alleles. Cord blood from children were analyzed for GAD65Ab-IA-2Ab simultaneously in a first screen. Samples with high binding levels (95th percentile) were reanalyzed individually for GAD65Ab and IA-2Ab in radiobinding assay calibrated with the WHO standard. The serum sample from the mother was analyzed for IA when levels were higher than normal in the child (cutoff at the 99th percentile). Insulin autoantibodies (IAA) was analyzed in a radiobinding assay as being standardized by Diabetes Autoantibody Standardization Program (DASP). Psychosocial questionnaires were filled out 2 months after birth. Questions on the mother's emotional well-being during pregnancy, specific concerns regarding the baby, and serious life events during pregnancy were asked in eight consecutive questions.

Logistic regression tested for factors associated with mothers filling in and returning the psychological questionnaires. Chi-square for proportions, and *t*-tests for means, tested whether there were significant differences in perinatal characteristics between newborns with increased IA levels and other newborns. Pearson correlations were examined for association between mother's and child's IA levels. Degree of worry and frequency of IA were compared using chi-square tests of trend. Multiple logistic regression examined whether life events during pregnancy were significant predictors of prevalence of high IA in cord blood when adjusting for other perinatal factors, such as sex of child, age of mother, birth weight, gestational age, mother's education, and country of birth.

RESULTS

The 2-month questionnaire was filled in and returned by 20,920 mothers. Older mothers [odds ratio (OR) = 1.04 (1.03–1.05) (95% CI); $P < 0.001$] and mothers giving birth to term singletons [OR = 0.78 (0.69–0.87); $P < 0.001$] were more likely to participate by completing the questionnaire.

In the children's cord blood higher than normal IA levels were detected for GAD65Ab ($N = 151$; 0.72%), IA-2Ab ($N = 17$; 0.08%), and IAA ($N = 128$; 0.61%). A total of 290 children (1.36%) had IA above normal levels (GAD65Ab: $N = 151$, 0.72%; IA-2Ab: $N = 17$; 0.08%; IAA: $N = 128$; 0.61%) with five children having high levels of both GAD65Ab and IA-2Ab and one child having high levels of both GAD65Ab and IAA. Higher than normal IA levels in the cord blood correlated strongly with IA levels in the mother (FIG. 1 A, B).

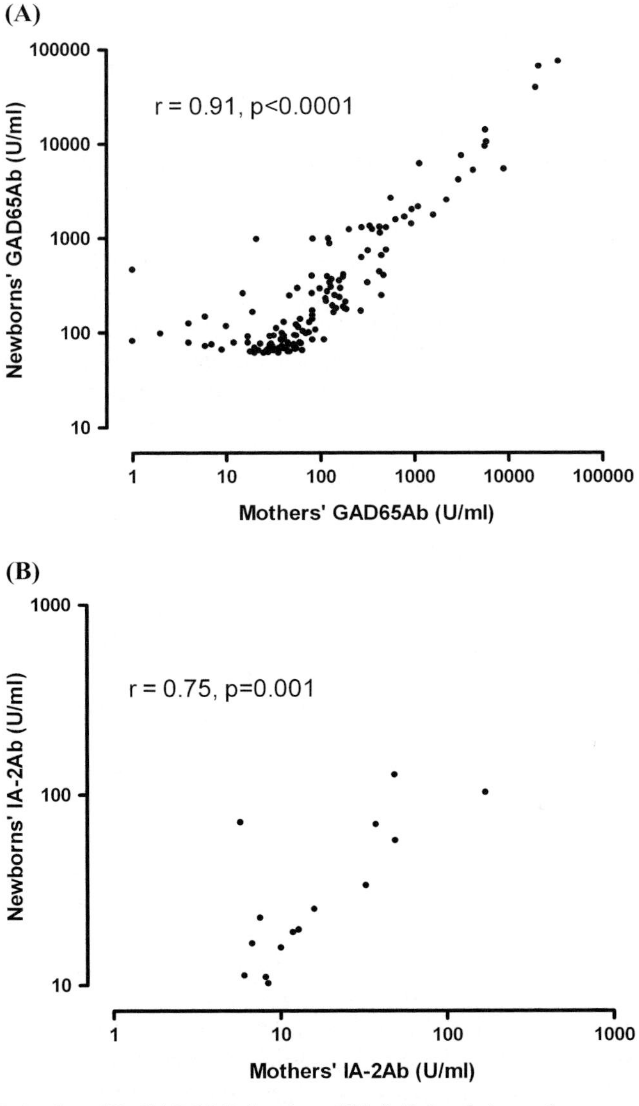

FIGURE 1. **A** and **B**. GAD65Ab levels and IA-2Ab levels in mother compared to child when child had higher than normal levels of GAD65Ab and IA-2Ab, respectively.

In boys, but not in girls a significantly larger proportion had high IA levels (59%) compared to normal levels (51.7%; $P = 0.02$). There were no other differences between children with high compared to normal IA levels regarding premature birth, mother's educational level, if the mother was born in Sweden, mother's age, child's birth weight, or if the child was large or small for gestational age.

The mothers' answers to questions on their emotional well-being during pregnancy show that 1.7% of the mothers who reported "more worried than usual" were more likely to have children with high IA levels in the cord blood compared to 1.3% of the mothers not reporting increased worries [OR = 1.30 (1.02–1.67), $P = 0.04$]. The association remained for mothers with HLA risk newborns [OR = 1.74 (1.07–2.83), $P = 0.025$], but not in mothers with non-HLA risk children [OR = 1.19 (0.88–1.59)].

The pregnant mothers' answers to four questions about worries related to the child indicated that newborns with the highest frequency of high IA levels were born to mothers who worried their child would be sick (test of trend: $P = 0.01$) or would not survive (test of trend: $P = 0.002$). When the mothers were very worried about their children's survival, the frequency of mothers with high IA positive newborns was significantly greater when the newborn had high-risk HLA (3.0%) compared to when they did not (1.3% [OR = 2.35 (1.31–4.20), $P = 0.004$]). Worries for a handicapped child or a child with malformations did not give significantly increased IA levels.

Mothers who had experienced serious life event during pregnancy also showed increased associations with IA in the child. After adjusting for perinatal factors "serious accident in the family" was associated with IA in the child [OR = 4.35 (2.25–8.39), $P < 0.0001$] regardless of the child's HLA risk. Also, mothers who reported "experienced violence" more frequently had children with high IA levels [OR = 3.95 (1.22–12.90), $P = 0.02$].

DISCUSSION

Worries and strong emotional experiences in the mother during pregnancy were associated with increased IA levels in the child's cord blood. Children with T1DM-HLA risk genotypes more often had increased IA levels. Early autoimmunity in children was found to be associated with a later diagnosis of T1DM,[6] but in another study being protective for later development of T1DM.[7] The prospective follow-up of the children will determine the significance of these early IA for the child's future risk of developing islet IA, T1DM, or both. The mechanisms by which IA develop during pregnancy in mothers reporting significant life events or increased stress remain to be determined.

ACKNOWLEDGMENTS

Members of the DiPiS study group are P. Almgren, B. Buveris-Svendburg, A. Carlsson, E. Cederwall, C. Cilio, H. Elding Larsson, J. Gerardsson, G. Hansson, S-A. Ivarsson, B. Jönsson, K. Kockum, K. Larsson, B. Lindberg, J. Neiderud, A. Nilsson, H. Rastkhani, and S. Sjöblad. We thank all the participating parents and children in the DiPiS study.

Our research is supported in part by the Swedish Research Council (Grant 14064), Juvenile Diabetes Research Foundation/Wallenberg Foundation, Swedish Childhood Diabetes Foundation, Swedish Diabetes Association, Nordisk Insulin Fund, National Institutes of Health (DK26190, DK63861), UMAS funds, and the Skåne Council Foundation for Research and Development.

REFERENCES

1. Robinson, N. *et al.* 1988. Psychosocial factors and the onset of type 1 diabetes. Diabetic Med. **6:** 53–58.
2. Sepa, A. *et al.* 2005. Psychological stress may induce diabetes-related autoimmunity in infancy. Diabetes Care **28:** 290–295.
3. Sepa, A., A. Frodi & J. Ludvigsson. 2005. Mothers' experiences of serious life events increase the risk of diabetes-related autoimmunity in their children. Diabetes Care **28:** 2394–2399.
4. Hägglöf, B. *et al.* 1991. The Swedish childhood diabetes study: indications of severe psychological stress as a risk factor for type 1 (insulin-dependent) diabetes mellitus in childhood. Diabetologia **34:** 579–583.
5. Thernlund, G.M. *et al.* 1995. Psychological stress and the onset of IDDM in children. Diabetes Care **18:** 1323–1329.
6. Lindberg, B. *et al.* 1999. Islet autoantibodies in cord blood from children who developed type I (insulin-dependent) diabetes mellitus before 15 years of age [see comments]. Diabetologia **42:** 181–187.
7. Koczwara, K., E. Bonifacio & A.G. Ziegler. 2004. Transmission of maternal islet antibodies and risk of autoimmune diabetes in offspring of mothers with type 1 diabetes. Diabetes **53:** 1–4.

Is It Dietary Insulin?

OUTI VAARALA

Laboratory for Immunobiology, Department of Viral Disease and Immunology, National Public Health Institute, Mannerheimintie 166, 00300 Helsinki, Finland

Department of Molecular and Clinical Medicine, Faculty of Health Sciences, Linköping University, 58185 Linköping, Sweden

ABSTRACT: In humans the primary trigger of insulin-specific immunity is a modified self-antigen, that is, dietary bovine insulin, which breaks neonatal tolerance to self-insulin. The immune response induced by bovine insulin spreads to react with human insulin. This primary immune response induced in the gut immune system is regulated by the mechanisms of oral tolerance. Genetic factors and environmental factors, such as the gut microflora, breast milk-derived factors, and enteral infections, control the development of oral tolerance. The age of host modifies the immune response to oral antigens because the permeability of the gut decreases with age and mucosal immune response, such as IgA response, develops with age. The factors that control the function of the gut immune system may either be protective from autoimmunity by supporting tolerance, or they may induce autoimmunity by abating tolerance to dietary insulin. There is accumulating evidence that the intestinal immune system is aberrant in children with type 1 diabetes (T1D). Intestinal immune activation and increased gut permeability are associated with T1D. These aberrancies may be responsible for the impaired control of tolerance to dietary insulin. Later in life, factors that activate insulin-specific immune cells derived from the gut may switch the response toward cytotoxic immunity. Viruses, which infect β cells, may release autoantigens and potentiate their presentation by an infection-associated "danger signal." This kind of secondary immunization may cause functional changes in the dietary insulin primed immune cells, and lead to the infiltration of insulin-reactive T cells to the pancreatic islets.

KEYWORDS: gut immune system; β cell autoimmunity; insulitis; enteral infections

Address for correspondence: Outi Vaarala, Laboratory for Immunobiology, Department of Viral Disease and Immunology, National Public Health Institute, Mannerheimintie 166, 00300 Helsinki, Finland. Voice: +358-9-47448463; fax: +358-9-47448281.
e-mail: outi.vaarala@ktl.fi

Ann. N.Y. Acad. Sci. 1079: 350–359 (2006). © 2006 New York Academy of Sciences.
doi: 10.1196/annals.1375.054

INTRODUCTION

Type 1 diabetes (T1D) is considered to be an autoimmune disease, in which insulin-secreting β cells are destroyed. Insulin autoantibodies (IAA) often appear as the first autoantibody in children who develop islet-cell autoimmunity,[1] suggesting that immune response to insulin may be the first event in the process toward β cell destruction. The importance of insulin as autoantigen is further supported by a study indicating that pancreatic-lymph-node-derived T cells in human T1D are reactive with insulin.[2] Also in an animal model of autoimmune diabetes, insulin was shown to be a driving autoantigen, because mice expressing insulin that had one amino acid change in B-chain did not develop autoimmune diabetes.[3]

As early as 1966, Grodsky *et al*. reported that immunization of rabbits with insulin led to extensive mononuclear cell infiltration in the islets of Langerhans, and to the development of diabetes mellitus.[4,5] In a nonobese diabetic (NOD)-mice model, insulin-reactive T cells have been shown to comprise the major population of T cells infiltrating the pancreatic islets.[6] Furthermore, insulin-reactive T cells are able to transfer autoimmune diabetes.[7]

Insulin-specific immunity is not restricted T1D, which has caused controversy about the use of IAA for prediction of T1D.[8] Our recent studies indicate that immunity to insulin is a common phenomenon in healthy children due to their dietary exposure to bovine insulin in cow milk (CM).[9–12] It is thus possible that the early immunization to CM insulin explains the findings of CM as a risk factor of T1D. This route of the primary immunization to insulin in humans implies a key role for the gut immune system in the regulation of insulin-specific immunity. The factors, which break the suppression of the insulin-specific immunity in the gut immune cells may thus be responsible for the autoimmune process leading to T1D.

Insulin-Specific Immunity Triggered by Dietary Insulin

The detection of antibodies to insulin has been a controversial issue.[8] The insulin-binding antibodies detected by liquid-phase radio-binding assay (RBA) are relatively specific for T1D. On the other hand, insulin-binding antibodies deteced by enzyme-linked solid-phase immunoassay (EIA) are not specific for T1D but detect sensitization to insulin.[9–12] The disease-related IAA show higher affinity and at least partly different epitope specificity than nondiabetes-related IAA.[8] Different epitopes of insulin are exposed in liquid-phase RBA than in the solid-phase EIA. Altogether the data imply that insulin-binding antibodies occur in healthy subjects without an increased risk of T1D.

Our studies show that infants who have been exposed to CM formulas before the age of 3 months, have higher levels of insulin-binding antibodies and T cell reactivity to insulin than infants who have been exclusively breastfed.[9–12] Both antibody and T cell response to bovine insulin showed to be cross-reactive with human insulin. We have identified an environmental trigger of insulin-specific immune response in humans, that is, dietary bovine insulin. Bovine insulin differs from human insulin by three amino acids. Immunogenic nature of bovine insulin in humans was recognized when bovine insulin was used for the treatment of diabetic patients. Bovine insulin induced high levels of insulin-binding antibodies, which declined when the patients were treated with less immunogenic porcine or human insulin.[13] As bovine insulin differs from human insulin it can be considered as a "modified self-antigen," which may escape tolerance induced to self-insulin in the thymus. Examples of the immunity against modified or cryptic epitopes of dietary and self-antigens are antibodies to modified wheat gliadin and autoantibodies to oxidized low-density lipoprotein (LDL) found in celiac disease and atherosclerosis, respectively.[14,15]

The induction of insulin-specific immunity by CM insulin is a physiological response to a new antigen encountered in the diet. Foreign dietary antigens induce a systemic antibody and T cell responses, which decline with age indicating the development of immune tolerance to food antigens.[16] Immune tolerance to dietary antigens does not always develop or it may be lost. Examples of pathology resulting from the loss of tolerance to dietary antigens are food allergies and celiac disease. It is of interest that in both diseases the target tissue is not restricted to the gut as the disease lesions are also found in other organs. In our follow-up study of children at increased genetic risk of T1D, the levels of bovine insulin-binding antibodies increased in the children who developed islet cell autoantibodies, whereas in the children who remained autoantibody negative, the levels remain stable or decreased in most cases.[10] This suggests that the children who develop islet cell autoimmunity may have a failure in tolerance induction to dietary insulin. We have asked whether children with T1D have aberrancies of the gut immune system that could be responsible for the dysregulation of tolerance to dietary insulin.

Immune Aberrancies of the Gut Immune System in T1D

The link between the gut immune system and T1D has been suggested by studies that have demonstrated that dietary factors modify the disease in animal models of autoimmune diabetes.[17,18] In Bio-breeding (BB) rats and NOD mice, a diet of hydrolyzed proteins decreased the incidence of the spontaneous autoimmune diabetes. A nondiabetogenic diet resulted in a switch to Th2-type cytokines from Th1-type response, which promotes cytotoxic activity, in the islet-infiltrating T cells. In NOD mice, islet-infiltrating lymphocytes express $\alpha4\beta7$-integrin, which is a homing receptor to the gut mucosa, and antibodies blocking this receptor prevent diabetes.[19–21] Furthermore, mesenterial lymphocytes transfer diabetes from NOD-mice to NOD/severe combined immunodeficient (SCID) mice.[22]

In humans, autoreactive T cells may originate from the gut immune system. For example, T cells derived from pancreas of a patient with T1D adhered to mucosal and pancreatic endothelium.[23] Autoreactive T cells from patients with T1D, expressed gut-associated homing receptor α4β7, whereas their tetanus toxoid-reactive T cells did not.[24] The expression of this gut-associated homing receptor has been shown in rotavirus specific T cells after oral antigen administration.[25] More direct evidence of aberrancies of the gut immune system in T1D comes from the studies performed in the intestinal biopsy samples taken from patients with T1D. We have found markers of intestinal immune activation in small intestinal biopsies taken from children with T1D.[26,27] The inflammation manifested as increased human-leukocyte-antigen (HLA) class II molecule, α4β7-integrin, intracellular adhesion molecule (ICAM)-1, interferon-γ (IFN-γ), interleukin-4 (IL-4), and IL-1β expression.[26,27] Scientists from Italy have reported similar kind of findings with increased numbers of intraepithelial CD3 cells and CD25 cells in lamina propria together with increased expression of ICAM-1 in intestinal biopsy samples from patients with T1D.[28] The Italian group demonstrated that stimulation of intestinal biopsy samples with wheat gliadin resulted in an expansion of CD3 and CD25 cells and an upregulation of ICAM-1 indicating that patients with T1D respond to wheat gliadin with intestinal inflammation though do not develop celiac disease.[28] This induction of inflammation to wheat gliadin may be due to the shared HLA risk genotype in celiac disease and T1D, namely DQ2 and DQ8.

Permeability of the Gut in T1D

Increased intestinal permeability to sugar molecules has been reported in patients with T1D already in the 1980s.[29] The studies on intestinal permeability in T1D are mostly based on the oral lactulose/mannitol test in which the ingested sugars are measured in urine. As the high levels of lactulose/mannitol are not found in all patients with T1D, the increased permeability may not be directly associated with the hyperglycemia-induced alterations in the mucosa, but could reflect a true aberrancies in these patients.[30–32] In a Finnish study, the increased permeability in lactulose/mannitol test was associated with the presence of HLA-DQB1*0201 allele in patients with T1D,[31] which supports the view that increased permeability associated with T1D is not due to metabolic disturbances but may be a fundamental feature in some patients. The increased permeability of the mucosal barrier leads to increased exposure of intestinal immune cells to antigenic load, which may change the functional stage of the immune system and break tolerance to oral antigens. It seems evident that children with T1D do show aberrancies of the gut immune system, which could favour the deviated immune response to oral antigens, such as dietary insulin.

Which Factors Modulate the Immune Response to Dietary Insulin?

The maturation of the gut plays a crucial role in the development of healthy immune response to dietary antigens. The development of human intestinum is slow when compared to the rodents: for example, the gut-closure occurs during the first 2 months of life in humans[33,34] and the number of IgA-positive plasma cells in the intestinum increase during the first months of life.[35] The increased permeability and impaired neutralizing effect of mucosal IgA allow oral antigens to pass the intestinal epithelial barrier resulting in increased amounts of antigens to be presented to the immune system. It is also of interest that the concentration of human insulin in breast milk seems to modulate the magnitude of antibody response to CM insulin in the infants (Tiittanen *et al.* unpublished data presented at IDS8 in Japan, 2005). It is thus possible that the immune response to dietary insulin could be affected by the age at introduction. Early CM exposure, that is, exposure before 2–3 months of life, has been reported to be a risk factor of T1D[36] and islet cell autoimmunity,[37] although not all studies have demonstrated the association.[38,39]

The use of hydrolyzed CM formula during the first 6–8 months of life in infants with genetic risk of T1D is tested in the prevention of T1D in the international TRIGR study, which is based on the pilot study suggesting that the intervention could decrease the risk of β cell autoimmunity.[40] In a FINDIA study the use of nonhydrolyzed CM formula with low insulin content is tested in the prevention of β cell autoimmunity. The FINDIA study specifically asks whether bovine insulin is the diabetogenic factor in CM. The results from the FINDIA pilot study with 40 children at genetic riks of T1D indicate that the removal of insulin in CM formula results in decreased levels of IgG-binding antibodies at the age of 3 months (FIG. 1) and even decreased levels of IgA-IAA at 12 months of age when compared to ordinary CM formula (FIG. 2). The basic character of immune system is the immunological memory; the lymphocyte population which has been induced against its antigen can be reactivated later when the same antigen is encountered again in a context of danger. Could

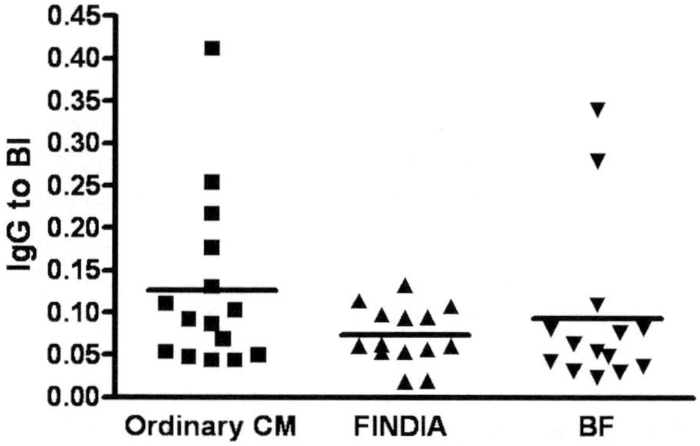

FIGURE 1. The levels of IgG antibodies to bovine insulin detected by EIA at 3 months of age in infants who received ordinary CM formula, FINDIA formula with low insulin content, or who were exclusively breastfed (BF).

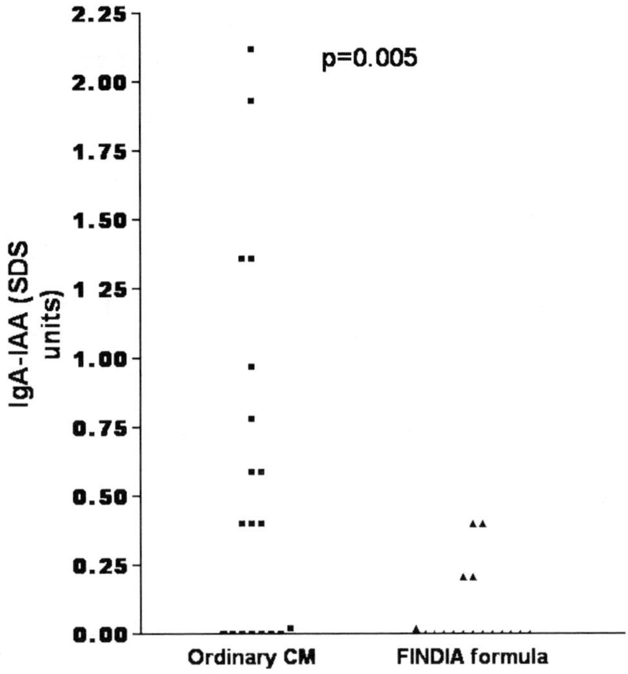

FIGURE 2. The levels of IgA antibodies to insulin detected by RBA at 12 months of age in infants who received ordinary CM formula or FINDIA formula with low insulin content.

other triggers of intestinal or pancreatic inflammation, such as virus infections or other dietary factors, reactivate the insulin-reactive lymphocytes and direct them to destroy the insulin-producing β cell?

Enterovirus and rotavirus infections have been associated with the development of islet cell autoimmunity.[41,42] Both viruses replicate in the gut and cause stimulation of the gut immune system. The enteric virus infections induce changes in the gut cytokine environment,[43] such as IFN-γ activation, and may activate the insulin-specific immune cells in the gut. Enteric virus infections may also increase the gut permeability and enhance the immunity to dietary insulin.[12]

The most intriguing options for the prevention of T1D are interventions targeted at the gut immune system. The colonization of gastrointestinal track with normal microflora is a necessity for the development of oral tolerance.[44] The composition of intestinal microflora varies between individuals and some disease-related differences have been demonstrated.[45–47] We have started the PRODIA study in which the use of probiotics, health-promoting intestinal bacteria, are tested in the prevention of β cell autoimmunity in children at genetic risk of T1D.[48] It is also evident that the composition of intestinal microflora differs between populations.[49] The changes in the microflora of

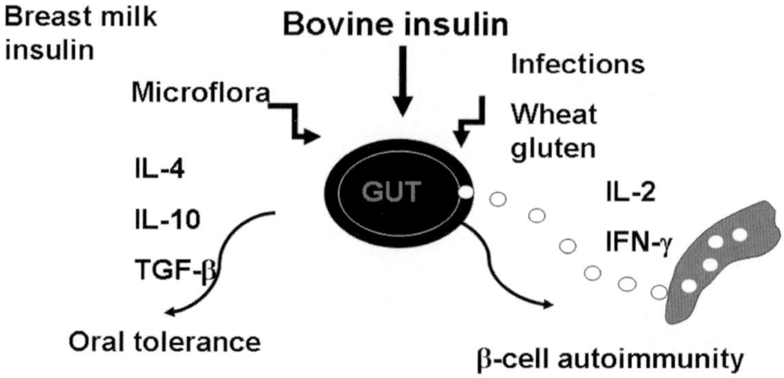

FIGURE 3. The hypothesis of the dietary insulin as a trigger of T1D. Intestinal inflammation caused by enteral infections or wheat gluten reactivates immunity to dietary insulin and β cell autoimmunity, whereas factors supporting the development of tolerance to dietary insulin, such as breast milk insulin and health-promoting microflora, protect from insulitis.

children with time may be associated with the changes in the incidence of T1D with time and the differences between the intestinal microflora between the populations may explain the differences in the incidence of T1D between different populations with similar genetic background.

The hypothesis that T1D is a disease of the gut immune system triggered by dietary insulin is illustrated in FIGURE 3. In the hypothesis the primary trigger of insulin-specific immunity is a modified self-antigen, that is, dietary bovine insulin, which breaks neonatal tolerance to self-insulin. The immune response spreads to react with self-insulin. This primary immune response is regulated by oral tolerance. Genetic factors and environmental factors, such as the gut microflora, breast milk-derived factors, dietary factors, such as wheat gluten, and enteral infections, control the development of oral tolerance. These factors may either be protective from autoimmunity by supporting tolerance, or they may enhance autoimmunity by abating oral tolerance to insulin and switching the insulin-specific immune response toward cytotoxic immunity. Later in life, factors which induce antigenic presentation of insulin in pancreatic islets may further activate insulin-specific immune cells derived from the gut. Viruses, which infect β cells, may release autoantigens and potentiate their presentation by an infection-associated "danger signal."[50] This kind of secondary immunization may cause functional changes in the dietary insulin primed immune cells, which leads to aggressive autoimmune attack against insulin-producing β cells.

REFERENCES

1. ZIEGLER, A.G. *et al.* 1999. Autoantibody appereance and risk for development of childhood diabetes in offspring of parents with type 1 diabetes. The 2-year analysis of the German BABYDIAB study. Diabetes **48:** 460–468.

2. KENT, S.C. *et al.* 2005. Expanded T cells from pancreatic lymph nodes of type 1 diabetic subjects recognize an insulin epitope. Nature **435:** 224–228.
3. NAKAYAMA, M. *et al.* 2005. Prime role for an insulin epitope in the development of type 1 diabetes in NOD mice. Nature **435:** 220–223.
4. GRODSKY, G.M. *et al.* 1966. Diabetes mellitus in rabbits immunized with insulin. Diabetes **15:** 579–585.
5. TORESON, W.E. *et al.* 1968. The histopathology of immune diabetes in the rabbit. Am. J. Pathol. **52:** 1099–1115.
6. WEGMANN, D.R. *et al.* 1994. Insulin-specific T cells are a predominant component of islet infiltrates in pre-diabetic NOD mice. Eur. J. Immunol. **24:** 1853–1857.
7. DANIEL, D. *et al.* 1995. Epitope specificity, cytokine production profile and diabetogenic activity of insulin-specific T cell clones isolated from NOD mice. Eur. J. Immunol. **25:** 1056–1062.
8. POTTER, K.N. & T.J. WILKIN. 2000. The molecular specificity of insulin autoantibodies. Diabetes Metab. Res. Rev. **16:** 338–353.
9. VAARALA, O. *et al.* 1998. Cow milk feeding induces antibodies to insulin in children- A link between cow milk and insulin-dependent diabetes mellitus. Scand. J. Immunol. **47:** 131–135.
10. VAARALA, O. *et al.* 1999. Cow's milk formula feeding induces primary immunization to insulin in infants at genetic risk for type 1 diabetes. Diabetes **48:** 1389–1394.
11. PARONEN, J. *et al.* 2000. The effect of cow milk exposure and maternal type 1 diabetes on cellular and humoral immunization to dietary insulin in infants at genetic risk for type 1 diabetes. Diabetes **49:** 1657–1665.
12. VAARALA, O. *et al.* 2002. The effect of coincident enterovirus infection and cow's milk exposure on immunization to insulin in early infancy. Diabetologia **45:** 531–534.
13. KURTZ, A.B. *et al.* 1980. Decrease of antibodies to insulin, proinsulin and contaminating hormones after changing treatment from conventional beef to purified pork insulin. Diabetologia **18:** 147–150.
14. MOLBERG, O. *et al.* 1998. Tissue transglutaminase selectively modifies gliadin peptides that are recognized by gut-derived T cells in celiac disease. Nat. Med. **4:** 713–717.
15. WITZTUM, J.L. 1994. The oxidation hypothesis of atherosclerosis. Lancet **344:** 793–795.
16. VAARALA, O. *et al.* 1995. Development of immune response to cow milk proteins in infants receiving cow milk formula or hydrolysed formula. J. Allergy Clin. Immunol. **96:** 917–923.
17. ELLIOTT, R.B. *et al.* 1998. Dietary prevention of diabetes in the non-obese diabetic mouse. Diabetologia **31:** 62–64.
18. SCOTT, F.W. *et al.* 1997. Potential mechanisms by which certain foods promote or inhibit the development of spontaneous diabetes in BB rats: dosage, timing, early effect on islet area, and switch in infiltrate from Th1 to Th2 cells. Diabetes **46:** 589–598.
19. HÄNNINEN, A. *et al.* 1996. Mucosa-associated (beta 7-integrinhigh) lymphocytes accumulate early in the pancreas of NOD mice and show aberrant recirculation behavior. Diabetes **45:** 1173–1180.
20. YANG, X.-D. *et al.* 1997. Involvement of β7 integrin and mucosal addressin cell adhesion molecule-1 (MAdCAM-1) in the development of diabetes in nonobese diabetic mice. Diabetes **46:** 1542–1547.

21. Hänninen, A. *et al.* 1998. Mucosal addressin is required for the development of diabetes in nonobese diabetic mice. J. Immunol. **160:** 6018–6025.
22. Jaakkola, I. *et al.* 2003. Diabetogenic T cells are primed both in pancreatic and gut-associated lymph nodes in NOD mice. Eur. J. Immunol. **33:** 3255–3264.
23. Hänninen, A. *et al.* 1993. Endothelial cell-binding properties of lymphocytes infiltrated into human diabetic pancreas. Implications for pathogenesis of IDDM. Diabetes **42:** 1656–1562.
24. Paronen, J. *et al.* 1997. Glutamate decarboxylase-reactive peripheral blood lymphocytes from patients with IDDM express gut-specific homing receptor $\alpha 4\ \beta 7$-integrin. Diabetes **46:** 583–588.
25. Rott, L.S. *et al.* 1997. Expression of mucosal homing receptor $\alpha 4\beta 7$ by circulating CD4+ cells with memory for intestinal rotavirus. J. Clin. Invest. **100:** 1204–1208.
26. Savilahti, E. *et al.* 1999. Jejuna of patients with insulin-dependent diabetes mellitus show signs of immune activation. Clin. Exp. Immunol. **116:** 70–77.
27. Westerholm-Ormio, M. *et al.* 2003. Immunologic activity in the small intestinal mucosa of pediatric patients with type 1 diabetes. Diabetes **52:** 2287–2295.
28. Auricchio, R. *et al.* 2004. In vitro-deranged intestinal immune response to gliadin in type 1diabetes. Diabetes **53:** 1680–1683.
29. Mooradian, A.D. *et al.* 1986. Abnormal intestinal permeability to sugars in diabetes mellitus. Diabetologia **29:** 221–224.
30. Carratù, R. *et al.* 1999. Altered intestinal permeability to mannitol in diabetes mellitus type 1. J. Pediatr. Gastroenterol. Nutr. **28:** 264–269.
31. Kuitunen, M. *et al.* 2002. Intestinal permeability to mannitol and lactulose in children with type 1 diabetes with the HLA-DQB1*02 allele. Autoimmunity **35:** 365–368.
32. Secondulfo, M. *et al.* 2004. Ultrastructural mucosal alterations and increased intestinal permeability in non-celiac, type I diabetic patients. Dig. Liver Dis. **36:** 35–45.
33. Catassi, C. *et al.* 1995. Intestinal permeability changes during the first month: effect of natural versus artificial feeding. Pediatr. Gastroenterol. Nutr. **21:** 383–386.
34. Kuitunen, M., E. Savilahti & A. Sarnesto. 1994. Human alpha-lactalbumin and bovine beta-lactoglobulin absorption in infants. Allergy **49:** 354–360.
35. Hacsek, G. *et al.* 1999. B-cell development in lamina propria of the large intestine: influence of age and T-cell densities. Acta Pathol. Microbiol. Scand. **107:** 661–666.
36. Knip, M. *et al.* 2005. Environmental triggers and determinants of type 1 diabetes. Diabetes **54**(Suppl 2)**:** S125–S136.
37. Kimpimäki, T. *et al.* 2001. Short-term exclusive breast-feeding predisposes young children with increased genetic risk of type 1 diabetes to progressive beta-cell autoimmunity. Diabetologia **44:** 63–69.
38. Norris, J.M. *et al.* 2003. Timing of initial cereal exposure in infancy and risk of islet autoimmunity. JAMA **290:** 1713–1720.
39. Ziegler, A.G. *et al.* 2003. Early infant feeding and risk of developing type 1 diabetes-associated autoantibodies. JAMA **290:** 1721–1728.
40. Akerblom, H.K. *et al.* 2005. Dietary manipulation of beta cell autoimmunity in infants at increased risk of type 1 diabetes: a pilot study. Diabetologia **48:** 829–837.

41. LÖNNROT, M. *et al.* 2000. Enterovirus infections as a risk factor for β-cell autoimmunity in a prospectively observed birth cohort: the Finnish Diabetes Prediction and Prevention Study. Diabetes **49:** 1314–1318.
42. HONEYMAN, M.C. *et al.* 2000. Association between rotavirus infection and pancreatic islet autoimmunity in children at risk of developing type 1 diabetes. Diabetes **49:** 1319–1324.
43. TOUGH, D., P. BORROW & J. SPRENT. 1996. Induction of bystander T cell proliferation by viruses and type I interferon *in vivo*. Science **272:** 1947–1950.
44. VAARALA, O. 2003. Immunological effects of probiotics with special reference to lactobacilli. Clin. Exp. Allergy **33:** 1634–1640.
45. BJORKSTEN, B. *et al.* 2001. Allergy development and the intestinal microflora during the first year of life. J. Allergy Clin. Immunol. **108:** 516–520.
46. KALLIOMAKI, M. *et al.* 2001. Distinct patterns of neonatal gut microflora in infants in whom atopy was and was not developing. J. Allergy Clin. Immunol. **107:** 129–134.
47. WATANABE, S. *et al.* 2003. Differences in fecal microflora between patients with atopic dermatitis and healthy control subjects. J. Allergy Clin. Immunol. **111:** 587–591.
48. LJUNGBERG, M. *et al.* 2006. Probiotics for the prevention of beta-cell autoimmunity in children at genetic risk of type 1 diabetes—PRODIA Study. Ann. N. Y. Acad. Sci. This volume.
49. BJORKSTEN, B. *et al.* 1999. The intestinal microflora in allergic Estonian and Swedish 2-year-old children. Clin. Exp. Allergy **29:** 342–346.
50. GALLUCCI, S. & P. MATZINGER. 2001. Danger signals: SOS to the immune system. Curr. Opin. Immunol. **13:** 114–119.

Probiotics for the Prevention of Beta Cell Autoimmunity in Children at Genetic Risk of Type 1 Diabetes—the PRODIA Study

MARTIN LJUNGBERG,[a] RIITA KORPELA,[b] JORMA ILONEN,[c] JOHNNY LUDVIGSSON,[a] AND OUTI VAARALA[a,d]

[a]*Division of Pediatrics and Diabetes Research Centre, Department of Molecular and Clinical Medicine, Linköping University, S-58 185 Linköping, Sweden*

[b]*Valio Ltd, 00037 Helsinki, Finland*

[c]*Department of Clinical Microbiology, University of Kuopio, Kuopio, Finland and Immunogenetics Laboratory, University of Turku, 20520 Turku, Finland*

[d]*Department of Viral Diseases and Immunology, National Public Health Institute, 00037 Helsinki, Finland*

ABSTRACT: The final aim of the PRODIA study is to determine whether the use of probiotics during the first 6 months of life decreases the appearance of type 1 diabetes mellitus (T1DM)-associated autoantibodies in children with genetic risk for T1DM. A pilot study including 200 subjects was planned to show whether the use of probiotics during the first 6 months of life is safe and feasible. The prevalence of autoantibodies among the study subjects at 6, 12, and 24 months of age was at levels close to the expected and the clinical follow-up did not either indicate problems in the feasibility of the study.

KEYWORDS: type 1 diabetes; probiotics; autoantibodies

INTRODUCTION

Type 1 diabetes mellitus (T1DM) is considered to be an autoimmune disease leading to destruction of the insulin-producing beta cells in pancreas. Interaction between genetic factors and environmental factors are believed to trigger the autoimmune response finally causing T1DM.[1] About 90% of the children

Address for correspondence: Martin Ljungberg, Centre of Clinical Experimental Research, Division of Pediatrics and Diabetes Research Centre, Department of Molecular and Clinical Medicine, Faculty of Health Sciences, Linköping University, S-581 85 Linköping, Sweden. Voice: +46-13-229538; fax: +46-13-127465.
e-mail: martin.ljungberg@imk.liu.se

**Ann. N.Y. Acad. Sci. 1079: 360–364 (2006). © 2006 New York Academy of Sciences.
doi: 10.1196/annals.1375.055**

developing T1DM carry high-risk genes (human leukocyte antigen [HLA] DQB1*0302 and/or HLA DQB1*0201), but less than 10% of the children with these risk genes actually develop T1DM.[2] A number of environmental factors have been suggested to be associated with T1DM. Early exposure to cow milk proteins and wheat gluten in the infant diet, as well as enteral virus infections, together with aberrant development and maturity of the gut immune system, are candidate risk factors.[3] Enterovirus and rotavirus infections have been associated with the appearance of beta cell autoantibodies.[4,5] In animal models the incidence of T1DM has been shown to be highest in a low microbial load environment.[6] Microbiotic colonization of the newborn infant's gut ecosystem by specific bacterial species may be important in the initial regulation of the developing immune system.[7] Development of T1DM has been associated with intestinal immune activation and enhanced immunity to food antigens.[8,9] Probiotics, defined as nonpathogenic cultures of living bacteria with a health-promoting effect,[10] have *in vitro* showed to activate monocytes, macrophages, and dendritic cells and thus influence the immune system.[11–13] Probiotics also have been shown to support the maturity of the gut immune system and could therefore support oral tolerance and protection against enteral virus infections, that is, risk factors of T1DM.[14] Beta cell autoantibodies occurring years before clinical onset of T1DM are predictive for the disease in individuals with genetic risk. The three major islet autoantibodies are those against glutamic acid decarboylase (GADA), tyrosine phosphatase (IA-2A), and insulin (IAA). Children developing T1DM are mostly positive for at least two of these markers.[15] The PRODIA study started in February 2003 at the Faculty of Health Sciences at Linköping University as a pilot study primarily to test feasibility and safety of the protocol. The final aim of a main study will be to determine whether the use of probiotics during the first 6 months of life decreases the appearance of beta cell autoantibodies in children with increased genetic risk for T1DM. Affected factors involved could be the reduced occurrence of enteral virus infections, enhanced maturation of the gut immune system, reduced immunization to dietary insulin, or induced immune regulation.

SUBJECTS AND METHODS

The PRODIA study was approved by the Research Ethics Committee at the Faculty of Health Sciences, Linköping University. PRODIA is a double-blind randomized placebo controlled study. Between February 2003 and June 2005 all parents to newborn infants at Linköping University Hospital were informed about the PRODIA pilot study. After informed consent by the parents, 1200 children were screened for HLA genotypes associated with risk for T1DM. HLA risk genotypes were defined as the presence of HLA-(DR3)-DQA1*05-DQB1*02 and/or (DR4)-DQB1*0302 haplotypes without protective haplotypes DQB1*06301 and DQB1*0301. When combined with HLA-(DR3)-DQA1* 05-DQB1*02 also DQB1*0603 and DQA1*0201-

DQB1*02 were considered protective. All children with risk genotype were randomized to receive either probiotics or placebo during the first 6 months of life. The probiotics, distributed once a day by parents at home in soluble capsules, consist of a cocktail of Lactobacillus rhamnosus GG (5×10^9 cfu), Lactobacillus rhamnosus LC705 (5×10^9 cfu), Bifidobacterium breve Bbi99 (2×10^8 cfu), and Propionibacterium freudenreichii ssp. Shermani JS (2×10^9 cfu). Blood samples are taken at 6, 12, and 24 months of age. Fecal samples are collected at home at 3 months intervals and the introduction of new foods is recorded. The diet of the children is not manipulated. We analyze the occurrence of beta cell autoantibodies (GAD, IA-2, and IAA) and measure monocyte and T cell-derived cytokines and chemokines in plasma and supernatants of *in vitro*-stimulated cells. We also study the expression of intracellular signal proteins (T bet, STAT-4, STAT-6, GATA-3) in peripheral blood mononuclear cells (PBMC). Expression of monocyte activation markers is analyzed in fresh whole blood and in whole blood stimulated with lipopolysaccharide (LPS) and lipoteichoic acid (LTA). The phytohemagglutinin (PHA) and IAA-induced T cell responses are studied. Microbiological analyses of feces samples are done to control incidence of enteral virus infections and compliance. Enterovirus infections are followed also by isolation of enterovirus RNA in blood samples and by serological tests. Venous blood samples were collected at 6, 12, and 24 months and measurements of beta cell autoantibodies GAD, IA-2, and IAA were done as previously described.[16] The cutoff for positivity was determined as 99th percentile level of autoantibodies in healthy 5-year-old children.

RESULTS

About 60% of the parents asked to participate gave their informed consent. As expected we found 264 children with risk genes among the tested infants. The dropout rate has been steady between 15% and 25%. TABLE 1 shows the detection of autoantibodies in various samples. One sample was detected positive for IAA at 6 months of age. No sample was detected positive at 12 months of age. However, at 24 months of age one sample was detected positive for GADA and another one for IA-2A. No sample was detected positive for more than one autoantibody.

TABLE 1. Positivity to autoantibodies in plasma samples at 6, 12, and 24 months of age

	GADA	IA-2A	IAA	Pos>1 a.a
Age	pos/tot	pos/tot	pos/tot	pos/tot
6 months	0/170	0/170	1/168	0/168
12 months	0/151	0/151	0/146	0/146
24 months	1/61	1/61	0/61	0/61

pos = positive; tot = total; a.a. = autoantibody

DISCUSSION

The PRODIA protocol seems to be feasible, although quite many parents do not want to participate and the dropout rate is quite high. We expected to find roughly a 2% prevalence of at least one of the measured autoantibodies at 24 months of age in the study group. In the Finnish Diabetes Prediction and Prevention (DIPP) study follow-up cohort a frequency of 2.9% of children were found persistently positive for IAA, 1.7% for GADA, and 1.2% for IA-2A at the same age.[17] The DIPP study was similarly based on genetic screening of general population, but the lower risk group of children selected based on the presence of (DR3)-DQA1*05-DQB1*02 haplotype was not included. This group with approximately half of the risk ratio to that of moderate risk group with (DR4)-DQB1*0302[18] covers around a third of PRODIA group, which is taken into account by lower expected autoantibody positivity. The detected number of autoantibodies, 1/168 for IAA at 6 months of age, 1/61 for GADA, and 1/61 for IA-2A at 24 months of age, is close to the expected and there is no evidence that the intervention would increase the appearance of beta cell autoimmunity in the children who participate in the PRODIA study. We conclude that the PRODIA study protocol seems to be safe and that the study protocol is feasible for the families. The mechanistic studies of the effect of probiotics on the development of the immune system and occurrence of enterovirus infections are ongoing.

ACKNOWLEDGMENTS

We are grateful to all the participating children and parents in the PRODIA study. Many thanks to the PRODIA team in Linköping: coordinator Anneli KR Johnsson, nurses Eva Isacsson and Ann-Marie Sandström, and laboratory technicians Gosia Smolinska and Ingela Johansson. Appreciation goes to Rosaura Casas PhD and Anna Lindström MSc in the PRODIA study group. This study was generously supported by Swedish Child Diabetes Foundation (Barndiabetesfonden), Swedish Research Council (K2002-72X-11242-08A and K2003-72X-14690-01A), Swedish Diabetes Association, and the Foundation for Strategic Research. Support from Valio Ltd. is very much appreciated.

REFERENCES

1. KIM, M.S. & C. POLYCHRONAKOS. 2005. Immunogenetics of type 1 diabetes. Horm. Res. **64:** 180–188.
2. BERZINA, L., A. SCTAUVERE-BRAMEUS, J. LUDVIGSSON & C.B. SANJEEVI. 2002. Newborn screening for high-risk human leukocyte antigen markers associated with insulin dependent diabetes mellitus: the ABIS study. Ann. N. Y. Acad. Sci. **958:** 312–316.

3. AKERBLOM, H.K., O. VAARALA, H. HYOTY, *et al.* 2002. Environmental factors in the etiology of type 1 diabetes. Am. J. Med. Genet. **115:** 18–29.
4. LONNROT, M., K. KORPELA, M. KNIP, *et al.* 2000. Enterovirus infection as a risk factor for beta-cell autoimmunity in a prospectively observed birth cohort: the Finnish Diabetes Prediction and Prevention Study. Diabetes. **49:** 1314–1318.
5. HONEYMAN, M.C., B.S. COULSON, N.L. STONE, *et al.* 2000. Association between rotavirus infection and pancreatic islet autoimmunity in children at risk of developing type 1 diabetes. Diabetes **49:** 1319–1324.
6. DELOVITCH, T. & B. SINGH. 1997. The nonobese diabetic mouse as a model of autoimmune diabetes: immune dysregulation gets the NOD. Immunity **7:** 727–738.
7. SALVINI, F., L. GRANIERI, L. GEMMELLARO & M. GIOVANNINI. 2004. Probiotics, prebiotics and child health: where are we going? J. Int. Med. Res. **32:** 97–108.
8. WESTERHOLM-ORMIO, M., O. VAARALA, P. PIHKALA, *et al.* 2003. Immunologic activity in the small intestinal mucosa of pediatric patients with type 1 diabetes. Diabetes **52:** 2287–2295.
9. VAARALA, O. 2002. The gut immune system and type 1 diabetes. Ann. N. Y. Acad. Sci. **958:** 39–46.
10. LIN, D. 2003. Probiotics as functional foods. Nutr. Clin. Pract. **18:** 497–506.
11. VECKMAN, V., M. MIETTINEN, S. MATIKAINEN, *et al.* 2003. Lactobacilli and streptococci induce inflammatory chemokine production in human macrophages that stimulates Th1 cell chemotaxis. J. Leukoc. Biol. **74:** 395–402.
12. POCHARD, P., P. GOSSET, C. GRANGETTE, *et al.*2002. Lactic acid bacteria inhibit TH2 cytokine production by mononuclear cells from allergic patients. J. Allergy Clin. Immunol. **110:** 617–623.
13. CHRISTENSEN, H.R., H. FROKIAER & J.J. PESTKA. 2002. Lactobacilli differentially modulate expression of cytokines and maturation surface markers in murine dendritic cells. J. Immunol. **168:** 171–178.
14. VAARALA, O. 2003. Immunological effects of probiotics with special reference to lactobacilli. Clin. Exp. Allergy **33:** 1634–1640.
15. KULMALA, P., K. SAVOLA, J.S. PETERSEN, *et al.* 1998. Prediction of insulin-dependent diabetes mellitus in siblings of children with diabetes. A population-based study. The Childhood Diabetes in Finland Study Group. J. Clin. Invest. **101:** 327–336.
16. HOLMBERG, H., O. VAARALA, V. SADAUSKAITE-KUEHNE, *et al.* 2006. Higher prevalence of autoantibodies to insulin and GAD65 in Swedish compared to Lithuanian children with type 1 diabetes. Diabetes Res. Clin. Pract. **72:** 308–314.
17. KIMPIMAKI, T., P. KULMALA, K. SAVOLA, *et al.* 2002. Natural history of beta-cell autoimmunity in young children with increased genetic susceptibility to type 1 diabetes recruited from the general population. J. Clin. Endocrinol Metab. **87:** 4572–4579.
18. NEJENTSEV, S., M. SJOROOS, T. SOUKKA, *et al.* 1999. Population-based genetic screening for the estimation of type 1 diabetes mellitus risk in Finland: selective genotyping of markers in the HLA-DQB1, HLA-DQA1 and HLA-DRB1 loci. Diabet. Med. **16:** 985–992.

Thiazolidinediones May Not Reduce Diabetes Incidence in Type 1 Diabetes

TOSHIKATSU SHIGIHARA,* YOSHIAKI OKUBO,* YASUHIKO KANAZAWA, YOICHI OIKAWA, AND AKIRA SHIMADA

Department of Internal Medicine, Keio University School of Medicine, 35 Shinanomachi, Shinjuku-ku, Tokyo 160-8582, Japan

* *These authors contributed equally to this work.*

ABSTRACT: Thiazolidinediones improve glycemic control by reducing insulin resistance. Some studies have demonstrated that troglitazone had a preventative effect on diabetes in NOD (non-obese diabetic) mice. One of the mechanisms proposed for the prevention of diabetes by thiazolidinediones is an effect on T-helper 1/T-helper 2 (Th1/Th2) balance. In this article, we attempted to clarify whether pioglitazone is also effective in preventing diabetes as compared to metformin, which has no immunological effect. Female NOD mice were administered pioglitazone or metformin orally, and the insulitis score, cytokines secreted from splenocytes, cytokine expression levels in the pancreas, and the incidence of diabetes after acceleration by cyclophosphamide were analyzed. We could not find any advantage of pioglitazone in preventing Th1 skewing and the development of diabetes over metformin. Therefore, further research should take place before the application of thiazolidinediones to human slowly progressive insulin-dependent diabetes mellitus (SPIDDM) patients.

KEYWORDS: thiazolidinedione; metformin; NOD (non-obese diabetic) mouse; slowly progressive insulin-dependent diabetes mellitus (SPIDDM)

INTRODUCTION

Thiazolidinediones are oral hypoglycemic agents that act as PPARγ agonists and ameliorate insulin resistance. Previously, it has been reported that some thiazolidinediones reduce the incidence of autoimmune diabetes in the NOD (non-obese diabetic) mouse,[1,2] an excellent model of human type 1 diabetes. Thiazolidinediones are thought to prevent autoimmune diabetes by suppressing interferon-γ (IFN-γ) mRNA expression and IFN-γ secretion, thereby preventing T-helper 1 (Th1) skewing of the Th1/Th2 balance observed at the onset of diabetes. Therefore, clinical application of thiazolidinediones to

Address for correspondence: Dr. Akira Shimada, 35 Shinanomachi, Shinjuku-ku, Tokyo 160-8582, Japan. Voice: +81-3-3353-1211; ext.: 62383; fax: +81-3-5269-3219.
e-mail: asmd@sc.itc.keio.ac.jp

Ann. N.Y. Acad. Sci. 1079: 365–368 (2006).
doi: 10.1196/annals.1375.056

human slowly progressive type 1 diabetic patients with residual β cell function to prevent insulin dependence has been anticipated. This article attempted to clarify whether oral administration of pioglitazone, the only thiazolidinedione available in Japan, is also effective in suppressing Th1 skewing and preventing diabetes in NOD mice compared with metformin, which improves insulin resistance but has no immunological effect, before clinical application.

METHODS

Four-week-old female NOD mice were purchased from CLEA Japan Inc. (Tokyo, Japan). They were kept under specific pathogen-free conditions in the animal facility of Keio University. Female NOD mice were divided into a pioglitazone group ($n = 10$) and metformin group ($n = 12$). Then, 0.1% pioglitazone admixture food or metformin dissolved in drinking water (200 mg/kg/day) was given orally from 4 weeks of age. At 30 weeks of age, mice were killed for evaluation of insulitis score, and measurement of cytokine secretion from splenocytes upon anti-CD3 antibody stimulation, cytokine mRNA expression in the pancreas, and number of GAD-reactive cytokine (IFN-γ or interleukin-4 [IL-4]) producing $CD4^+$ splenocytes. Evaluation of insulitis was performed by scoring at least 30 islets from each mouse, and the degree of insulitis was assessed as three stages (no insulitis, peri-insulitis, intrainsulitis). Measurement of cytokine secretion from splenocytes after stimulation by anti-CD3 antibody for 48 h was performed by ELISA as previously described,[3] as well as measurement of pancreatic mRNA expression levels by semiquantitative RT-PCR, and measurement of numbers of GAD65-reactive cytokine-producing $CD4^+$ splenocytes by intracellular cytokine staining as previously described.[3] Then 23- and 27-week-old nondiabetic NOD mice that were given 0.01% pioglitazone or 200 mg/kg metformin were injected with 200 mg/kg cyclophosphamide intraperitoneally (i.p.). Urinary glucose analysis was performed daily, and the incidence of diabetes was assessed at 14 days after injection of cyclophosphamide.

RESULTS

Regarding insulitis score and cytokine responses of splenocytes after polyclonal stimulation at 30 weeks of age, there was no significant difference between the pioglitazone and metformin groups, although the pioglitazone group tended to have a higher insulitis score and higher IFN-γ (and lower IL-4) production (TABLE 1). Moreover, higher IFN-γ and lower IL-10 mRNA expression levels in the pancreas were observed in the pioglitazone group as compared to the metformin group (TABLE 1). There was no significant difference in the number of GAD65-reactive cytokine-producing $CD4^+$ splenocytes and the incidence of diabetes at 14 days after acceleration with cyclophos-

TABLE 1. Insulitis score, cytokine profiles, and cytokine expression levels

	Pioglitazone	Metformin	*P* value
Insulitis score (%)			
No insulitis	14	37	–
Peri-insulitis	44	16	–
Intra-insulitis	42	47	–
Cytokine profile after anti-CD3 Ab stimulation (48 hours' stimulation)			
IFN-γ (ng/ml)	2.5 ± 0.3	2.2 ± 0.2	NS
IL-4 (pg/ml)	5.7 ± 2.3	8.4 ± 3.5	NS
IL-10 (ng/ml)	1.5 ± 0.2	1.1 ± 0.3	NS
mRNA expression in pancreas (vs. β- actin)			
IFN-γ	4.1 ± 1.1	0.2 ± 0.1	<0.05
IL-4	3.0 ± 1.0	2.5 ± 1.5	NS
IL-10	3.2 ± 0.8	20.3 ± 7.2	<0.05
GAD65 reactive CD4+ T cells (72 hours' stimulation)			
IFN-γ (/50,000 CD4+ T cells)	0	311	–
IL-4 (/50,000 CD4+ T cells)	30	241	–

Data are shown as mean or mean ± SE. *P* values were calculated by unpaired *t* test where appropriate. NS = not significant.

phamide between the two groups; the incidence of diabetes was 60% in the pioglitazone group and 67% in the metformin group.

DISCUSSION

Our study revealed no significant advantage of pioglitazone over metformin in reducing the incidence of diabetes in NOD mice. It has been demonstrated that troglitazone and rosiglitazone, other thiazolidinediones, prevented autoimmune diabetes in NOD mice.[1] Troglitazone is thought to possess an anti-inflammatory property in addition to amelioration of insulin resistance. Giorgini *et al.* reported that troglitazone reduced proinflammatory cytokines, such as TNF-α and IFN-γ *in vitro*.[4] Augstein *et al.* showed that troglitazone reduced IFN-γ expression in splenic T cells in NOD mice.[2] Therefore, it has been hypothesized that thiazolidinediones prevent autoimmune diabetes by suppressing the Th1 skewing of the Th1/Th2 balance seen at the onset of diabetes in NOD mice. On the other hand, metformin is another oral hypoglycemic agent that decreases insulin resistance, but it is reported to have no effect of reducing the incidence of diabetes in NOD mice.[5] In this study, we examined the cytokine profiles of NOD mice given pioglitazone or metformin, and showed that mice fed pioglitazone had a higher insulitis score, higher IFN-γ (and lower IL-4) production, and higher IFN-γ mRNA expression in the pancreas. The discrepancy between the results of previous studies and ours may derive from the structural difference between pioglitazone and troglitazone (or rosiglitazone), the concentration of the agents, or the timing and duration of treatment. Because of its favorable effect on NOD mice previously reported, clinical application of thiazolidinediones in islet-associated autoantibody positive patients with residual β cell function has been planned. However, as no favorable effect of pioglitazone compared to metformin in suppressing the incidence of diabetes was seen in the present study, we conclude that further investigation should take place before using pioglitazone as a drug to prevent insulin dependence in slowly progressive type 1 diabetes in humans.

REFERENCES

1. BEALES, P.E. & P. POZZILLI. 2002. Thiazolidinediones for the prevention of diabetes in the non-obese diabetic (NOD) mouse: implications for human type 1 diabetes. Diabetes Metab. Res. Rev. **18:** 114–117.
2. AUGSTEIN, P., A. DUNGER, *et al.* 2003. Prevention of autoimmune diabetes in NOD mice by troglitazone is associated with modulation of ICAM-1 expression on pancreatic islet cells and IFN-γ expression in splenic T cells. Biochem. Biophys. Res. Commun. **304:** 378–384.
3. SHIGIHARA, T., A. SHIMADA, *et al.* 2005. CXCL10 DNA vaccination prevents spontaneous diabetes through enhanced beta cell proliferation in NOD mice. J. Immunol. **75:** 8401–8408.
4. GIORGINI, A.E., P.E. BEALES, *et al.* 1999. Troglitazone exhibits immunomodulatory activity on the cytokine production of activated human lymphocytes. Horm. Metab. Res. **31:** 1–4.
5. BEALES, P.E., A.E. GIORGINI, *et al.* 1997. Metformin does not alter diabetes incidence in the NOD mouse. Horm. Metab. Res. **29:** 261–263.

Mechanisms Mediating Anti-CD3 Antibody Efficacy

Insights from a Mathematical Model of Type 1 Diabetes

DANIEL L. YOUNG, SAROJA RAMANUJAN, HUUB T.C. KREUWEL, CHAN CHUNG WHITING, KAPIL G. GADKAR, AND LISL K.M. SHODA

Entelos Inc., Foster City, California 94404, USA

ABSTRACT: Anti-CD3 antibody therapy, a promising clinical approach for the treatment of type 1 diabetes (T1D), was investigated using a mathematical model of T1D in the female nonobese diabetic (NOD) mouse. Analyses of model simulation results indicate that, in addition to the known direct effects of anti-CD3 antibody on T lymphocytes, two additional mechanisms are required for sustained disease remission: (*a*) rapid regrowth of healthy β cells following clearance of islet inflammation and (*b*) enhanced regulatory T cell activity and/or phenotypic changes in antigen presenting cells (APCs) that promote a stable regulatory environment in the pancreas.

KEYWORDS: diabetes remission; β cells; antigen presenting cells; 145-2C11; systems biology; glucose control

INTRODUCTION

Although anti-CD3 antibody therapy has yielded positive outcomes in human type 1 diabetes (T1D) clinical trials,[1,2] complete disease remission was not seen in humans as it was in the nonobese diabetic (NOD) mouse, a preclinical animal model of spontaneous T1D. To elucidate the critical mechanism(s) mediating anti-CD3-induced remission in NOD mice, we investigated the actions of anti-CD3 therapy using a mathematical model of T1D in the female NOD mouse.

Address for correspondence: Lisl K.M. Shoda, Ph.D., Entelos Inc., 110 Marsh Drive, Foster City, CA 94404. Voice: 650-572-5400; fax: 650-572-5401.
e-mail: shoda@entelos.com

Ann. N.Y. Acad. Sci. 1079: 369–373 (2006). © 2006 New York Academy of Sciences.
doi: 10.1196/annals.1375.057

RESEARCH DESIGN AND METHODS

The actions of the anti-CD3 antibody, 145-2C11, were quantitatively represented and examined in a large-scale, mathematical model of T1D pathogenesis in the NOD mouse. This model, the T1D PhysioLab platform (Entelos, Inc., Foster City, CA), comprises differential and algebraic equations that mathematically represent cellular functions and biochemical interactions in pancreatic lymph node, pancreatic islet, and blood compartments. The following cell types are modeled: conventional $CD4^+$ T cells (including Th1, Th2, and adaptive regulatory $CD4^+$ T cells), innate regulatory T cells (iTregs, including $CD4^+$ $CD25^+$ and natural killer T cells [NKT]), $CD8^+$ T cells, B lymphocytes, endothelial cells, dendritic cells, macrophages, and pancreatic β cells. For each cell type, functions important for disease pathogenesis were modeled, such as cellular activation, turnover (e.g., proliferation, apoptosis), traffic between the pancreatic lymph node and islets, mediator secretion, contact-mediated functions (e.g., antigen presentation, β cell killing), and insulin secretion and glucose regulation.

Quantitative data on cell populations, functions, and mediator activities obtained from published *in vivo* and *in vitro* studies were used to estimate parameter values in the model. Disease outcome data for certain interventions (exogenous interleukin-10 (IL-10), anti-CD8 antibody, anti-CD3 antibody, LipCl2MDP, and anti-B7.1 + anti-B7.2 antibodies) were used to further constrain and calibrate the model. The resulting model was validated by verifying the agreement between simulation results and reported data not used in model development, namely, the therapeutic responses in female NOD mice to exogenous transforming growth factor-β (TGF-β), anti-CD40L antibody, and exendin-4 treatments. Additionally, eliminating $CD4^+$ T cells, $CD8^+$ T cells, or B lymphocytes reproduced diabetes protection as reported in the literature.

To quantitatively address the impact of data uncertainty and/or heterogeneity in the biology of female NOD mice, multiple virtual NOD mice were created in the T1D PhysioLab platform. Each virtual NOD mouse represents distinct biological specifications or hypotheses, specified by unique parameter value combinations, while still reproducing known characteristics of T1D pathogenesis. As the regulatory $CD4^+$ $CD25^+$ T cell subset is thought to be important for anti-CD3 efficacy in diabetic NOD mice,[3] this study investigated that effect in three virtual NOD mice with differing regulatory T cell functions.

To simulate the effect of anti-CD3 antibody treatment in the virtual NOD mice, direct effects of the drug on $CD3^+$ T cells were assessed from the literature and represented mathematically in the model, incorporating the pharmacokinetics for different routes of administration (intraperitoneal or intravenous), as well as the reported functional antibody half-life.[4] The dose-dependent direct effects of anti-CD3 antibody on activation, proliferation, and apoptosis of T cell subsets in blood, pancreatic lymph node, and islet compartments were modeled. In addition, differential effects on conventional T cells versus iTregs and on naïve versus activated T cells were implemented.

RESULTS

Published anti-CD3 antibody protocols tested in NOD mice (for review, see Ref. 5) were simulated in virtual NOD mice to test the predictive value of each virtual mouse, as well as to determine critical mechanisms mediating anti-CD3 disease protection. For anti-CD3 treatment of prediabetic mice, effects on disease progression in the three virtual NOD mice matched reported findings, yielding disease protection following a single anti-CD3 antibody injection 1 day after birth, and an increasing delay in diabetes onset for treatments starting between 4 and 12 weeks of age administered for 5 consecutive days.

To reproduce the reported efficacy of anti-CD3 treatment of diabetic NOD mice,[6,7] two novel hypothesized mechanisms of anti-CD3 activity were required in addition to the known effects of anti-CD3 antibody on T lymphocytes. The first mechanism concerns the ability of the residual β cell mass of diabetic NOD mice to restore normoglycemia. In all virtual NOD mice tested, the clearance of islet infiltration resulting from the direct effects of anti-CD3 antibody alone was not sufficient to restore normoglycemia, due to reduced mass and glucose-induced exhaustion of the remaining β cells. Analysis of simulation results demonstrated that even transient restoration of normoglycemia would require additional recovery of β cell mass, β cell function, or a combination of the two. For example, a 2.25-fold increase in β cell proliferation enabled by the clearance of inflammation was required to restore normoglycemia in all virtual NOD mice, provided that newly generated β cells exhibited healthy insulin-producing capabilities.

The second hypothesized mechanism required for sustained disease remission concerns the character of the pancreatic insulitis following cessation of anti-CD3 administration. Consistent with experimental data,[6,7] model results indicated that insulitis declined during treatment of recent onset diabetic virtual NOD mice yet returned following cessation of treatment. Without a treatment-induced change in the character (e.g., destructive versus regulatory) of this infiltrate, disease remission was only transient, suggesting a requirement for altered infiltrate character. This notion is in agreement with experimental data showing that increased TGF-β-dependent $CD4^+$ $CD25^+$ T cells might contribute to sustained remission following anti-CD3 antibody treatment.[3] Simulation results indicated that sustained disease remission was attained in virtual mice with either enhanced iTreg functionality and/or a therapy-induced increase in the ratio of *suppressive* to *inflammatory* antigen presenting cells (APCs) (FIG. 1). Such a change in the APC ratio corresponds to a qualitative change in the cytokine-production and T cell priming pattern of the APCs, and resulted in preferential priming of regulatory T cells versus inflammatory Th1-like T cells. These results suggest that long-term remission following anti-CD3 antibody treatment reflects a more tolerant insulitis resulting from enhanced iTreg activity and/or suppressive APC contributions.

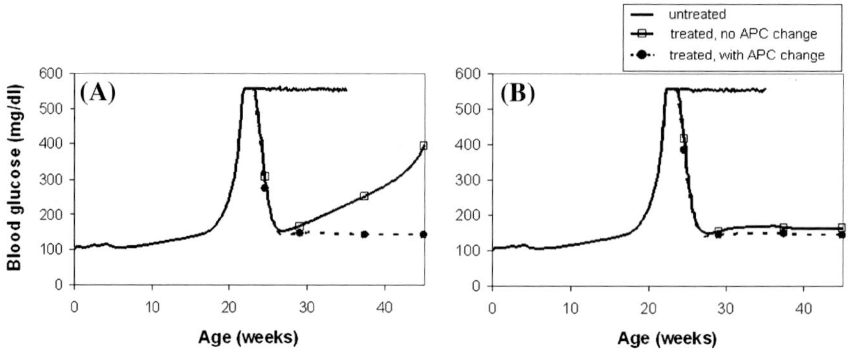

FIGURE 1. Predicted responses to anti-CD3 treatment in virtual NOD mice. (**A**) Blood glucose responses to anti-CD3 treatment are depicted in the first virtual NOD mouse, which has low regulatory T cell activity. An altered APC phenotype (circles) is required for sustained disease remission following anti-CD3 antibody administration. (**B**) Responses to anti-CD3 treatment are depicted in the second virtual NOD mouse, which has higher regulatory T cell activity due to colocalization of regulatory T cells with activated T cells in the pancreatic lymph node. No change in the APC phenotype is required for sustained disease remission (squares). Responses (not shown) in the third virtual NOD mouse, in which regulatory T cells have increased cytokine production and cell–cell contact effects, resemble those shown in panel (B).

DISCUSSION

Analysis of a mathematical model of T1D pathogenesis in female NOD mice showed that in addition to the known direct effects of anti-CD3 antibody on T cells, sustained remission required: (*a*) rapid β cell recovery and (*b*) a more regulatory pancreatic infiltrate, resulting from either greater iTreg activity and/or a switch in APC phenotype. These hypotheses could be verified by experimental characterization of β cell activity (e.g., proliferation, insulin secretion) following anti-CD3 treatment and measurement of iTreg activity and APC phenotypic changes to elucidate which mechanism(s) foster suppressive infiltration and sustained remission. The mechanisms promoting such changes in regulatory cells are unclear; however, it has been suggested that clearance of pathogenic T cells from inflamed tissues could enable recovery of regulatory activities.[8] Elucidation of the mechanisms critical for anti-CD3-mediated remission in mice could lead to more targeted treatments and the enhancement of anti-CD3 antibody therapy in humans.

ACKNOWLEDGMENTS

We thank the American Diabetes Association's Scientific Advisory Board: Drs. Mark Atkinson, Jeff Bluestone, George Eisenbarth, Diane Mathis, and

Aldo Rossini, for their guidance of this work. This work was funded by the American Diabetes Association.

REFERENCES

1. Herold, K.C., S.E. Gitelman, U. Masharani, *et al.* 2005. A single course of anti-CD3 monoclonal antibody hOKT3{gamma}1(Ala-Ala) results in improvement in C-peptide responses and clinical parameters for at least 2 years after onset of type 1 diabetes. Diabetes **54:** 1763–1769.
2. Keymeulen, B., E. Vandemeulebroucke, A.G. Ziegler, *et al.* 2005. Insulin needs after CD3-antibody therapy in new-onset type 1 diabetes. N. Engl. J. Med. **352:** 2598–2608.
3. Belghith, M., J.A. Bluestone, S. Barriot, *et al.* 2003. TGF-beta-dependent mechanisms mediate restoration of self-tolerance induced by antibodies to CD3 in overt autoimmune diabetes. Nat. Med. **9:** 1202–1208.
4. Hayward, A.R. & M. Shreiber. 1989. Neonatal injection of CD3 antibody into nonobese diabetic mice reduces the incidence of insulitis and diabetes. J. Immunol. **143:** 1555–1559.
5. Shoda, L.K., D.L. Young, S. Ramanujan, *et al.* 2005. A comprehensive review of interventions in the NOD mouse and implications for translation. Immunity **23:** 115–126.
6. Chatenoud, L., E. Thervet, J. Primo & J.F. Bach. 1994. Anti-CD3 antibody induces long-term remission of overt autoimmunity in nonobese diabetic mice. Proc. Natl. Acad. Sci. USA **91:** 123–127.
7. Chatenoud, L., J. Primo & J.F. Bach. 1997. CD3 antibody-induced dominant self tolerance in overtly diabetic NOD mice. J. Immunol. **158:** 2947–2954.
8. Ruprecht, C.R., M. Gattorno, F. Ferlito, *et al.* 2005. Coexpression of CD25 and CD27 identifies $FoxP3^+$ regulatory T cells in inflamed synovia. J. Exp. Med. **201:** 1793–1803.

Why Diabetes Incidence Increases—A Unifying Theory

JOHNNY LUDVIGSSON

Department of Molecular and Clinical Medicine, Division of Pediatrics, Faculty of Health Sciences, Linköping University, SE- 581 85 Linköping, Sweden

ABSTRACT: There is a wide spectrum within the diabetes syndrome. Type 1 diabetes may have a slow progression with good residual insulin secretion and without autoantibodies, while phenotypic type 2 diabetes may have autoantibodies. A single patient may have traits of both types of diabetes. Their incidence increases in parallel. The etiology is mainly unknown, but environmental factors play an important role in genetically predisposed individuals. The search for just one single cause of manifest diabetes may be confusing. Different mechanism may be important in different parts of the world. Furthermore, certain mechanisms may lead to islet inflammation while other/additional mechanisms may increase insulin demand and cause insulin deficiency with manifestation of clinical diabetes. Several hypothesis of etiology may fit different parts of the disease process. Thus, increased hygiene may contribute to an imbalance of the immune system, facilitating autoimmune reactions when virus infections, or proteins like cow's milk or gluten, provoke. Increased insulin demand because of rapid growth, or insulin resistance caused by stress, infections, puberty, etc., lead to β cell stress, antigen presentation and may cause both an autoimmune reaction in genetically predisposed individuals, and insulin deficiency leading to manifest diabetes in individuals who have lost β cell function. Vitamins may modulate the immune process, but we know too little to give vitamin substitution. However, we do know that low physical exercise, obesity, and stress, increases insulin demand resulting in insulin deficiency. Now we can therefore intervene to prevent the diabetic syndrome.

KEYWORDS: islet inflammation; preclinical diabetes; type 1 diabetes; type 2 diabetes; LADA; etiology; hypothesis; autoimmunity; insulin resistance

Address for correspondence: Johnny Ludvigsson, M.D., Ph.D., Division of Pediatrics, and Diabetes Research Centre, Department of Molecular and Clinical Medicine, Faculty of Health Sciences, Linköping University, SE-581 85 Linköping, Sweden. Voice: +46-13-221333; fax: +46-13-148265.
e-mail: johnny.ludvigsson@lio.se

**Ann. N.Y. Acad. Sci. 1079: 374–382 (2006). © 2006 New York Academy of Sciences.
doi: 10.1196/annals.1375.058**

Both type 1 and type 2 diabetes increases rapidly,[1–3] almost epidemically. Both types of the disease end up with a lack of insulin, at least in relation to the need, with similar consequences for metabolism and in the long run, negative effects on the body, late complications. Based on the different phenotypes and seemingly different etiology they are regarded as different diseases, even though there are mixed forms with unclear borders. Thus autoimmune signs in phenotypic type 2 diabetes has been called LADA (Latent Autoimmune Diabetes in the Adults)[4] or SPIDDM (Slowly Progressive Insulin Dependent Diabetes Mellitus).[5] Phenotypic type 2 diabetes in children have quite often autoantibodies[6] and have been called type 1.5 or double diabetes.[7] Evidently there is a wide spectrum within the diabetes syndrome.

The two main types of the disease increase in parallel but the incidence and prevalence differs in different parts of the world. Although difficult to prove, it is natural to expect different disposition to the two main forms of diabetes in different parts of the world. Because of the climate and living circumstances, people in certain areas of the world have had little reason to store food for future colder seasons when no plants grow, but they could just move to another place when food in the area had been consumed (nomads). Such people, especially in the warmer areas of the world, have had good reasons to develop a metabolism allowing them to starve for a day or two while seeking food, and hypoglycemia during their moving around to find food at another place would have been deleterious. Thus they have developed a metabolism with a low tendency to get hypoglycemia and good efficiency to store energy. Insulin resistance has become a survival factor. No wonder that these populations get a dramatic increase of obesity and type 2 diabetes when they find food in abundance without needing to walk/move (exercise)! In other parts of the world the people have had to face a colder climate. Winters without growing fruits or plants have made it necessary for them to collect and store food for future needs. As farmers at a certain locality, the need to survive starvation for some days now and then have become less common. Such people have needed less insulin resistance and may have a low tendency to get obesity and type 2 diabetes, unless they almost completely avoid exercise, with dysregulation of appetite and fat storage, and increase their energy intake abnormally. However, these people, typically Caucasians, have needed a good immune system to survive when they have been attacked by viruses and bacteria while they were living in cold and wet houses, as they have not been able to build big, tempered, clean houses until recently. No wonder that their very strong immune systems tend to lose balance now and then when there is lack of duties or occupation. Sometimes the immune system then react abnormally strong towards ridiculous enemies like foreign antigens from birch or cats, allergic reactions, and sometimes the system goes wrong and reacts against own tissue, autoimmune reactions. These tendencies believed to be characterized by Th2 and Th1 deviation, respectively, may seem contrary, but it is not surprising that with the decreasing use of the immune system both types of deviations may occur in the same population, or even in the same individual.[8]

In addition to the speculations mentioned above serious efforts are made to identify the cause of diabetes. Regarding type 2 diabetes this does not look very difficult. Most people, even scientists, probably accept the idea that lack of exercise causes not only less energy consumption but also decreasing insulin sensitivity, loss of appetite regulation, perhaps abnormal fat distribution, etc. Modern discoveries like the endocannabinoid system[9] and increasing awareness of fat cells taking part in a communication or hormonal system cast light on the cause of the so-called Metabolic Syndrome and type 2 diabetes. Almost everybody agrees that although different people and different populations have more or less the same genetic predisposition to Metabolic Syndrome and type 2 diabetes, these problems would be prevented by less energy intake, less stress that causes insulin resistance, and more physical exercise.

Type 1 diabetes looks worse. We want to find one single cause, the same for the whole world, for example, one virus like the one causing polio, or one nutritional factor like gluten causing celiac disease, or the lack of one vitamin like vitamin D causing rickets. When there are good arguments for each and different etiological parameters we get confused. Epidemiology does not seem to solve the problem, and making worldwide collaborative efforts to find a common cause might even cause further confusion. Nobody would agree that broken legs in children should have the same cause in all parts of the world. Adding completely different populations from different parts of the world in a mix would probably lead to a situation where falling from downhill skiing does not seem to be a cause of broken legs in Africa, and football (soccer) does not seem to play a role in girls under the age of 6 years in Greenland, etc. But as broken legs or cancer may depend on different contributing causes, type 1 diabetes may depend on, and most probably does depend on, different causes.

Several Good Hypotheses

The *Hygiene hypothesis*[10] may certainly be relevant as increased hygiene causes lack of occupation for the strong immune system, once built for heavier tasks. In addition, increased hygiene changes the gut bacterial flora that might influence the maturation of the immune system.[11] Certain viruses will become less frequent leading to decreasing immunity in the population,[12] which facilitates dangerous damage of tissue when such a virus attacks, even though we should not necessarily expect to find the virus, suggested by the *Polio hypothesis*.[12] But it is quite plausible that sporadic cases of diabetes are caused by virus attacks (*The Virus hypothesis*) as several viruses are capable of damaging the pancreas and also the islets.[13,14] Or, at least the virus may mimic autoantigens or cause so much damage that autoantigens are presented, enough to facilitate or initiate an autoimmune process in genetically predisposed individuals.

But how does this fit with the increasing evidence of the *Diet Hypothesis*, saying that dietary factors or intake of *toxic agents*, such as nitrite/nitrate, play an important role in the development of type 1 diabetes. As an organizer of a

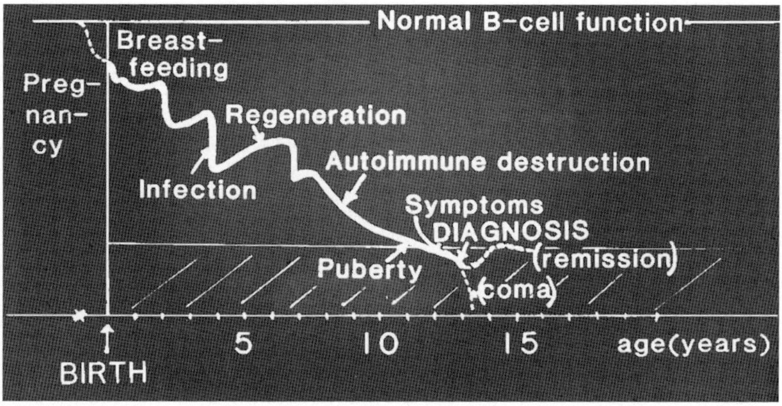

FIGURE 1. After a long disease process, influenced by many environmental factors, some individuals may develop manifest diabetes. Hypothetical picture presented at Nordic symposium on diabetes epidemiology outside Linköping 1981.

Nordic symposium in 1981 on the epidemiology of type 1 diabetes I presented a slide (FIG. 1) that was followed by studies by one of the participants at the symposium showing that *breastfeeding* seems to play a role in the risk of getting diabetes.[15] Later on it has been proposed that breastfeeding as such has no influence on the risk of getting diabetes, but rather that the early introduction of cow's milk does (*the Cow's Milk hypothesis*)[16]; but still several studies do support the hypotheses that breastfeeding in itself may well play a protective role and there are several good explanations why. However, early introduction of cow's milk probably also plays a role in the development of type 1 diabetes. Introduction of antigenic bovine insulin via cow's milk in food has been shown to increase an immune reaction, which later on may turn into an autoimmune reaction against own insulin secretion.[17] Introduction of other components in cow's milk might also play a role[18,19] and cause immune reactions in genetically predisposed individuals, facilitated by the lack of immune regulation because of modern hygiene and disturbed maturation of the immune system, etc. The increased nutritional load by early consumption of cow's milk might also contribute to increased β cell stress, increased antigen presentation, and thereby autoimmunity in predisposed individuals.[20,21] While the role of cow's milk has been seen mainly in the Nordic countries[22] this influence has not been evident in other areas[23] where other nutrients have been suspected. The introduction of *gluten*, either too early or too late, seems to be dangerous[24] while the introduction during a time window between 4 and 6 months of age seems to be the best for the body. This fact is the same as for celiac disease where too early introduction of gluten causes the disease[25] but also too late introduction, proven in the Swedish national experiment: When gluten introduction was postponed from 4 months of age to 6 months of age between

1984 and 1996 the world's already highest incidence of celiac disease became threefold higher, then falling dramatically back to its earlier incidence when gluten introduction from the age of 4 months was reallowed/recommended.[25]

Islet Autoimmunity or Clinical Diabetes?

Of course, we long for the driving antigen like gluten in celiac disease, but there are good reasons why so far no single dietary antigen has been identified. Research on celiac disease is concentrating on factors causing a reasonably well-defined disease process, inflammation in the gut, defined by biopsies, irrespective of whether there are any clinical consequences for the individual patient or not. In diabetes, however, we are almost ashamed of searching for the cause of islet inflammation, but we only count the consequence, clinical manifestation of diabetes, the metabolic end disaster seen only in a minority of those with islet autoimmunity. This makes the picture much more complicated and could be compared with the search for "The One Cause" of symptoms of celiac disease, such as depression, or infertility, or kidney disease, or retarded growth, or all these symptoms. There is no reason to expect one single cause of all these clinical manifestations in some of those individuals who have inflammation in the gut because of celiac disease. With the same kind of argumentation there is no reason to expect one single factor to explain both the development of the islet inflammation, usually autoimmune, and why some sporadic individuals get serious lack of insulin.

The β Cell Stress Hypothesis

Lack of insulin may become pronounced when the need increases. During periods with rapid growth the demand for insulin is great, and one would therefore expect that the β cells have to work hard to produce insulin. If the immune system is prone to react against insulin overload, for example, because of earlier sensitization caused by dietary introduction of bovine insulin, one would not be surprised that increased insulin production during, for example, early rapid growth or during puberty stimulates the autoimmune process. Furthermore, the great need for insulin may well cause relative insulin insufficiency, high glucose and glucose toxicity, and finally manifest clinical diabetes. As rapid weight gain in young children is becoming more common one would expect to see more cases of islet autoimmunity, and initially relative, and later absolute, lack of insulin in younger children, which fits both with the *Accelerator hypothesis*[26] and the increased tendency to get clinical presentation at younger ages.[27] In addition, not only is insulin presentation increased when the β cells work harder to produce more insulin, but also other antigens are presented in increased amounts, for example, glutamic acid decarboxylase (GAD)[21] and probably tyrosinfosfatase (IA-2). Therefore, it would be natural to find more autoimmune reactions also toward these and similar antigens. If there is an inflammation in the islets with infiltration of mononuclear cells one can expect some β cells to die, and also some other islet cells, and antibodies against a wide range of antigens would be expected islet cell antibodies (ICA). When the inflammation is heavy and cell death widespread, these ICA react not only against β cell antigens but also against other islet cells, a phenomenon that has been shown to be more predictive for future clinical diabetes than when the ICA are β cell specific.

However, β cell stress may be caused not only by the increased need to cover metabolic needs related to growth. Increased stimulation of the β cells by regular overfeeding might stimulate the cells too much in some individuals. Thus, our increasing consumption of sucrose might play a role in the spread of the disease. With increasing insulin resistance β cell stress will increase further. Any infections may cause insulin resistance and may contribute to such β cell stress.[28] Psychological stress may cause insulin resistance and thereby β cell stress and diabetes-associated autoimmunity in certain individuals.[29,30] Psychological mechanisms might even influence the immune balance and could therefore work in two ways to promote islet inflammation and the development of diabetes. Puberty not only leads to increased growth but also an increase of stress and sex hormones causing insulin resistance and it is natural that the breakdown of the system will occur during puberty. All this fits into the *Accelerator hypothesis* or our proposed somewhat wider β *cell stress hypothesis*.

Protective Agents

But where does vitamin D deficiency fit? There are several good arguments that vitamin D deficiency plays a role for the development of type 1 diabetes.[31] Of course, vitamin D deficiency may in many ways contribute to immune imbalance as well as exaggerated hygiene can. Maybe lack of other vitamins also can contribute to increased risk of getting disturbed immune balance like vitamin C.[32] Vitamins like nikotinamid (vitamin B) may also protect the β cells during the ongoing inflammation. This does not mean that we know what doses are to be recommended and it would be hazardous to give general high dose recommendations as high doses might well give unexpected side effects on other organs, for example cancer by too much vitamin E[33] or nephrocalcinosis by too much vitamin D.[34]

A Unifying Theory

Several mechanisms mentioned above, such as increased hygiene and vitamin D deficiency, may cause a labile immune system, while certain viruses, dietary bovine insulin, or toxic agents may initiate an autoimmune reaction, facilitated if the immune system is labile, and mainly in genetically predisposed individuals. That will cause islet inflammation, which in the majority of cases probably recovers spontaneously at a level when the number of functioning β cells is sufficient to produce enough insulin. In some individuals, however, either the insulin production becomes extremely poor, or the demand for insulin because of growth, weight, stress, or low physical exercise, insulin resistance becomes too high. Relative lack of insulin causes increasing blood glucose, increasing β cell stress, glucose toxicity, β cell death, and further promotion of the autoimmune process. Diabetes becomes manifest, in those cases with pronounced islet inflammation and rapid β cell loss called type 1 diabetes; in others it becomes manifest with slight islet autoimmunity and less rapid β cell loss called LADA or SPIDDM, and in the great majority of adults without detectable autoimmunity, it is called type 2 diabetes.

In our effort to explain why islet inflammation develops, we may continue our efforts to identify the most specific factors. Research on the immune mechanisms sometimes seems to dig deeper and deeper tunnels without finding any light at the end, and it can be questioned whether increased knowledge on communication between individual soldiers or companies, or detailed knowledge on weapons really facilitates the peace process or prevents civil war. Perhaps we also need more research on why the leaders, the central nervous system, allow such mistakes as civil wars. But, on the other hand, new knowledge on immune regulation might also open up for interventions and unfortunately we do not know whether we are digging deep or still just in the superficial layer.

In any case islet inflammation or "preclinical diabetes" is one thing and manifests diabetes is another, which is sometimes caused because of low insulin production due to poor function or death of β cells, and sometimes because of too high need for insulin. Thus, insulin resistance or increased insulin demand because of growth, etc. may well play an important role in the clinical manifestation not only of type 2 diabetes but also of type 1 diabetes, and it is possible that increased β cell stress stimulates or sometimes even initiates the autoimmune islet disease.

Prevention of Diabetes Is Already Possible

More knowledge is needed to explain why islet autoimmunity develops in humans. Additional knowledge is needed to explain why some people get diabetes, with or without foregoing islet autoimmunity, and why many with islet autoimmunity do not. We still need more intervention trials to prevent islet autoimmunity and/or diabetes. What doses of vitamin D and/or other vitamins are best to improve immune balance and/or protect β cells? When and how much cow's milk should be given to children? How can the immune system be regulated or occupied in a peace process decreasing the present tendency to deviate either toward allergic or autoimmune, or both abnormal reactions. Can insulin sensitizers decrease β cell stress and thereby prevent islet autoimmunity? While searching for new knowledge, but not necessarily The One Cause, we could already now use existing knowledge to prevent diabetes, irrespective of islet autoimmunity and irrespective of disagreement of type 1, 2, 1.5, or any other form of the diabetes syndrome. We must not wait for prevention of all cases! Every single case that can be prevented is wonderful for that child or adult! By changing our lifestyle we *will* decrease β cell stress and the relative lack of insulin. That will, without question, reduce type 2 diabetes and most likely also type "<2" diabetes.[35]

REFERENCES

1. KARVONEN, M., M. VIIK-KAJANDER, E. MOLTCHANOVA, *et al.* 2000. Incidence of childhood type 1 diabetes worldwide. Diabetes Mondiale (DiaMond) Project Group. Diabetes Care **23:** 1516–1526.
2. ZIMMET, P., K.G. ALBERTI & J. SHAW. 2001. Global and societal implications of the diabetes epidemic. Nature **13:** 782–787.
3. SINGH, R., J. SHAW & P. ZIMMET. 2004. Epidemiology of childhood type 2 diabetes in the developing world. Pediatr. Diabetes **5:** 154–168.
4. ZIMMET, P.Z., T. TUOMI, I.R. MACKAY, *et al.* 1994. Latent autoimmune diabetes mellitus in adults (LADA): the role of antibodies to glutamic acid decarboxylase in diagnosis and prediction of insulin dependency. Diabet. Med. **11:** 299–303.
5. KOBAYASHI, T., T. MARUYAMA, A. SHIMADA, *et al.* 2002. Insulin intervention to preserve beta cells in slowly progressive insulin-dependent (type 1) diabetes mellitus. Ann. N. Y. Acad. Sci. **958:** 117–130.
6. BROOKS-WORREL, B.M., C.J. GREENBAUM, J.P. PALMER, *et al.* 2004. Autoimmunity to islet proteins in children diagnosed with new-onset diabetes. J. Clin. Endocrinol. Metab. **89:** 2222–2227.
7. LIBMAN, I.M. & D.J. BECKER. 2003. Coexistence of type 1 and type 2 diabetes mellitus: "double" diabetes? Pediatr. Diabetes **4:** 110–113.
8. CARDWELL, C.R., M.D. SHIELDS, D.J. CARSON, *et al.* 2003. A meta-analysis of the association between childhood type 1 diabetes and atopic disease. Diabetes Care **26:** 2568–2574.
9. BOYD, S.T. & B.A. FREMMING. 2005. Rimonabant—a selective CB1 antagonist. Ann. Pharmacother. **9:** 684–690.
10. KOLB, H. & R.B. ELLIOT. 1994. Increasing incidence of IDDM a consequence of improved hygiene. Diabetologia **37:** 729.
11. ROOK, G.A. & L.R. BRUNET. 2005. Microbes, immunoregulation, and the gut. Gut **54:** 317–320.
12. VISKARI, H., J. LUDVIGSSON, R. UIBO, *et al.* 2005. Relationship between the incidence of type 1 diabetes and maternal enterovirus antibodies: time trends and geographical variation. Diabetologia **48:** 1280–1287.
13. YOON, J.W., M. AUSTIN, T. ONODERA, *et al.* 1979. Isolation of a virus from the pancras of a child with diabetic ketoacidosis. N. Engl. J. Med. **200:** 1173–1179.
14. HYOTY, H. 2004. Environmental causes: viral causes. Endocrinol. Metab. Clin. North. Am. **33:** 27–44.
15. BORCH-JOHNSEN, K., G. JONER, T. MANDRUP-POULSEN T, *et al.* 1984. Relation between breast-feeding and incidence rates of insulin-dependent diabetes mellitus. A hypothesis. Lancet **2:** 1083–1086.
16. SAUKKONEN, T., S.M. VIRTANEN, M. KARPPINEN, *et al.* 1998. Significance of cow's milk protein antibodies as risk factor for childhood IDDM: interactions with dietary cow's milk intake and HLA-DQB1 genotype. Childhood Diabetes in Finland Study Group. Diabetologia **41:** 72–78.
17. VAARALA, O., P. KLEMETTI, S. JUHELA, *et al.* 2002. Effect of coincident enterovirus infection and cow's milk exposure on immunisation to insulin in early infancy. Diabetologia **45:** 531–534.

18. Elliot, R.B., H. Wassmuth, J. Hill, *et al.* 1996. Diabetes and cow's milk. Sardinian IDDM Study Groups. Lancet **348:** 1657.
19. Dosch, H.M. 1993. The possible link between insulin dependent (juvenile) diabetes mellitus and dietary cow milk. Clin. Biochem. **26:** 307–308.
20. Johansson, C., U. Samuelsson & J. Ludvigsson. 1994. A high weight gain early in life is associated with an increased risk of type 1 (insulin-dependent) diabetes mellitus. Diabetologia **37:** 91–94.
21. Kampe, O., A. Andersson, E. Bjork, *et al.* 1989. High-glucose stimulation of 64000-Mr islet cell autoantigen expression. Diabetes **38:** 1326–1328.
22. Kimpimaki, T., M. Erkkola, S. Korhonen, *et al.* 2001. Short term exclusive breastfeeding predispose young children with increased genetic risk of Type 1 diabetes to progressive beta-cell autoimmunity. Diabetologia **44:** 63–69.
23. Scott, F.W., J.M. Norris & H. Kolb. 1996. Milk and type 1 diabetes. Diabetes Care **19:** 379–383.
24. Ziegler, A.G., S. Schmid, D. Huber D, *et al.* 2003. Early infant feeding and risk of developing type 1 diabetes-associated autoantibodies. JAMA **290:** 1721–1728.
25. Ivarsson, A., L.A. Persson, L. Nystrom, *et al.* 2000. Epidemic of celiac disease in Swedish children. Acta Paediatr. **89:** 165–171.
26. Wilkin, T.J. 2002. Diabetes mellitus: type 1 or type 2? The accelerator hypothesis. J. Pediatr. **141:** 449–450.
27. Pundziute-Lycka, A., G. Dahlquist, B. Urbonaite, *et al.* 2004. Time trend of childhood type 1 diabetes incidence in Lithuania and Sweden, 1983-2000. Acta. Paediatr. **93:** 1519–24.
28. Ludvigsson, J. & A.O. Afoke. 1989. Seasonality of type 1 (insulin-dependent) diabetes mellitus: values of C-peptide, insulin antibodies and haemoglobin A1c show evidence of a more rapid loss of insulin secretion in epidemic patients. Diabetologia **32:** 84–91.
29. Sepa, A., J. Wahlberg, O. Vaarala, *et al.* 2005. Psychological stress may induce diabetes-related autoimmunity in infancy. Diabetes Care **28:** 290–295.
30. Sepa, A., A. Frodi & J. Ludvigsson. 2005. Mothers' experiences of serious life events increase the risk of diabetes-related autoimmunity in their children. Diabetes Care **28:** 2394–2399.
31. Mathieu, C. & K. Badenhoop. 2005. Vitamin D and type 1 diabetes mellitus: state of the art. Trends Endocrinol. Metab. **16:** 261–266.
32. Al-Zuhair, H. & H.E. Mohamed. 1998. Vitamin C attenuation of the development of type 1 diabetes mellitus by interferon-alpha. Pharmacol. Res. **38:** 59–64.
33. Walsh, P.C. 2005. Effects of long-term vitamin E supplementation on cardiovascular events and cancer: a randomized controlled trial. J. Urol. **174:** 1823–1824.
34. Alon, U.S. 1997. Nephrocalcinosis. Curr. Opin. Pediatr. **9:** 160–165.
35. Wilkin, T., J. Ludvigsson, C. Greenbaum C, *et al.* 2004. Future interventions trials in type 1 diabetes. Diabetes Care **27:** 996–997.

Overcoming the Challenges Now Limiting Islet Transplantation

A Sequential, Integrated Approach

ANTONELLO PILEGGI,[a,b] LORENZO COBIANCHI,[a,c]
LUCA INVERARDI,[a,d] AND CAMILLO RICORDI[a,b]

[a]*Cell Transplant Center, Diabetes Research Institute, University of Miami Leonard M. Miller School of Medicine, Miami, Florida 33136, USA*

[b]*Dewitt Family Department of Surgery, Division of Cellular Transplantation, University of Miami Leonard M. Miller School of Medicine, Miami, Florida 33136, USA*

[c]*Istituto di Chirurgia Generale Epatopancreatica, Dipartimento di Scienze Chirurgiche, Universita' degli Studi di Pavia, IRCCS Policlinico 'San Matteo,' 27100 Pavia, Italy*

[d]*Department of Microbiology and Immunology, University of Miami Leonard M. Miller School of Medicine, Miami, Florida 33136, USA*

ABSTRACT: **Steady improvements in islet cell processing technology and immunosuppressive protocols have made pancreatic islet transplantation a clinical reality for the treatment of patients with Type 1 diabetes mellitus (T1DM). Recent trials are showing that improved glycemic metabolic control, prevention of severe hypoglycemia, and better quality of life can be reproducibly achieved after transplantation of allogeneic islets in patients with unstable T1DM. Despite these encouraging results, challenges ahead comprise obtaining adequate islet cells for transplant, enhancing islets engraftment, sustaining β cell mass and function over time, and defining effective immune interventions, among others. In order to overcome the current hurdles to the widespread application of islet transplantation there is a need for implementation of integrated, sequential therapeutic approaches.**

KEYWORDS: **diabetes; islet transplantation; β cell replacement; insulin; stem cells; cytoprotection; immune intervention; immunosuppression; tolerance; bioengineering; pancreas**

Address for correspondence: Camillo Ricordi, M.D., Diabetes Research Institute, Miller School of Medicine, University of Miami, 1450 NW 10th Avenue (R-134), Miami, FL 33136. Voice: 305-243-5275; fax: 305-243-4404.
e-mail: ricordi@miami.edu

Ann. N.Y. Acad. Sci. 1079: 383–398 (2006). © 2006 New York Academy of Sciences.
doi: 10.1196/annals.1375.059

INTRODUCTION

Transplantation of allogeneic islets represents a viable therapeutic option for the treatment of patients with type 1 diabetes mellitus (T1DM).[1] Steady progress in islet isolation and purification techniques and the use of novel immunosuppressive protocols in recent years have allowed for increased success of islet transplantation trials worldwide.[2,3] Improved glycemic metabolic control (i.e., mean amplitudes of glucose excursions throughout the day, glycated hemoglobin) and prevention of severe hypoglycemia can be reproducibly achieved after transplantation of allogeneic islets, even when a suboptimal islet mass is transplanted.[4–13] Additional benefits of the transplant include improved diabetes quality of life and reduced fear of hypoglycemia when exogenous insulin is required to maintain glycemic values within a normal range, suggesting that restoration of β cell function may dramatically impact the overall management of diabetes.[14–16] Insulin independence can be achieved by transplanting sufficient islet numbers, and generally requires that more than one islet preparation per recipient is transplanted as either sequential or pooled islet preparations.[5,17]

The transplantation procedure is currently performed with a minimally invasive approach using interventional radiology techniques. It consists of a percutaneous, transhepatic cannulation of the portal vein, through which islets are infused into the recipient's liver.[18–22] This technique is associated with low morbidity and can be repeated, when additional islets are required to achieve insulin independence.[20,21,23,24]

Current challenges to the widespread application of islet transplantation for the treatment of a large number of patients with T1DM are multifold and require that an integrated, sequential approach be implemented in order to overcome them. For instance, improvement of islet cell viability by induction of cytoprotection through the use of extracellular matrices may be of assistance in improving the mass of viable islets implanted, but may trigger an immune response that will accelerate graft loss through rejection and/or autoimmunity recurrence. Additionally, even when adequate islet numbers are available for implantation, it is highly desirable to be able to induce long-term graft survival by the use of efficient immune interventions aiming at minimizing untoward effects of immunosuppressive drugs and possibly to achieve tolerance to the implanted tissue. This article will review the possible areas of intervention toward this important goal.

Obtaining Adequate Islet Cells

The need for high numbers of islets (generally obtained from more than one donor pancreas) to achieve insulin independence after transplantation represents a major drawback in light of the shortage of pancreata from the deceased, multiorgan donors. The number and quality (namely, viability and function)

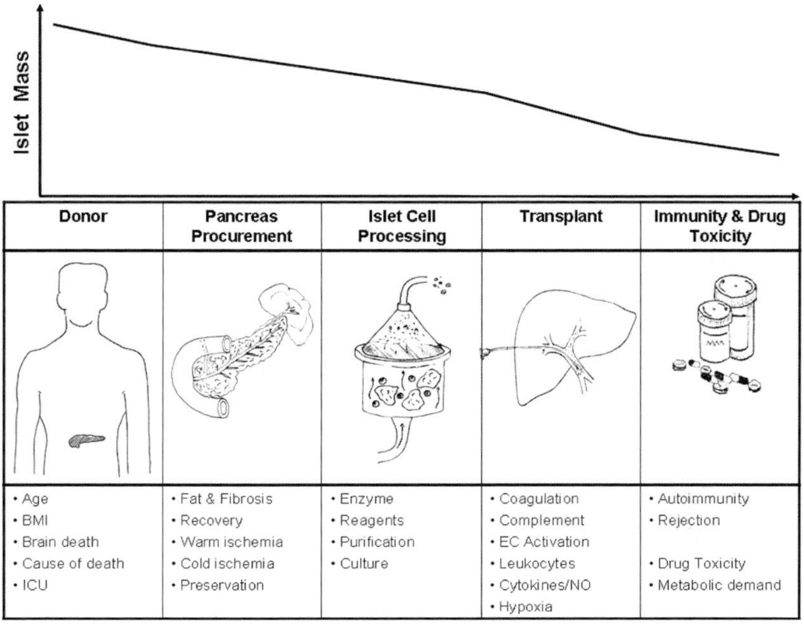

FIGURE 1. Factors influencing islet graft mass.

of islets obtained from a donor pancreas depend on the combination of many variables, including donor characteristics, organ recovery and preservation, islet isolation and purification processes, and culture conditions. Interventions targeting any (independently or simultaneously) of the aforementioned steps may be of assistance in preventing loss of viable islet mass for transplantation and in improving the success rate of islet transplantation from a single donor organ (TABLE 1).

Donor Interventions

Current underuse of deceased donor pancreata still represents an area for intervention.[25] Improved pancreas use has been successfully obtained following the implementation of organ sharing regional networks.[26] Implementation of a more aggressive management of the donor during hospital stay may contribute to reducing organ injury, therefore allowing for the recovery of higher islet quality and yield.[27,28] Broadening donor selection criteria that include "marginal" organs such as those obtained from elderly donors and donation after cardiac death may contribute to the expansion of the donor pool.[29–32] This will be possible after the definition of more stringent donor and recipient selection criteria to improve the success rate of human islet cell processing and to overcome potential competition with whole pancreas transplant programs.[33,34]

TABLE 1. Areas for interventions

1. **Obtaining adequate islet cells**
   (a) Donor interventions
      (i) Expanding the pancreas donor pool
         1. Improving deceased donor organ donation
         2. Elderly donors
         3. Donation after cardiac death
         4. Living donors
      (ii) Pancreas procurement
      (iii) Pancreas preservation
   (b) Islet cell processing
      (i) Pancreas dissociation
      (ii) Islet purification
      (iii) Islet culture
   (c) Alternative sources
      (i) Xenogeneic islets
      (ii) Stem cells
      (iii) Islet regeneration
2. **Improving islet transplantation techniques**
   (a) Prevention of islet cell infusion-related complications
   (b) Alternative implantation sites
3. **Favoring islet engraftment**
   (a) Islet cytoprotection
   (b) Reduction of inflammation
   (c) Sustaining β cell mass and function overtime
4. **Immune interventions**
   (a) Novel immunosuppression protocols
   (b) Immunomodulation
   (c) Tolerance induction
5. **Monitoring graft function**
6. **Immune monitoring**

For instance, the use of pancreata from high body mass index (BMI) donors is generally associated with better islet yields,[35–38] but they are commonly considered "not optimal" for whole pancreas transplantation.[39] It is noteworthy that ideal donor characteristics may be similar for both vascularized pancreas and islet cell transplantation, and that implementation of fair allocation criteria between the two therapeutic approaches might contribute to improve the success rate of islet transplantation. Furthermore, use of living donors for islet grafts has been recently proposed[40] and may represent a viable option in the near future when effective immune interventions for tolerance induction will be available.[2]

Pancreas Procurement and Preservation

Improved surgical methods for the recovery of donor pancreata with careful dissection using the no-touch isolation technique, prompt cooling of the gland, and excision of the gland before the liver, have been associated with increased success rate of islet isolation processing.[41] Development of customized preservation solutions for human pancreata and the use of oxygenated perfluorochemicals may provide higher oxygen availability and reduce cold ischemic damage to the gland, therefore resulting in improved islet recovery.[29,32,42–48] Indeed, the use of the two-layer method (TLM) has been recognized as the gold standard for pancreas preservation as it allows for the recovery of higher islet numbers even after extended cold ischemia, from marginal donors and after cardiac death.[29,32,42–47]

Islet Cell Processing and Culture

Steady improvements in the processing of human islet cell products have been introduced in recent years, and they have allowed for increasing efficiency and success rate. The process consists of a mechanically enhanced enzymatic digestion of the pancreas followed by purification on density gradients.[2,49] The efficiency of this process highly depends on the quality of the organ, the protocols used for isolation and purification, and the experience of the center. The Food and Drug Administration considers islet cell products as *somatic cell therapy* under the category of Investigational New Drugs until a Biological License Application will be issued for large-scale treatment of patients with T1DM.[50] Current good manufacturing practice (cGMP) and strict quality control and assurance policies are therefore required at each Islet Cell Processing Facility (ICPF) in order to warrant that high standards of reproducibility and sterility of the final cell product characteristics are obtained for clinical use. This imposes a burden on the center and requires a substantial institutional commitment and investment. The use of regional ICPF that isolate and distribute islet cell products for transplantation at remote sites has proven effective in maximizing the use of donor pancreata for islet transplantation while reducing the costs of manufacturing.[6,26,51]

The introduction of the automated method has permitted large-scale human islet isolation for transplantation, and is currently recognized as the gold standard technique.[49] Availability of improved enzyme blends has further contributed to obtain larger islet yields to meet the requirements for transplantation.[52] Numerous technological improvements have been introduced toward the standardization of the procedures and enhancement of the isolation process.[53–57] The use of the semiautomated method for large-scale islet purification on density gradients[58,59] and implementation of an additional purification step for low purity fractions after standard purification have been of assistance in increasing the efficiency of the process, therefore maximizing use of donor organs and of resources.[60]

Assessment of human islet preparations prior to transplantation is a fundamental step to characterize the quality of the final cell product for clinical use. Besides exclusion of adventitious potential (i.e., endotoxin, mycoplasma, and bacterial contamination), it is required to characterize islet cell viability and potency.[50] The limitation of the methods used for product release in recent years has been well recognized, and has led to the quest for more sensitive tests predictive of clinical islet outcome.[61–63] Selective assessment of β cell fractional viability in human islet preparations has been shown to predict *in vivo* performance in experimental conditions,[60] and may be of assistance in discriminating between islet preparation that are suitable for transplant and those that should be discarded. The unique cytoarchitecture of human islets[64,65] and the proportion of endocrine cell subsets composing the clusters[61,64,65] may have implications for function and engraftment. Availability of novel sophisticated techniques for islet cell assessment will be of assistance in improving our discriminative power in the near future.

Culturing human islets offers a window of opportunity for potential interventions aiming at preserving islet mass and at conferring cytoprotection to the graft. Islet culture prior to transplantation can be considered in order to allow sufficient time to perform potency testing, achieve therapeutic levels of immunosuppressive drugs in the recipients, arranging admission and access to radiology suite for the patients, and also shipping islets to distant transplantation centers.[5,8] Optimization of culture protocols for human islets with improved oxygen availability and customized media formulations to prevent oxidative stress while providing proper nutrients and extracellular matrices may allow for improved quality of islet cell products for transplantation, and reduce immunogenicity.[66–75]

Attractive approaches to overcome the shortage of human islets for transplantation include the use of alternative, unlimited sources of insulin-producing cells such as stem cells, xenogeneic islets, as well as induction of islet regeneration. Porcine and human insulin differ for a single amino acid and pig islets could be readily available in large amounts for transplantation into humans. The main limitation to the use of xenogeneic islets is the immune response to the transplanted tissue. Promising results in xenogeneic islet transplantation into nonhuman primates have been recently reported suggesting that porcine islets can restore glycemic control in diabetic recipients.[76,77] Development of safe immune intervention and/or immmunoisolation treatments that are clinically applicable may lead to the use of porcine islets transplantation for T1DM in the near future.

Generation of human pancreatic β cells from multipotent stem cells form either adult or embryonic stem cells could be of assistance to obtain unlimited tissue for transplantation. Development of protocols that allow for the efficient expansion and differentiation of progenitor stem cells into competent insulin-producing cells *in vitro* is promising, although both efficiency and quality of insulin-producing cells appear suboptimal at the present time.[78–80] Modulation of the self-regenerative potential of β cells in the adult pancreas also represents an interesting approach for intervention. Restoration of β cells mass in the diabetic pancreas under appropriate stimuli and in combination with effective immunointervention protocols to prevent autoimmunity recurrence might result eventually in a cure of the disease.[81]

Improving Islet Transplantation Techniques

Islet transplantation is currently performed by percutaneous, intrahepatic infusion of all the islets into the recipient's liver. The technique is associated with relatively low morbidity.[19–24] Development of implantation approaches that reduce the risk of portal hypertension subsequent to islet embolization into the liver (i.e, the bag technique) and sealing of the catheter tract with collagenase/thrombin paste or coils to prevent bleeding have been instrumental to this aim.[19,20] Surgical access (laparotomy or laparoscopy) can be used in patients at risk of bleeding or with anatomical variation of the hepatic vascular tree.[5,12] Alternative sites for islets transplantation have been proposed to reduce risks of bleeding and favor engraftment in the absence of islet-blood contact. Transplantation of islets into the omental pouch has been successfully performed in experimental models.[82] The use of subcutaneous, prevascularized devices may represent an appealing alternative due to the ease of implantation, biopsy, and removal of a well-confined bioartificial pancreas.[83]

Favoring Islet Engraftment

Recent clinical trials are showing that insulin independence can be achieved after allogeneic islet transplantation when sufficient islet numbers are implanted. This is generally obtained after the infusion of more than one islet preparation per recipient (approximately >12,000 IEQ/kg).[4–13] Islet embolization into the recipient's liver and the generation of nonspecific inflammation soon after transplantation may lead to lack of engraftment and/or functional impairment of a substantial mass of the implanted islets, contributing to the observed high islet mass requirements to obtain insulin independence. Notably, islet cells may actively participate in the generation of inflammation in the transplant microenvironment also because of their proinflammatory potential: expression of tissue factor, monocyte chemoattractant protein-1, Toll-like receptors, and CD40 (among others), which can be induced by stress-mediated pathways.[66,84–86] An instant blood-mediated inflammatory reaction (IBMIR) characterized by activation of the coagulation and complement cascades, leukocyte and macrophage recruitment at the site of implantation, platelet deposition, and islet cell death may contribute to islet cell functional impairment and loss of mass.[87,88] The consequent generation of oxidative mediators, including nitric oxide (NO), proinflammatory cytokines, and chemokines produced by activated endothelial cells in the implant microenvironment may further amplify this process and lead to a stronger specialized immune response later on. Methods that favor islet engraftment by modulating islet cell resistance to the noxious stimuli and/or the level of inflammation at the transplant site may result in long-term insulin independence after transplantation of a reduced number of islets, possibly improving the donor-to-recipient ratio to 1:1.[89,90] Induction of islet cytoprotection to reduce and/or prevent the negative effects of noxious stimuli may be achieved by multiple means, including preconditioning of the graft in culture prior to transplantation and/or treatment of the recipients in the peritransplant period. Several approaches have been proposed toward this goal, including the use of a number of cytoprotective regimens via pharmacological administration, gene therapy, gene silencing, protein transduction domains, among others.[68,90–95] Potential candidate molecules that have been used in experimental studies include 17-β-estradiol, nicotinamide, metal protoporphyrins, glucagon-like peptide-1 (GLP-1), etc.,[67,90,96–100] that may be used during isolation, added in the culture media or administered to the recipient as they may avoid or partially prevent the effects of oxidative stress and proinflammatory cytokines early after transplant, therefore maximizing islet engraftment. Understanding the molecular mechanisms involved in islet cell dysfunction and death following islet transplantation may provide the basis for targeted interventions to maximize islet cytoprotection in the transplantation setting. In particular, modulation of intracellular stress-mediated signaling pathways, such as mitogen-activated protein kinases (MAPK p38), c-Jun NH(2)-terminal kinase (JNK), and nuclear factor-κB may be targets of molecular interventions in the near future.[73–75,101,102] Inhibition of MAPK p38 and JNK pathways of signal transduction, for instance, have been shown to reduce islets cytokine production, reduce islet cell apoptosis, and improve graft function after transplantation in relevant experimental models.[75,101]

The outcomes of recent clinical trials are showing that progressive decline in graft function is commonly observed in islet transplant recipients treated with steroid-sparing immunosuppression and sirolimus-tacrolimus-based maintenance therapy.[5,103] Although persistent graft function can be measured in these patients for a long term (detectable basal and stimulated c-peptide), insulin is required in order to sustain good glycemic control, with ~10% of the patients free from exogenous insulin at 5 years.[103] The causes of this phenomenon are not completely understood, and it is conceivable that combination of multiple factors contribute to it: (*a*) engraftment of a suboptimal islet mass that may undergo exhaustion due to (*b*) high metabolic demand in the hyperglycemic liver microenvironment and (*c*) toxicity due to the relatively high levels of immunosuppressive drugs in the liver; and (*d*) immune response (rejection and recurrence of autoimmunity).[3,104–106] It is conceivable that cytoprotective approaches that favor the engraftment and maintenance of islet mass after transplantation may allow for sustained function long term.

Immune Interventions

The introduction of novel, more powerful immunosuppressive protocols for human islet transplantation has allowed for the unprecedented results of recent clinical trials. Human islet transplantation based on maintenance treatment with sirolimus and tacrolimus has shown engraftment and sustained function, but has been associated with progressive decline of graft function over time.[5,103] Also, currently available immunosuppressive drugs can cause untoward side effects associated with acute and chronic treatment, including islet β cells toxicity.[106–108]

Interestingly, the use of antibody treatment targeting the CD40–CD154 costimulation pathway in pancreatectomized nonhuman primates recipients of allogeneic islets showed improvement of intrahepatic islet graft function over time,[109,110] suggesting that the use of targeted immunomodulatory treatments void of systemic and/or organ-specific toxicity may be of assistance in sustaining islet graft function long term without the need for chronic immunosuppression.[2]

Immune isolation of islet grafts has been proposed as a strategy to eliminate the need for chronic immunosuppression and to allow long-term graft survival. Development of adequate technologies able to overcome the limited availability of oxygen and nutrients while scavenging oxidative radical in encapsulated islets to maintain islet mass after transplantation may prove a viable therapeutic approach.[2]

The ultimate goal of immune interventions is the induction of donor-specific tolerance.[2] Numerous approaches have been explored in experimental models that justify a cautious optimism for a clinical application.[111] The use of donor-derived marrow cells combined with short-term preconditioning of the recipient to achieve stable hematopoietic chimerism represents an appealing strategy toward this goal.[112]

Monitoring Graft Function

There is no consensus on the best means to monitor islet graft function. The primary end points of current clinical trials rely on measures of insulin requirements, HbA1c, mean amplitude of glycemic excursion, and basal c-peptide levels. The use of metabolic tests that are time consuming and cumbersome to perform (i.e., glucose tolerance test, mixed meal test, clamp studies) is limited to selected time points during the follow-up, and therefore they can detect graft dysfunction when a substantial islet mass has been already lost, preventing timely rescue interventions. Development of novel and easier methods to measure islet graft function and β cell mass over time will be extremely useful for the monitoring of islet engraftment, islet cell plasticity, and functionality after transplantation. They may also be of assistance in guiding timely interventions to prevent loss of mass.

Immune Monitoring

Monitoring of immune function at the follow-up may be of assistance in determining the efficacy of the immunotherapy treatment used and detecting episodes of rejection or recurrence of autoimmunity that could guide targeted interventions to prevent graft loss. Availability of novel analytical tools for the monitoring of immune function represents an exciting area of investigation as it will allow to shed more light on the mechanisms of immune response to islet allografts in the clinical settings. Monitoring of immune cell phenotypes, assessment of *in vitro* proliferative responses of recipient cells to donor antigens, and expression of cytotoxic lymphocyte genes (i.e., granzyme and perforin) may be of assistance in detecting reactivation of immunity and implement "rescue" treatments in a timely manner.[113] Additionally, monitoring of autoantibody levels and the use of tetramers to determine autoreactive lymphocytes may allow identifying reactivation of autoimmunity to islet antigens.

CONCLUSIONS

The success of recent clinical trials for allogeneic islet transplantation is showing that the β cell replacement therapy for the treatment of patients with diabetes is a reality. Steady progress has been achieved in recent years in islet cell isolation technology and immune therapies that justify optimism. Current challenges to the widespread application of this therapeutic approach to larger cohorts of patients that would benefit from the restoration of β cell function require implementation of a sequential, integrated approach combining multiple interventions.

ACKNOWLEDGMENTS

This study was supported by the National Institutes of Health/National Center for Research Resources (U42 RR016603, M01RR16587); Juvenile Diabetes Research Foundation International (No. 4–2000–946); National Institutes of Health/National Institute of Diabetes and Digestive and Kidney Diseases (5 R01 DK55347, 5 R01 DK056953, R01 DK025802); State of Florida; a contract for support of this research sponsored by Congressman Bill Young and funded by a special congressional out of the Navy Bureau of Medicine and Surgery, is currently managed by the Naval Health Research Center, San Diego, California; and the Diabetes Research Institute Foundation (available at www.diabetesresearch.org).

REFERENCES

1. RICORDI, C. 2003. Islet transplantation: a brave new world. Diabetes **52:** 1595–1603.
2. RICORDI, C. & T.B. STROM. 2004. Clinical islet transplantation: advances and immunological challenges. Nat. Rev. Immunol. **4:** 259–268.

3. PILEGGI, A., R. ALEJANDRO & C. RICORDI. 2006. Islet transplantation: steady progress and current challenges. Curr. Opin. Organ Transplant. **11:** 7–13.
4. RYAN, E.A. *et al.* 2005. {beta}-Score: an assessment of {beta}-cell function after islet transplantation. Diabetes Care **28:** 343–347.
5. FROUD, T. *et al.* 2005. Islet transplantation in type 1 diabetes mellitus using cultured islets and steroid-free immunosuppression: miami experience. Am. J. Transplant. **5:** 2037–2046.
6. GOSS, J.A. *et al.* 2004. Development of a human pancreatic islet-transplant program through a collaborative relationship with a remote islet-isolation center. Transplantation **77:** 462–466.
7. HERING, B.J. *et al.* 2005. Single-donor, marginal-dose islet transplantation in patients with type 1 diabetes. JAMA **293:** 830–835.
8. HERING, B.J. *et al.* 2004. Transplantation of cultured islets from two-layer preserved pancreases in type 1 diabetes with anti-CD3 antibody. Am. J. Transplant. **4:** 390–401.
9. FRANK, A. *et al.* 2004. Transplantation for type I diabetes: comparison of vascularized whole-organ pancreas with isolated pancreatic islets. Ann. Surg. **240:** 631–643.
10. WARNOCK, G.L. *et al.* 2005. Improved human pancreatic islet isolation for a prospective cohort study of islet transplantation vs best medical therapy in type 1 diabetes mellitus. Arch. Surg. **140:** 735–744.
11. GEIGER, M.C. *et al.* 2005. Evaluation of metabolic control using a continuous subcutaneous glucose monitoring system in patients with type 1 diabetes mellitus who achieved insulin independence after islet cell transplantation. Cell Transplant. **14:** 77–84.
12. PILEGGI, A. *et al.* 2005. Twenty Years of Clinical Islet Transplantation at the Diabetes Research Institute—University of Miami. UCLA Immunogenetics Center. Los Angeles, CA.
13. O'CONNELL P.J. *et al.* 2006. Clinical islet transplantation in type 1 diabetes mellitus: results of Australia's first trial. Med. J. Aust. **184:** 221–225.
14. POGGIOLI, R. *et al.* 2006. Quality of life after islet transplantation. Am. J .Transplant. **6:** 371–378.
15. JOHNSON, J.A. *et al.* 2004. Reduced fear of hypoglycemia in successful islet transplantation. Diabetes Care **27:** 624–625.
16. BARSHES, N.R. *et al.* 2005. Health-related quality of life after pancreatic islet transplantation: a longitudinal study. Transplantation **79:** 1727–1730.
17. MARKMANN, J.F. *et al.* 2003. Insulin independence following isolated islet transplantation and single islet infusions. Ann. Surg. **237:** 741–749; discussion 749–750.
18. ALEJANDRO, R. & D.H. MINTZ. 1988. Experimental and clinical methods of islet transplantation. *In* Transplantation of the Endocrine Pancreas in Diabetes Mellitus. R. van Schilfgaarde & M.A. Hardy, Eds.: 217–223. Elsevier Science. New York.
19. BAIDAL, D.A. *et al.* 2003. The bag method for islet cell infusion. Cell Transplant. **12:** 809–813.
20. FROUD, T. *et al.* 2004. Use of D-STAT to prevent bleeding following percutaneous transhepatic intraportal islet transplantation. Cell Transplant. **13:** 55–59.
21. GOSS, J.A. *et al.* 2003. Pancreatic islet transplantation: the radiographic approach. Transplantation **76:** 199–203.

22. CASEY, J.J. *et al.* 2002. Portal venous pressure changes after sequential clinical islet transplantation. Transplantation **74:** 913–915.
23. OWEN, R.J. *et al.* 2003. Percutaneous transhepatic pancreatic islet cell transplantation in type 1 diabetes mellitus: radiologic aspects. Radiology **229:** 165–170.
24. VENTURINI, M. *et al.* 2005. Technique, complications, and therapeutic efficacy of percutaneous transplantation of human pancreatic islet cells in type 1 diabetes: the role of US. Radiology **234:** 617–624.
25. KRIEGER, N.R. *et al.* 2003. Underutilization of pancreas donors. Transplantation **75:** 1271–1276.
26. KEMPF, M.C. *et al.* 2005. Logistics and transplant coordination activity in the GRAGIL Swiss-French multicenter network of islet transplantation. Transplantation **79:** 1200–1205.
27. ECKHOFF, D.E. *et al.* 2004. Enhanced isolated pancreatic islet recovery and functionality in rats by 17beta-estradiol treatment of brain death donors. Surgery **136:** 336–345.
28. ROSENDALE, J.D. *et al.* 2003. Aggressive pharmacologic donor management results in more transplanted organs. Transplantation **75:** 482–487.
29. RICORDI, C. *et al.* 2003. Improved human islet isolation outcome from marginal donors following addition of oxygenated perfluorocarbon to the cold-storage solution. Transplantation **75:** 1524–1527.
30. MARKMANN, J.F. *et al.* 2003. The use of non-heart-beating donors for isolated pancreatic islet transplantation. Transplantation **75:** 1423–1429.
31. MATSUMOTO, S. & K. TANAKA. 2005. Pancreatic islet cell transplantation using non-heart-beating donors (NHBDs). J. Hepatobiliary Pancreat. Surg. **12:** 227–230.
32. MATSUMOTO, S. *et al.* 2003. Improved islet yields from Macaca nemestrina and marginal human pancreata after two-layer method preservation and endogenous trypsin inhibition. Am. J. Transplant. **3:** 53–63.
33. RIS, F. *et al.* 2004. Are criteria for islet and pancreas donors sufficiently different to minimize competition? Am. J. Transplant. **4:** 763–766.
34. O'GORMAN, D. *et al.* 2005. Multi-lot analysis of custom collagenase enzyme blend in human islet isolations. Transplant. Proc. **37:** 3417–3419.
35. BRANDHORST, D. *et al.* 1994. Body mass index is an important determinant for human islet isolation outcome. Transplant. Proc. **26:** 3529–3530.
36. BRANDHORST, H. *et al.* 1995. Body mass index of pancreatic donors: a decisive factor for human islet isolation. Exp. Clin. Endocrinol. Diabetes **103**(Suppl2): 23–26.
37. MATSUMOTO, I. *et al.* 2004. Improvement in islet yield from obese donors for human islet transplants. Transplantation **78:** 880–885.
38. LAKEY, J.R. *et al.* 1996. Variables in organ donors that affect the recovery of human islets of Langerhans. Transplantation **61:** 1047–1053.
39. HUMAR, A. *et al.* 2004. The impact of donor obesity on outcomes after cadaver pancreas transplants. Am. J. Transplant. **4:** 605–610.
40. MATSUMOTO, S. *et al.* 2005. Insulin independence after living-donor distal pancreatectomy and islet allotransplantation. Lancet **365:** 1642–1644.
41. LEE, T.C. *et al.* 2004. Procurement of the human pancreas for pancreatic islet transplantation. Transplantation **78:** 481–483.
42. BRANDHORST, H. *et al.* 1995. Comparison of histidine-tryptophane-ketoglutarate (HTK) and University of Wisconsin (UW) solution for pancreas perfusion prior to islet isolation, culture and transplantation. Transplant. Proc. **27:** 3175–3176.

43. Noguchi, H. *et al.* 2006. Modified two-layer preservation method (M-Kyoto/PFC) improves islet yields in islet isolation. Am. J. Transplant. **6:** 496–504.
44. Fraker, C.A., R. Alejandro & C. Ricordi. 2002. Use of oxygenated perfluorocarbon toward making every pancreas count. Transplantation **74:** 1811–1812.
45. Kuroda, Y. *et al.* 1988. A new, simple method for cold storage of the pancreas using perfluorochemical. Transplantation **46:** 457–460.
46. Tsujimura, T. *et al.* 2004. Influence of pancreas preservation on human islet isolation outcomes: impact of the two-layer method. Transplantation **78:** 96–100.
47. Tsujimura, T. *et al.* 2004. Short-term storage of the ischemically damaged human pancreas by the two-layer method prior to islet isolation. Cell Transplant. **13:** 67–73.
48. Avila, J.G. *et al.* 2003. Improvement of pancreatic islet isolation outcomes using glutamine perfusion during isolation procedure. Cell Transplant. **12:** 877–881.
49. Ricordi, C. *et al.* 1988. Automated method for isolation of human pancreatic islets. Diabetes **37:** 413–420.
50. Wonnacott, K. 2005. Update on regulatory issues in pancreatic islet transplantation. Am. J. Ther. **12:** 600–604.
51. Goss, J.A. *et al.* 2002. Achievement of insulin independence in three consecutive type-1 diabetic patients via pancreatic islet transplantation using islets isolated at a remote islet isolation center. Transplantation **74:** 1761–1766.
52. Linetsky, E. *et al.* 1997. Improved human islet isolation using a new enzyme blend, liberase. Diabetes **46:** 1120–1123.
53. Lakey, J.R. *et al.* 2001. Serine-protease inhibition during islet isolation increases islet yield from human pancreases with prolonged ischemia. Transplantation **72:** 565–570.
54. Lakey, J.R. *et al.* 1997. Development of an automated computer-controlled islet isolation system. Transplant. Proc. **29:** 1956.
55. Lakey, J.R. *et al.* 1999. Intraductal collagenase delivery into the human pancreas using syringe loading or controlled perfusion. Cell Transplant. **8:** 285–292.
56. Fraker, C. *et al.* 2004. The use of multiparametric monitoring during islet cell isolation and culture: a potential tool for in-process corrections of critical physiological factors. Cell Transplant. **13:** 497–502.
57. Goto, M. *et al.* 2004. Refinement of the automated method for human islet isolation and presentation of a closed system for in vitro islet culture. Transplantation **78:** 1367–1375.
58. Lake, S.P. *et al.* 1989. Large-scale purification of human islets utilizing discontinuous albumin gradient on IBM 2991 cell separator. Diabetes **38**(Suppl. 1): 143–145.
59. Alejandro, R. *et al.* 1990. Isolation of pancreatic islets from dogs. Semiautomated purification on albumin gradients. Transplantation **50:** 207–210.
60. Ichii, H. *et al.* 2005. Rescue purification maximizes the use of human islet preparations for transplantation. Am. J. Transplant. **5:** 21–30.
61. Ichii, H. *et al.* 2005. A novel method for the assessment of cellular composition and Beta-cell viability in human islet preparations. Am. J. Transplant. **5:** 1635–1645.
62. Street, C.N. *et al.* 2004. Islet graft assessment in the Edmonton Protocol: implications for predicting long-term clinical outcome. Diabetes **53:** 3107–3114.

63. Barnett, M.J. *et al.* 2004. Variation in human islet viability based on different membrane integrity stains. Cell Transplant. **13:** 481–488.
64. Brissova, M. *et al.* 2005. Assessment of human pancreatic islet architecture and composition by laser scanning confocal microscopy. J. Histochem. Cytochem. **53:** 1087–1097.
65. Cabrera, O. *et al.* 2006. The unique cytoarchitecture of human pancreatic islets has implications for islet cell function. Proc. Natl. Acad. Sci. USA **103:** 2334–2339.
66. Moberg, L. *et al.* 2002. Production of tissue factor by pancreatic islet cells as a trigger of detrimental thrombotic reactions in clinical islet transplantation. Lancet **360:** 2039–2045.
67. Moberg, L. *et al.* 2003. Nicotinamide inhibits tissue factor expression in isolated human pancreatic islets: implications for clinical islet transplantation. Transplantation **76:** 1285–1288.
68. Pileggi, A. *et al.* 2005. Prolonged allogeneic islet graft survival by protoporphyrins. Cell Transplant. **14:** 85–96.
69. Inverardi, L. *et al.* 1997. Human mixed lymphocyte-islet cultures: the influence of heterologous proteins on islet immunogenicity. Transplant. Proc. **29:** 2066.
70. Kuttler, B., A. Hartmann & H. Wanka. 2002. Long-term culture of islets abrogates cytokine-induced or lymphocyte-induced increase of antigen expression on beta cells. Transplantation **74:** 440–445.
71. Pinkse, G.G.M. *et al.* 2006. Integrin signaling via RGD peptides and anti-{beta}1 antibodies confers resistance to apoptosis in islets of Langerhans. Diabetes **55:** 312–317.
72. Noguchi, H. *et al.* 2005. Cell permeable peptide of JNK inhibitor prevents islet apoptosis immediately after isolation and improves islet graft function. Am. J. Transplant. **5:** 1848–1855.
73. Abdelli, S. *et al.* 2004. Intracellular stress signaling pathways activated during human islet preparation and following acute cytokine exposure. Diabetes **53:** 2815–2823.
74. Bottino, R. *et al.* 2004. Response of human islets to isolation stress and the effect of antioxidant treatment. Diabetes **53:** 2559–2568.
75. Matsuda, T. *et al.* 2005. Inhibition of p38 pathway suppresses human islet production of pro-inflammatory cytokines and improves islet graft function. Am. J. Transplant. **5:** 484–493.
76. Hering, B.J. *et al.* 2006. Prolonged diabetes reversal after intraportal xenotransplantation of wild-type porcine islets in immunosuppressed nonhuman primates. Nat. Med. **12:** 301–303.
77. Cardona, K. *et al.* 2006. Long-term survival of neonatal porcine islets in nonhuman primates by targeting costimulation pathways. Nat. Med. **12:** 304–306.
78. Murtaugh, L.C. *et al.* 2003. Notch signaling controls multiple steps of pancreatic differentiation. Proc. Natl. Acad. Sci. USA **100:** 14920–14925.
79. Dor, Y. *et al.* 2004. Adult pancreatic beta-cells are formed by self-duplication rather than stem-cell differentiation. Nature **429:** 41–46.
80. Bonner-Weir, S. & G.C. Weir. 2005. New sources of pancreatic beta-cells. Nat. Biotechnol. **23:** 857–861.
81. Ogawa, N. *et al.* 2004. Cure of overt diabetes in NOD mice by transient treatment with anti-lymphocyte serum and exendin-4. Diabetes **53:** 1700–1705.

82. Movahedi, B. *et al.* 2003. Laparoscopic approach for human islet transplantation into a defined liver segment in type-1 diabetic patients. Transpl. Int. **16:** 186–190.
83. Pileggi, A. *et al.* 2006. Reversal of diabetes by pancreatic islet transplantation into a subcutaneous, neovascularized device. Transplantation **81:** 1318–1324.
84. Piemonti, L. *et al.* 2002. Human pancreatic islets produce and secrete MCP-1/CCL2: relevance in human islet transplantation. Diabetes **51:** 55–65.
85. Klein, D. *et al.* 2005. A functional CD40 receptor is expressed in pancreatic beta cells. Diabetologia **48:** 268–276.
86. Vives-Pi, M. *et al.* 2003. Evidence of expression of endotoxin receptors CD14, toll-like receptors TLR4 and TLR2 and associated molecule MD-2 and of sensitivity to endotoxin (LPS) in islet beta cells. Clin. Exp. Immunol. **133:** 208–218.
87. Johansson, H. *et al.* 2005. Tissue factor produced by the endocrine cells of the islets of Langerhans is associated with a negative outcome of clinical islet transplantation. Diabetes **54:** 1755–1762.
88. Moberg, L. 2005. The role of the innate immunity in islet transplantation. Ups. J. Med. Sci. **110:** 17–55.
89. Ricordi, C. *et al.* 2005. Requirements for success in clinical islet transplantation. Transplantation **79:** 1298–1300.
90. Pileggi, A. *et al.* 2004. Protecting pancreatic beta-cells. IUBMB Life. **56:** 387–394.
91. Pileggi, A. *et al.* 2001. Heme oxygenase-1 induction in islet cells results in protection from apoptosis and improved in vivo function after transplantation. Diabetes **50:** 1983–1991.
92. Pastori, R.L. *et al.* 2004. Delivery of proteins and peptides into live cells by means of protein transduction domains: potential application to organ and cell transplantation. Transplantation **77:** 1627–1631.
93. Klein, D. *et al.* 2004. Delivery of Bcl-XL or its BH4 domain by protein transduction inhibits apoptosis in human islets. Biochem. Biophys. Res. Commun. **323:** 473–478.
94. Fenjves, E.S. *et al.* 2004. Adenoviral gene transfer of erythropoietin confers cytoprotection to isolated pancreatic islets. Transplantation **77:** 13–18.
95. Curran, M.A. *et al.* 2002. Efficient transduction of pancreatic islets by feline immunodeficiency virus vectors1. Transplantation **74:** 299–306.
96. Contreras, J.L. *et al.* 2002. Cytoprotection of pancreatic islets before and early after transplantation using gene therapy. Kidney Int. **61:** 79–84.
97. Contreras, J.L. *et al.* 2001. Cytoprotection of pancreatic islets before and soon after transplantation by gene transfer of the anti-apoptotic Bcl-2 gene. Transplantation **71:** 1015–1023.
98. Contreras, J.L. *et al.* 2002. 17beta-Estradiol protects isolated human pancreatic islets against proinflammatory cytokine-induced cell death: molecular mechanisms and islet functionality. Transplantation **74:** 1252–1259.
99. Contreras, J.L. *et al.* 2002. Simvastatin induces activation of the serine-threonine protein kinase AKT and increases survival of isolated human pancreatic islets. Transplantation **74:** 1063–1069.
100. D'Amico, E. *et al.* 2005. Pancreatic beta-cells expressing GLP-1 are resistant to the toxic effects of immunosuppressive drugs. J. Mol. Endocrinol. **34:** 377–390.
101. Matsuda, T. *et al.* 2005. Silymarin protects pancreatic beta-cells against cytokine-mediated toxicity: implication of c-Jun NH2-terminal kinase and janus

kinase/signal transducer and activator of transcription pathways. Endocrinology **146:** 175–185.
102. Paraskevas, S. *et al.* 1999. Activation and expression of ERK, JNK, and p38 MAP-kinases in isolated islets of Langerhans: implications for cultured islet survival. FEBS Lett. **455:** 203–208.
103. Ryan, E.A. *et al.* 2005. Five-year follow-up after clinical islet transplantation. Diabetes **54:** 2060–2069.
104. Shapiro, A.M. *et al.* 2005. The portal immunosuppressive storm: relevance to islet transplantation? Ther Drug Monit. **27:** 35–37.
105. Desai, N.M. *et al.* 2003. Elevated portal vein drug levels of sirolimus and tacrolimus in islet transplant recipients: local immunosuppression or islet toxicity? Transplantation **76:** 1623–1625.
106. Fernandez, L.A. *et al.* 1999. The effects of maintenance doses of FK506 versus cyclosporin A on glucose and lipid metabolism after orthotopic liver transplantation. Transplantation **68:** 1532–1541.
107. Molinari, M. *et al.* 2005. Sirolimus-induced ulceration of the small bowel in islet transplant recipients: report of two cases. Am. J. Transplant. **5:** 2799–2804.
108. Cure, P. *et al.* 2004. Alterations of the female reproductive system in recipients of islet grafts. Transplantation **78:** 1576–1581.
109. Kenyon, N.S. *et al.* 1999. Long-term survival and function of intrahepatic islet allografts in rhesus monkeys treated with humanized anti-CD154. Proc. Natl. Acad. Sci. USA **96:** 8132–8137.
110. Kenyon, N.S. *et al.* 1999. Long-term survival and function of intrahepatic islet allografts in baboons treated with humanized anti-CD154. Diabetes **48:** 1473–1481.
111. Stratta, R.J. *et al.* 2003. Kidney and pancreas transplantation at Wake Forest University Baptist Medical Center. Clin. Transp. 229-245.
112. Inverardi, L. *et al.* 2004. Targeted bone marrow radioablation with 153Samarium-lexidronam promotes allogeneic hematopoietic chimerism and donor-specific immunologic hyporesponsiveness. Transplantation **77:** 647–655.
113. Han, D. *et al.* 2004. Assessment of cytotoxic lymphocyte gene expression in the peripheral blood of human islet allograft recipients: elevation precedes clinical evidence of rejection. Diabetes **53:** 2281–2290.

Index of Contributors

OHIO